Pediatric Trauma Resuscitation Manual (PTRM) for Primary Care Providers

Neha Thakur Rai
Editor

Pediatric Trauma Resuscitation Manual (PTRM) for Primary Care Providers

Springer

Editor
Neha Thakur Rai
Department of Pediatrics
Dr. Ram Manohar Lohia Institute of Medical Sciences
Lucknow, Uttar Pradesh, India

ISBN 978-981-95-4978-8   ISBN 978-981-95-4979-5 (eBook)
https://doi.org/10.1007/978-981-95-4979-5

This Springer imprint is published by the registered company Springer Nature Singapore Pte Ltd.
The registered company address is: 152 Beach Road, #21-01/04 Gateway East, Singapore 189721, Singapore

Foreword

In the fast-paced and unpredictable environment of the emergency department, a critically injured child presents a unique and formidable challenge. The physiological, anatomical, and psychological differences between children and adults mean that pediatric trauma resuscitation demands a specialized and confident approach. For every emergency doctor and nurse, the ability to act decisively and correctly in these moments is not just a skill—it is a moral imperative.

Dr. Neha Thakur Rai's *Pediatric Trauma Resuscitation Manual for Primary Care Providers* is a powerful and much-needed resource that directly addresses this critical need. This book is a testament to the fact that effective pediatric care is a right, not a luxury. Dr. Rai has distilled the complexities of pediatric trauma into a clear, actionable, and systematic module that can be readily applied in any emergency setting. She has successfully created a comprehensive and easy-to-navigate guide, empowering frontline healthcare professionals to deliver life-saving care without hesitation.

This module is an invaluable tool that will undoubtedly enhance the skills and confidence of emergency doctors and nurses everywhere. It provides a clear roadmap for initial assessment, airway management, fluid resuscitation, and stabilization, ensuring that the critical "golden hour" is utilized to its fullest potential. By demystifying pediatric trauma, Dr. Rai has not only created a learning module but also a catalyst for improved patient outcomes.

I do not doubt that this module will become an indispensable resource for primary care providers across India. It will not only enhance the quality of care for countless children but also provide physicians with the confidence to face one of the most stressful situations in medicine. Dr. Rai's work is a beacon of hope, illuminating the path forward for better pediatric care and ensuring that every child has a fighting chance.

ICMR – Dr AS Paintal Distinguished Scientist Chair
Editor In Chief IJMR

Prof (Dr.) Piyush Gupta
MD, FIAP, FNNF, FAMS, FRCPCH

Preface

Delivering immediate, effective care to an injured child is one of the most demanding tasks in medicine. It requires not only rapid action but also a specialized understanding of pediatric physiology—an area often underserved by existing training materials, especially for those working on the frontline in Primary Care settings across India.

This module, *Pediatric Trauma Resuscitation Manual (PTRM) for Primary Care Providers*, was born from a collaborative commitment by both doctors and nurses to address this critical gap. It is a practical, evidence-based compendium designed specifically for Primary Care Providers (PCPs), including doctors, nurse practitioners, and paramedical staff, who serve as the critical first responders in the trauma chain. We recognize the immense challenge faced by PCPs. You are often the sentinel at the gateway of care, requiring you to make swift, life-saving decisions with limited resources. This book is engineered to be your shield of specialized knowledge and your guide to confident action in those high-stakes moments.

The core purpose of this module is a call to action aimed at standardizing and elevating the quality of pediatric trauma care outside of major trauma centers. We focus on practical application, ensuring you are prepared to manage the critical first hour—the golden hour—of resuscitation. The chapters within are meticulously structured to bridge the gap between complex theory and immediate clinical need. You will find focused, accessible guidance on Pediatric Biomechanics and Physiology, Initial Critical Assessment, and Mastering the rapid primary and secondary surveys. Airway, Breathing, and Circulation (ABC) Management: Practical strategies for fragile pediatric airways, thoracic trauma, and managing shock/fluid resuscitation. The health of our nation is intrinsically tied to the well-being of its children. By mastering the principles in this module, you are not merely treating injuries; you are safeguarding the future.

We offer this collaborative work with the deepest respect for your commitment and resolve. May these pages empower you to stand confidently in the vanguard of pediatric trauma care, ensuring a brighter, safer tomorrow for the young souls entrusted to your care.

Dr Ram Manohar Lohia Institute of Medical Sciences
Lucknow, India

Neha Thakur Rai

Acknowledgments

The successful creation of the *Pediatric Trauma Resuscitation Manual (PTRM) for Primary Care Providers* is the result of the dedication, mentorship, and collective expertise of numerous individuals. We wish to express our profound gratitude to those who championed this project from concept to completion.

My sincere gratitude goes to my PTRM Faculty who took out time from their busy schedule and helped me create this module. Special thanks to *Dr. Aaditya Katyal* for his tireless efforts and unwavering commitment in developing this module.

I am profoundly indebted to my mentors, whose guidance shaped the scope and quality of this module: *Prof. CM Singh*, Director, Dr Ram Manohar Lohia Institute of Medical Sciences, for providing institutional support, mentorship, and guidance. *Dr. Sagar Galwankar, CEO of INDUSEM*, for his invaluable mentorship and for providing the platform and encouragement necessary to pursue this vital educational mission. *Dr. Prashant Mahajan* and *Dr. Jabeen Fayyaz* for their expert guidance, critical insights, and collaborative spirit, which significantly enriched the clinical depth and academic rigor of the content. *Prof. MC Misra, Prof. Sanjeev Bhoi,* and *Prof. Samir Misra* for their insightful mentorship and support, lending their vast experience to ensure this module meets the highest standards of emergency care education.

A special thanks to *Arun Varghese, Nurse Coordinator*, whose dedicated organizational skills and clinical perspective ensured seamless collaboration between the authors and maintained the practical focus essential for our nursing readership.

Finally, I extend my heartfelt appreciation to my parents, *Usha Thakur* and *Pramod Kumar Thakur*, for their lifelong support, encouragement, and understanding, which provided the foundation and personal resilience required to undertake a project of this magnitude.

I am also indebted to the following experts in the field of Pediatrics, Emergency Medicine and Trauma who have given valuable advice in the development of the manual.

Prof. (Dr.) Piyush Gupta Ex Principal University College of Medical Sciences, New Delhi, India
Prof. (Dr.) Dheeraj Shah Principal University College of Medical Sciences, New Delhi, India
Prof. MC Misra ATLS Chair India Ex Director AIIMS New Delhi, India
Prof. Samir Misra Prof Trauma Surgery and Incharge CASD KGMU, Lucknow India
Prof. (Dr.) Sanjeev Bhoi, Head ,WHO CCET, SEAROProf and Head Emergency Medicine AIIMS New Delhi, Delhi, India
Dr. Sagar Galwankar, Director for Research in Emergency Medicine Florida State University College of Medicine USA
Dr. Prashant Mahajan Chair, Department of Emergency Medicine Professor Departments of Emergency Medicine and Pediatrics University of Michigan Ann Arbor Michigan, USA
Prof. (Dr.) Prerna Batra Prof Pediatrics University College of Medical Sciences, and GTB Hospital New Delhi, India
Prof. (Dr.) Abhijeet Saha Prof Pediatrics Lady Hardinge Medical College New Delhi, India
Prof. AK Goel Prof and Head Department of Pediatrics AIIMS Raipur, India

Neha Thakur Rai

Contents

The Evolution of Pediatric Trauma Care: A Global Challenge and Call to Action

1

Arvind Kumar Singh and Neha Thakur Rai

Learning Objectives

By the end of this chapter, the reader should be able to:

- Describe the global burden and disparities in pediatric trauma care, with particular emphasis on the challenges faced by low- and middle-income countries (LMICs), including infrastructure gaps, delayed access to care, and lack of pediatric-specific training.
- Explain the historical evolution of pediatric trauma systems, including the contributions of key pioneers, policy frameworks like the Platt Report and EACH Charter, and the transition from adult-centric to child-centered trauma care models.
- Identify the essential roles and responsibilities of primary care providers (PCPs) in pediatric trauma management, including assessment, stabilization, decision-making for referral, and the application of trauma-informed and family-centered care approaches.
- Evaluate current innovations and emerging technologies—such as simulation training, telemedicine, and artificial intelligence—and their impact on improving pediatric trauma outcomes, especially in resource-constrained settings.
- Formulate strategic recommendations for improving pediatric trauma systems globally, including the development of standardized protocols, investment in

A. K. Singh
Department of Community Medicine, Dr Ram Manohar Lohia Institute of Medical Sciences, Lucknow, Uttar Pradesh, India

N. T. Rai (✉)
Department of Pediatrics, Dr. Ram Manohar Lohia Institute of Medical Sciences, Lucknow, Uttar Pradesh, India

N. T. Rai (ed.), *Pediatric Trauma Resuscitation Manual (PTRM) for Primary Care Providers*, https://doi.org/10.1007/978-981-95-4979-5_1

capacity building, creation of trauma registries, ethical integration of AI, and promotion of community-based injury prevention and education.

Introduction

The World Health Organization's 2004 estimate of approximately 262,000 child deaths from road traffic accidents worldwide highlights the global magnitude of this issue. Alarmingly, in India alone, the number of child fatalities in road traffic accidents surged by 10.54% within a single year, climbing from 14,875 in 2021 to 16,443 in 2022, demonstrating a rapidly worsening situation. Given that pediatric trauma often necessitates hospitalization and emergency surgical intervention, the need for specialized care is paramount. A pediatric PCP's role extends beyond addressing physical injuries; it requires a holistic approach that encompasses empathetic communication, psychological support to mitigate the trauma's impact on the child's mental well-being, assessment of social support networks, and active engagement of family and friends in the care process.

Lerner et al. have accurately observed the historical lack of specialized protocols tailored to the unique vulnerabilities of children in trauma care. While the Advanced Trauma Life Support (ATLS) course, initiated in the United States in 1978, has significantly contributed to standardizing trauma assessment globally, adherence to these protocols in pediatric trauma centers remains inconsistent. The contemporary medical landscape offers a plethora of advanced technologies, including robotics and artificial intelligence, which hold immense potential for enhancing patient safety and outcomes. However, the disparity in pediatric trauma care quality across the globe is profound. Developed nations have specialized trauma centers equipped with advanced technologies, whereas low-resource settings often rely on integrated trauma management centers that treat children as small adults, neglecting their distinct physiological and psychological needs. A report published in Nature concludes that while theoretically 70% of children could access a pediatric trauma center (PTC) within an hour by air, in practice, over 80% receive their initial trauma care elsewhere. Consequently, there is an urgent need to address these disparities through specialized, evidence-based training programs that equip PCPs with the skills and knowledge required to provide optimal care for pediatric trauma patients. This includes not only procedural competency but also the development of a child-centered, trauma-informed approach to care.

Case Scenario

Ten-year-old Venkatesh was brought to the emergency unit of a primary care facility by his parents after falling down a flight of stairs at home. He was crying in pain, clutching his right forearm, which was markedly swollen and red. His parents were panicked and incoherent, each blaming the other for not watching him closely enough. They pleaded for someone to do something quickly.

Ravi, a junior emergency technician, was on duty with Priya, a final-year nursing student posted in the emergency unit for clinical training. There was no doctor present at the time. Ravi began assessing the child, but Venkatesh was inconsolable—kicking, screaming, and refusing to be touched. Priya attempted to calm him and asked the parents about any history of loss of consciousness, bleeding from the nose or ears, or seizures, but they were too distressed to provide clear answers.

They tried to check vital signs, but Venkatesh did not allow a blood pressure cuff or pulse oximeter near him. Ravi considered giving an analgesic but was unsure of the correct dose for a child. They referred to a wall chart for weight-based drug calculation, but there was no scale available to weigh the child. Attempts to secure intravenous access failed due to the child's agitation.

With no splinting material, sedation protocol, or clear pediatric trauma algorithm to follow, Ravi and Priya felt helpless. A crowd of bystanders gathered around, and the parents began raising their voices, demanding immediate transfer to a bigger hospital. As the situation spiraled, Priya found herself emotionally overwhelmed—torn between wanting to help the child and not knowing what the safest next step was without formal supervision or structured guidelines.

Reflective Questions

1. What immediate non-pharmacological strategies can be used to reduce distress in a pediatric trauma patient in such a setting?
2. How can a PCP decide when to stabilize and when to refer a child in the absence of a physician?
3. What basic pediatric trauma assessment skills should every emergency PCP be trained in to handle such situations safely?

History of Pediatric Nursing Practice

An English nurse, Catherine Jane Wood (1841–1930), has considerable work in establishment of specialized hospitals for children and is considered a pioneer of pediatric nursing. She established a new hospital known as "The House of Relief for Children with Chronic Diseases of the Joints" in 1867.

One of the oldest documents that could be traced for beneficence of children visiting hospitals within the United Kingdom during the mid-twentieth century was the report on "Welfare of Sick Children in Hospital (Ministry of Health, 1959)," also known as the "Platt Report." The same period also marks establishment of the first pediatric ICU at Children's Hospital of Gothenburg, Sweden, in 1955 by Goran Haglund. The Platt Report summarized that the hospitals designed for adults had no play area for children and the children were bound by strict routines meant for adult patients. The entry of parents was restricted. The report's recommendations included unrestricted access to parents while children were ill. In 1988, Leiden charter from the European Association for Children in Hospital (EACH) was introduced, which formalized the Platt Report recommendations internationally through creation of

Convention on the Rights of the Child. Subsequently, the recommendations of this report and charter paved path for development of child trauma wards in hospital.

In 1960s in the United States, the thought of establishing trauma centers for civilians like the medical centers for military casualties emerged. Several studies were conducted that established the belief that establishment of trauma care systems could improve the mortality in nonmilitary accidents also. Initially, the pediatric trauma care units developed within these centers were meant for adults. Almost at all places in the world, work on dedicated pediatric trauma units started only after the adult trauma centers started. The earliest evidence of establishment of dedicated pediatric trauma centers in the United States dates to early 1970s in Boston, Ann Arbor, Baltimore, Washington DC, Toronto, and Brooklyn.

A society of pediatric nurses was formed in 1992 with Margaret Shandor "Marge" Miles as the founder president. Miles' main research was in the field of family-centered nursing which evolved in the 1980s. In recent years, initiatives like the National Pediatric Readiness Project (NPRP) have been instrumental in enhancing pediatric trauma care. The NPRP provides a framework for emergency departments to ensure preparation for pediatric emergencies, emphasizing the importance of pediatric readiness in improving outcomes for injured children. The National Pediatric Readiness Project (NPRP) is a comprehensive, multiphase quality improvement program designed to standardize and elevate the level of emergency care provided to children in all US emergency departments, by ensuring the availability of essential guidelines and resources.

Global Perspectives

Traumatic injuries constitute a significant global health crisis, impacting both developed and developing nations, particularly low- and middle-income countries (LMICs). Alarmingly, over 95% of childhood injury-related deaths, encompassing both intentional and unintentional causes, occur within LMICs. This disproportionate burden is attributed to a confluence of factors, including higher population, weaker safety regulations, and mortality rates nearly double those observed in developed countries. Furthermore, the burden of disability-adjusted life years (DALYs) in LMICs is almost three times greater, signifying a profound and long-lasting impact on children's well-being. The World Health Organization (WHO) estimates that a staggering 50% of children hospitalized for unintentional injuries will endure lifelong disabilities, signifying the severity of the issue. Compounding this concern, a recent study revealed that children in India face a risk of death from traumatic injury more than 22 times higher than their counterparts in the United States, even after adjusting for injury severity. Notably, this elevated risk is most pronounced among children with seemingly less severe injuries, suggesting systemic deficiencies in early management. A critical challenge in LMICs is the lack of organized trauma systems, which often results in injured children being transported by untrained individuals. This leads to significant delays in care and compromised initial treatment, exacerbating the severity of injuries. Moreover, pediatric-specific trauma training is severely limited. A systematic review identified only 16 trauma curricula utilized in LMICs, with a mere two focusing specifically on pediatric trauma. This glaring gap in targeted education stresses the urgent need for specialized training programs to equip healthcare professionals in LMICs with the necessary skills to effectively manage pediatric trauma cases.

Several organizations play pivotal roles in shaping pediatric trauma care. The World Health Organization (WHO) champions integrated public health strategies, encompassing injury prevention, first aid, hospital care, disability limitation, and rehabilitation. Notably, the WHO emphasizes the critical importance of readily available, qualified pediatric critical care teams for managing severely injured children. Beyond the WHO, the Pediatric Trauma Society is dedicated to developing optimal care guidelines, fostering education, promoting research, and advocating for improved hospital practices. Additionally, the International Trauma Life Support (ITLS) pediatric course provides essential training to PCPs on the principles of accurate assessment and effective management of young trauma patients.

Advancements and Innovations in Pediatric Trauma

Technological advancements are playing a key role in pediatric trauma, improving efficiency and quality of care. A vital component of pediatric trauma training involves simulation training which allows PCPs to safely practice complex procedures. This immersive approach has demonstrated a marked improvement in PCPs' confidence, clinical reasoning, and preparedness for real-world pediatric trauma situations. Telemedicine also plays an important role in low resource settings by providing expert consultation and support to PCPs in remote or underserved areas. By facilitating guidance through specialists, telemedicine technologies positively influence the management of pediatric trauma cases. Trauma registries, such as the National Trauma Data Bank, serve as invaluable tools for collecting comprehensive data, identifying trends, and informing evidence-based practice. These registries enable continuous performance improvement by tracking outcomes and guiding policy development. Considerable progress in standardized pediatric trauma protocols, including Advanced Trauma Life Support (ATLS) and Pediatric Advanced Life Support (PALS), has improved pediatric patient assessment and management. These protocols provide guidelines and frameworks for rapid evaluation and intervention, which are essential for minimizing morbidity and mortality in pediatric patients. ATLS emphasizes a structured approach to initial trauma assessment and management, while PALS specifically addresses the unique physiological needs of pediatric patients, ensuring appropriate pediatric-specific resuscitation and stabilization techniques. PCP research and evidence-based practice directly translate to improved patient care and safety.

Current Challenges and Barriers

Despite significant advancements in pediatric trauma, many challenges continue to persist worldwide. A critical issue is the gap in pediatric trauma training and education, particularly in low- and middle-income countries (LMICs). The lacunae in existence of structured training programs and PCP courses in such regions compromise the capacity of healthcare systems to effectively manage pediatric trauma cases in such countries. Resource constraints and infrastructure limitations further widen the gaps in global trauma care. Limited access to advanced medical technologies, shortages of trained personnel, and inadequate hospital facilities in LMICs contribute to poorer outcomes for pediatric trauma patients compared to their counterparts in developed regions. Pediatric trauma PCPs undergo significant psychological burdens, including high stress, burnout, and secondary stress stemming from frequent exposure to severely injured children and emotionally charged caregivers. Overcoming these barriers through targeted education initiatives, infrastructure improvements, and robust emotional support systems is crucial for the continued advancement and global standardization of pediatric trauma practices.

Current Policies Supporting Pediatric Trauma Care Globally

Pediatric trauma is a huge global public health issue and demands the development of strong prevention programs and child protection policies. The Global Initiative for Children's Surgery (GICS) by Abdelbasit E Ali et al. has proposed a comprehensive pediatric trauma care initiative for reducing the mortality and morbidity in pediatric trauma, specifically targeting low- and middle-income countries (LMICs). This initiative stresses structured collaboration with relevant organizations and local stakeholders to address all facets of trauma care, including first aid, prehospital primary trauma care, hospital care, ATLS, diagnostic capabilities, surgical interventions, rehabilitation, registry, research, and auditing. PCPs should play the central role when talking about policy change and improvement in pediatric trauma care. They have primary knowledge about the challenges and needs within existing trauma systems of their country and region. By actively participating in policy development, engaging in research, and collaborating with interdisciplinary teams, PCPs can significantly influence the creation and implementation of guidelines that improve outcomes.

Recommendations for Policy Reforms at National and Global Levels

1. *Establishment of Standardized Pediatric Trauma Care Protocols:* There is urgent need for enforcement of uniform pediatric trauma care guidelines globally. This would ensure equal, high-quality treatment across all healthcare settings, regardless of location or limited resources.

2. *Investment in Comprehensive Capacity Building:* Funding for training programs that train PCPs, particularly in low resource, should be increased. The training programs must focus on development of specialized skills and knowledge required for effective pediatric trauma management.
3. *Develop and Utilize Robust Data Collection and Research Systems:* Comprehensive trauma registries to collect data on pediatric injuries should be established and maintained so that evidence-based research is boosted, and subsequent policy decisions are based on such research.
4. *Optimize Resource Allocation for Pediatric Trauma Care through Strong Political Will:* Dedicated funding and resources to strengthen pediatric trauma care infrastructure, including the provision of essential equipment, adequate staffing, and accessible rehabilitation services, must be ensured.
5. *Community Engagement and Education:* No public health program can succeed without community engagement. Public awareness campaigns focusing on injury prevention and timely medical intervention in pediatric trauma cases should be designed and propagated.

Role of Digital Health, Artificial Intelligence (AI), and Future Technologies

Digital health is rapidly changing pediatric training, hospital care, and rehabilitation settings. Newer approaches are being developed for patient engagement, education, and rehabilitation. These technologies include mobile learning applications, virtual and augmented reality, simulation games, robotic devices (like robot companions and robotic nurses), telemedicine platforms, automated assessment tools, and wearable devices (like smartwatches and rings). Artificial intelligence (AI) is also rapidly integrating into healthcare, providing applications like automated triage, continuous patient monitoring with critical alarms, diagnostic assistance, and clinical decision-making. In pediatric emergency medicine, AI-enhanced socially assistive robots (SARs) are being developed to personalize support experiences and mitigate discomfort during painful procedures.

Strategic Recommendations for Improving Global Pediatric Trauma Outcomes

1. *Integrate Technological Innovations into Patient Management:* Adoption and integration of AI and digital health tools into pediatric trauma care would lead to improvement in diagnostic accuracy, would facilitate real-time patient monitoring, and would deliver personalized treatment plans.
2. *Invest in Research:* Prioritize and fund research studies to evaluate the efficacy of emerging technologies in pediatric trauma settings. This should establish a robust evidence base for implementation and optimization of such technologies into the national healthcare systems.

3. *Develop Comprehensive Technology Training Programs:* Designing and implementation of specialized training in innovative technologies should make PCPs proficient in the use of technology and bring out their potential benefits.
4. *Collaborative Partnerships:* Partnerships between high-income and LMICs for facilitating exchange of knowledge, resources, and best practices in pediatric trauma care should be encouraged.
5. *Ethical Considerations:* Prioritize and address ethical considerations related to the integration of AI and digital health, ensuring patient privacy, data security, and equitable access to technological advancements. For example, an important ethical consideration would be if harm occurs to a patient by a robot nurse, in this case, who is to be blamed: the head nurse, the treating physician, the hospital, the manufacturer, the coder, or someone else?

Case Resolution

Priya quickly realized that Venkatesh's intense distress was the biggest obstacle to any meaningful assessment. Instead of insisting on procedures right away, she stepped back and shifted her approach. Sitting down beside him to avoid appearing intimidating, she spoke gently and used age-appropriate, reassuring words. She handed him a pen and asked if he could squeeze it to show how strong he was—an attempt at distraction that slowly eased his crying. She also requested the parents to speak softly and hold his other hand, turning the chaotic scene into a more controlled and comforting environment.

As Venkatesh began to calm down slightly, Ravi managed to count his respiratory rate and palpate his pulse. Priya performed a quick visual survey of his injuries and observed significant swelling over the right forearm, with tenderness and reduced movement, suggestive of a possible fracture. There were no signs of bleeding from the nose or ears, and Venkatesh was alert and responding—ruling out, for now, any obvious signs of head trauma.

Pain management was the next priority. With no scale available and the child too agitated for accurate weighing, they turned to the pediatric dosing chart on the wall, which provided age-based ranges. For a 10-year-old, the chart recommended 250–500 mg of paracetamol. After verifying with the parents that Venkatesh had no known allergies or previous adverse drug reactions, Priya administered an appropriate dose of oral paracetamol syrup—the only pediatric analgesic available at the facility.

While waiting for the medication to take effect, Ravi and Priya improvised a splint using folded cardboard and gauze. They gently supported the forearm in a neutral position, wrapped it securely, and fashioned a sling from a clean cloth to immobilize the limb. Though it wasn't textbook perfect, it provided the necessary support to minimize further pain and movement.

With limited diagnostic tools and no imaging facility at hand, they knew referral was the appropriate next step. Venkatesh was stable, alert, and slightly more settled, but his injury required radiological evaluation and possibly orthopedic management. They documented their assessment and the interventions provided and arranged for ambulance transport to the nearest tertiary care center, calling ahead to ensure preparedness on arrival.

Throughout the ordeal, Priya and Ravi remained composed, made clear decisions based on basic trauma principles, and used their training to adapt to the limitations of their setting. Despite the absence of a physician, they prioritized non-pharmacological calming techniques, applied basic pediatric assessment skills, and made an informed judgment on when to stabilize and when to refer—ensuring Venkatesh received timely and safe care.

Key Messages

- Pediatric trauma is a major public health issue, particularly in low- and middle-income countries (LMICs), where over 95% of childhood injury deaths occur.
- LMICs face significant challenges, including a lack of dedicated pediatric trauma facilities, inadequate training, limited resources, and compromised initial care, leading to higher mortality and disability rates compared to developed nations.
- There is a critical gap in pediatric-specific trauma training, especially in LMICs, with limited structured programs and curricula.
- Pediatric trauma requires specialized care due to children's unique physiological and psychological needs, which are often overlooked in adult-centric trauma systems.
- The evolution of pediatric trauma care includes pioneering figures like Catherine Jane Wood and landmark reports like the Platt Report, which highlighted the need for child-centered hospital environments.
- Organizations like the WHO, Pediatric Trauma Society, and ITLS play crucial roles in advocating for improved care, developing guidelines, and providing training.
- Digital health, AI, and simulation training are transforming pediatric trauma, improving assessment, management, and patient outcomes.
- Pediatric trauma PCPs face significant psychological challenges, including burnout and secondary traumatic stress, requiring institutional support.
- The article recommends standardized care protocols, capacity building, data collection, resource allocation, and community engagement to improve pediatric trauma care globally.
- The integration of AI and digital health raises ethical concerns regarding patient privacy, data security, and equitable access, demanding careful consideration and policy development.

Bibliography

1. Abdur-Rahman L O vAABRH. Pediatric trauma care in Africa: the evolution and challenges. Semin Pediatr Surg. 2012; 21(2): p. 111-15.
2. Auerbach M RLAAGMKJBKCMSK. In situ pediatric trauma simulation: assessing the impact and feasibility of an interdisciplinary pediatric in situ trauma care quality improvement simulation program. Pediatr Emerg Care. 2014; 30(12): p. 884-91.
3. Botelho F TPMDCLZKRLea. Pediatric trauma primary survey performance among surgical and non-surgical pediatric providers in a Brazilian trauma center. Trauma Surg Acute Care Open. 2020; 5(1).
4. Chandran A HAAPAC. The global burden of unintentional injuries and an agenda for progress. Epidemiol Rev. 2010;(32): p. 110-120.
5. EACH European Association for Children in Hospital. The EACH Charter.
6. EMSC Innovation and Improvement Center. National Pediatric Readiness Project.
7. Epstein D, BJ. A History of Pediatric Critical Care Medicine. Pediatr Res. 2005; 58: p. 987-96.
8. Goddard A JEEL. Trauma-informed care for the pediatric nurse. J Pediatr Nurs. 2022; 62: p. 1-9.
9. Isabelle R JSENea. Exploring the perspectives of health care professionals on digital health technologies in pediatric care and rehabilitation. Journal of NeuroEngineering and Rehabilitation. 2024; 21.
10. James P Marcin HSSFea. Impact of Tele-Emergency Consultations on Pediatric Interfacility Transfers. Pediatrics. 2023; 6(2).
11. Jane A Rivas JBSBYSTENMLS. Paediatric trauma education in low- and middle-income countries: A systematic literature review. Journal of Global Health. 2022; 12: 04078.
12. Joan E, Shook M, Thomas H, Chun M, Gregory P, Conners M. Management of Pediatric Trauma.
13. Kiragu AW DSWBSSMMST. Pediatric Trauma Care in Low- and Middle-Income Countries: A Brief Review of the Current State and Recommendations for Management and a Way Forward. Pediatr Intensive Care. 2017; 6(1): p. 52-59.
14. Lorenzo DS ACGTea. Artificial Intelligence in Pediatric Emergency Medicine: Applications, Challenges, and Future Perspectives. Biomedicines. 2024; 12(6): p. 1220.
15. Margie Peden, Kayode Oyegbite, Joan Ozanne-Smith, et al. World report on child injury prevention. Geneva: World Health Organization & UNICEF. 978 92 4 156357 4.
16. Melhado CG, YBK, RKea. Pediatric Readiness and Trauma Centers: History, Relevance, and Practical Application. Curr Trauma Rep. 2023; 9.
17. Morrison W WJPC. Pediatric trauma systems. Crit Care Med. 2002; 30(11 Suppl): p. 448-56.
18. SR S. The ongoing and worldwide challenge of pediatric trauma. Int J Crit Illn Inj Sci. 2012; 2: p. 111-3.
19. Stas Amato KCEDea. Pediatric trauma mortality in India and the United States: A comparison and risk-adjusted analysis. Journal of Pediatric Surgery. 2023; 58(1): p. 99-105.
20. Wu HP. Pediatric trauma—a global public health issue: What and who should we focus on in pediatric injury prevention. Pediatrics and Neonatology. 2021; 62(6): p. 579-80.

Triage and Transport of Pediatric Trauma Victims

2

P. Rabeesh Kumar and Romit Saxena

Learning Objectives

By the end of this chapter, the reader should be able to:

- *Understand the unique features of pediatric trauma patients* and apply appropriate triage methods and initial assessment techniques tailored to children's physiological and emotional needs.
- *Explain the core components of triage*, including categorization, prioritization, and decision-making based on severity and available resources.
- *Recognize the importance of safe pediatric transport*, and identify different transport types and modes based on clinical condition and logistical factors.
- *Describe the role of primary care providers (PCPs)* in pediatric trauma triage and transport, including stabilization, communication, documentation, and coordination of care.

Introduction

Pediatric trauma refers to injuries in children that result from various incidents such as falls, motor vehicle accidents, burns, or drowning. Their unique physiological, anatomical, and developmental differences provide with challenges that necessitates need for tailored management. Pediatric trauma especially traumatic brain injury, anoxia, and hemorrhage contributes to mortality within 24 h to presentation

P. Rabeesh Kumar
Nursing Officer, JIPMER, Pondicherry, India

R. Saxena (✉)
Department of Pediatrics, Maulana Azad Medical College and Associated LN Hospital, New Delhi, India

N. T. Rai (ed.), *Pediatric Trauma Resuscitation Manual (PTRM) for Primary Care Providers*, https://doi.org/10.1007/978-981-95-4979-5_2

to pediatric emergency. Timely and accurate triage in pediatric emergency department (ED) is crucial for prioritizing critically ill children and optimizing resource allocation. Various triaging tools have been developed to assess the severity of illness and predict outcomes such as short-term mortality including IMNCI, PREM, ETAT, ESI, PAT, and IAP ALS. Each of these tools utilizes different physiological parameters, clinical assessments, and scoring methodologies to classify patients according to their risk level. The accuracy and predictive value of these tools, however, vary based on population demographics, disease burden, and healthcare system constraints.

Case Scenario

An 11-year-old boy is brought to the emergency department after being struck by an electric pole while riding his bicycle without a helmet. On arrival, he is unresponsive, with irregular breathing, a GCS of 7, and delayed capillary refill. Using the Pediatric Assessment Triangle, the triage nurse identifies respiratory failure and shock. The child is intubated, given fluid boluses, and placed on spinal precautions. A head CT reveals intracranial hemorrhage. The nurse coordinates with the transport team and facilitates a time-sensitive transfer to a pediatric trauma center with neurosurgical capability.

Reflective Questions

1. What are key indicators of respiratory failure and shock that PCPs can identify using the Pediatric Assessment Triangle (PAT)?
2. How can PCPs initiate airway and circulation management in an unresponsive child when advanced tools are unavailable?
3. What critical information should be documented and communicated during a pediatric trauma transfer?

Why Is Pediatric Trauma and Triaging Different from Adults?

This is elucidated in Table 2.1.

Triage and Initial Evaluation in Pediatric Trauma Victims

Triage prioritizes patient treatment according to the seriousness of their condition. In pediatric trauma, triage focuses on quickly identifying life-threatening conditions while providing rapid interventions to stabilize the patient. The goal is to identify which pediatric patients need immediate care, who can wait, and who are stable enough to transfer to a specialized facility. Triaging tools often assign color-coded labels as per patient's sickness level (red, yellow, green, black) or a number (1–5).

Table 2.1 Unique aspects of child's anatomy and physiology

Physiological changes	1. Children have less blood volume. 2. Hypothermia develops easily as they have up to 3 times BSA as adults, with proportionally large heads. 3. Intracranial pressure (ICP) is lower and ranges not well defined as per age. Also, BP nomograms are considerably different at different ages. 4. Glucose cerebral metabolism is 2/third of adult value then rapidly increases to 5 years of age, before decreasing to adult value, through adolescence.
Anatomical changes	1. *Thinner and more pliable cranial bones:* The pediatric skull is softer and more flexible, allowing for deformation under impact. This pliability, while offering some protection, makes invasive intracranial pressure (ICP) monitoring more challenging. Basal skull fractures are also relatively common in this age group. 2. *Larger head-to-body ratio:* In children, the head is disproportionately large and heavy compared to the torso, supported by relatively weak neck muscles and ligaments. As a result, during falls or motor vehicle incidents, the head often strikes the ground first, increasing the risk of head injury. 3. *Weaker cervical support structures:* The cervical ligaments and paraspinal muscles in children are less developed, and the craniocervical junction is particularly vulnerable. This predisposes them to a spectrum of injuries, including fractures with or without subluxation, ligamentous injuries, and *spinal cord injury without radiographic abnormality (SCIWORA)*. 4. *High and anterior larynx with a narrow airway:* The pediatric larynx is positioned higher and more anteriorly, with the cricoid cartilage forming the narrowest portion of the airway. Even minimal swelling or obstruction can significantly compromise airflow, leading to rapid airway deterioration. 5. *Cartilaginous and compliant chest wall:* The flexible thoracic cage readily transmits external forces to underlying organs. Consequently, pulmonary contusions are common, while rib fractures may be absent despite significant internal injury. 6. *Larger solid organs with limited abdominal protection:* Children possess proportionally larger solid organs, reduced intraperitoneal fat, and weaker abdominal musculature. These features make them more susceptible to solid organ injuries in cases of blunt abdominal trauma.

Effective triage ensures that resources are appropriately allocated, prioritizing the sickest children for immediate care first. There are many triaging tools for pediatric triage as Taiwan Triage and Acuity Scale (TTAS) which is a 5-point scale, but most scales dwell upon initial and primary assessment and can include the following components:

(a) *Airway and Breathing Assessment*: Checking for airway patency, assessing the adequacy of breathing, intervening if there is any obstruction or breathing difficulty, and providing supplemental oxygen
(b) *Circulation*: Check blood pressure, heart rate, and capillary refill and intervene accordingly, depending upon presence of shock (compensated/hypotensive)
(c) *Neurological Status*: Use tools like the Pediatric Glasgow Coma Scale (Table 2.2) and AVPU to determine the child's level of consciousness and intervene as needed.

Table 2.2 Pediatric Glasgow Coma Scale

Response	Child 1–5 years	Infant (<1 year)	Score
Eye opening	Spontaneous	Spontaneous	4
	To speech	To speech	3
	To pain only	To pain only	2
	No response	No response	1
Best verbal response	Oriented, appropriate	Coos and babbles	5
	Confused	Irritable cries	4
	Inappropriate words	Moans to pain	3
	Incomprehensible sounds	Moans to pain	2
	No response	No response	1
Best motor response	Obeys command	Moves spontaneously and purposefully	6
	Localizes painful stimulus	Withdraws to touch	5
	Withdraws in response to pain	Withdraws in response to pain	4
	Flexion in response to pain	Abnormal flexion to pain	3
	Extension in response to pain	Abnormal extension posture to pain	2
	No response	No response	1

[a] Adapted from James H. E. (1986). Neurologic evaluation and support in the child with an acute brain insult. *Pediatric annals*, *15* (1), 16–22

(d) *Exposure:* Additional assessments of blood sugar, rashes, and other relevant investigations help in triaging. The presence of point-of-care tests such as blood glucose and INR helps in triaging as per the clinical condition.
(e) *Mechanism of Injury (MOI)*: Understanding how the injury occurred (e.g., fall, car accident) helps predict the severity of injuries.

Cardiorespiratory Arrest

At any point during triaging if the child is noticed to be pulseless and apneic, cardiorespiratory resuscitation needs to be initiated depending upon age, witnessed/unwitnessed arrest, and number of rescuers. Prior to resuscitation, the rescuer should assess for scene safety. For example, you would not want to start resuscitation on a road traffic accident victim, in the middle of the road. Also, there is a need to activate emergency response system for additional hands, and for bringing equipment such as bag and mask, and defibrillator.

Initial Assessment and Triaging

Based on initial triaging, the patient resource allocation and treatment is prioritized. However, it is important to remember that children can improve and deteriorate with time. Hence, a child triaged yellow can throw a seizure and have altered sensorium and become red in the emergency room. Hence, regular monitoring and watchful expectancy of signs is important.

Evaluate➔Identify➔Intervene sequence: This sequence needs to be followed at each step:

The signs and symptoms and physiological signs (as assessed by monitoring or as shown on the monitor) need to be conglomerated to identify and categorize the physiological state. On the basis of the physiological state, the treatment needs to be tailored and escalated.

Pediatric Assessment Triangle (PAT)

This triaging tool helps in rapid evaluation to assess critically ill or injured children. It emphasizes assessment of appearance of the child at presentation, breathing and color (Fig. 2.1).

1. *Appearance*: Observing the child's mental status, interaction with the environment, and muscle tone. A child who is limp, lethargic, or nonresponsive needs immediate attention.
2. *Work of Breathing*: Check for increased respiratory effort, abnormal breath sounds, and body posture indicating respiratory distress (e.g., nasal flaring, retractions).
3. *Circulation to Skin*: Assess the skin's color, temperature, and capillary refill. Pale, mottled, or cyanotic skin may indicate poor circulation, shock, or hypoxia.

Based on the PAT, the patient can be triaged as per the following physiological status (Table 2.3).

An example of how to use a triaging tool is elucidated below (Table 2.4).

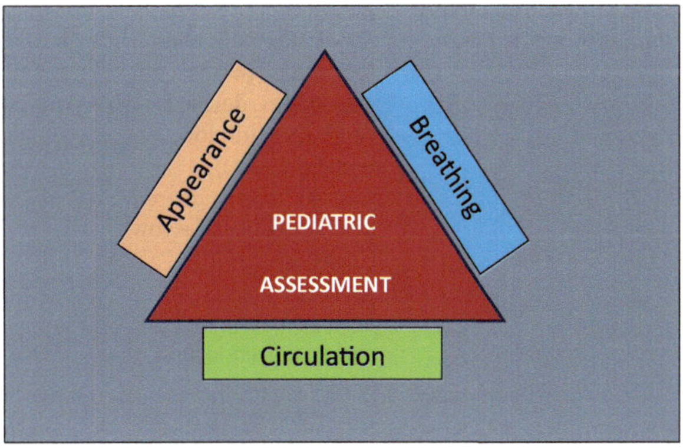

Fig. 2.1 Pediatric Assessment Triangle

Table 2.3 Physiological status categorization as per initial assessment

Components of PAT	Stable	Respiratory insufficiency[a,b]	Circulatory insufficiency[a,c]	Primary or secondary brain dysfunction[a,d]
Appearance/ consciousness	Normal	Abnormal	Abnormal	Abnormal
Breathing (WoB)	Normal	Abnormal	Normal	Normal >> Abnormal
Circulation/ color	Normal	Normal	Abnormal	Normal >> Abnormal

[a]During resuscitation or assessment if the patient becomes pulseless or apneic, cardiopulmonary resuscitation should be started
[b]Respiratory insufficiency can be further categorized into respiratory distress or failure: In both cases, supplemental oxygen with non-rebreather mask at 10–15 L is needed. In case of failure, additional airway stabilization may be needed
[c]Circulatory insufficiency can be further due to ventilatory-circulation mismatch resulting in compensated or decompensated shock. It is important to know the normal values of heart rate/BP in children as per age
[d]Neurological dysfunction: This can be due to cortical or brainstem dysfunction. Increased intracranial pressure can result, which needs additional stabilizing measures
At each step, the PCP would need to escalate to the doctor on duty and the team needs to manage the same

Table 2.4 Illustration of use of triaging categorization as per triaging tools

Category	Criteria	Example	Action
Red—Immediate This category includes critically ill or injured patients who require immediate lifesaving interventions. Without rapid treatment, these patients are at imminent risk of death, but they have a chance of survival with appropriate care.	*Airway compromise:* The patient has difficulty breathing and requires airway management or assisted ventilation. *Severe respiratory distress*: Signs of hypoxia (e.g., cyanosis, gasping) *Shock:* Poor circulation (e.g., weak pulses, cool extremities, delayed capillary refill, low blood pressure) *Unconscious or altered mental status:* Glasgow Coma Scale (GCS) score ≤8, unresponsiveness, or altered consciousness *Severe trauma:* Life-threatening injuries such as severe head trauma, massive bleeding, or penetrating injuries	A child with severe head injury, unresponsive, and irregular breathing after a road accident A patient in shock with weak pulses and cool, pale skin due to major blood loss	Immediate lifesaving treatment such as airway management, fluid resuscitation, and emergency surgery Rapid transport to a trauma facility with specialized care

(continued)

Table 2.4 (continued)

Category	Criteria	Example	Action
Yellow—Delayed Patients in this category are stable for the moment but require urgent medical care. Their condition is not immediately life-threatening, but if left untreated, they could deteriorate over time. They can wait for a limited period for treatment without significant risk of death.	*Stable airway and breathing*: Adequate breathing but may have injuries that need attention *Stable circulation*: No signs of shock, but injuries may require monitoring (e.g., fractures, moderate blood loss) *Moderate injuries*: May have fractures, moderate head injuries, or abdominal trauma without signs of major internal bleeding *Responsive*: Patient is alert or responding to commands but may have pain or discomfort.	A child with a fractured limb who is in pain but has stable vital signs A patient with moderate head injury (e.g., concussion) and mild confusion but no signs of severe brain trauma	Provide necessary interventions like splinting, IV fluids, and pain management. Treatment can be delayed briefly while red category patients receive immediate attention, but these patients should be monitored closely for deterioration.
Green—Minor This category includes patients with minor injuries that do not pose an immediate threat to life. They are walking wounded and can wait for medical care for an extended period without risk of their condition worsening. These patients may also be able to assist in their own care or move to safety independently.	*Walking and talking*: Patients are conscious, alert, and able to move on their own. *Minor injuries*: Superficial wounds, abrasions, bruises, or minor fractures that do not impair mobility or vital functions *No immediate risk to life*: Normal respiratory and cardiovascular status	A child with minor cuts and bruises after a bicycle accident A patient with a sprained ankle or minor burn, stable, and alert.	Provide basic first aid (e.g., bandaging, wound cleaning) and reassurance These patients can be treated after red and yellow patients receive care or can be directed to walk-in clinics or minor injury units for treatment.

(continued)

Table 2.4 (continued)

Category	Criteria	Example	Action
Blue—Expectant (Palliative Care) The blue category is assigned to patients whose injuries are so severe that survival is unlikely, even with the best possible care. These patients are not expected to survive due to the extent of their injuries, and resources are generally focused on other patients who have a better chance of survival. Comfort care is provided to these patients to ease pain and suffering.	*Massive traumatic injuries*: Extensive head trauma, crushing injuries, or multiple severe internal injuries *Agonal breathing*: Signs of impending death, including gasping breaths or no effective respiratory effort *Very low Glasgow Coma Scale (GCS)*: Severe brain damage with a GCS score of 3, indicating no meaningful brain activity *Non-survivable conditions*: Incompatible with life, such as large open head wounds, decapitation, or catastrophic brain injury	A patient with catastrophic head injury and no response to pain stimuli, with no chance of recovery A child with severe crushing injuries involving multiple organs and expected to die despite advanced interventions	Focus on palliative care: Keep the patient comfortable, control pain, and provide emotional support to the patient and family. Prioritize resources for patients in the red and yellow categories.
Black—Deceased The black category is for patients who are already deceased or whose injuries are incompatible with life. These patients show no signs of life and have no chance of resuscitation.	*No pulse and no breathing*: The patient has no signs of life, and all efforts to resuscitate have failed. *Non-survivable injuries*: Injuries that result in immediate death or conditions such as massive head trauma, decapitation, or severe burns involving most of the body	A child found pulseless and apneic at the scene of a traumatic event with massive injuries A patient with severe thermal burns covering more than 90% of the body surface area	Confirm death and record vital details. Notify the family and provide support. Preserve the body for further examination by medical examiners.

Triaging in Trauma

Certain characteristics need to be considered specifically when triaging children with trauma, high risk factors which necessitate up-triaging and urgent interventions, are categorized in Table 2.5.

Table 2.5 Factors associated with high-risk injuries in pediatric trauma

Major physiological factors	Major anatomical factors	Mechanism of injury factors
Assess signs of shock, altered mental status, and abnormal respiratory or circulatory function.	Determine the type and extent of injuries, such as fractures, head injuries, or internal organ damage.	Understanding the MOI helps predict injury patterns (e.g., a high-speed car crash may cause spinal injury or internal bleeding).
Glasgow Coma Scale (GCS) ≤ 13—when the low score is attributable to a traumatic head injury Systolic blood pressure (SBP) <70 mmHg in children younger than 7 years & <80 mmHg in children aged 7–14 years Respiratory compromise—defined as a respiratory rate <20 breaths/min in infants under 1 year, or requiring ventilatory support	Any visible penetrating injuries on the head or neck, torso or extremities proximal to the elbow or knee Pelvic fractures Open or depressed skull fracture Two or more proximal long bone fractures Flail chest Crushed, degloved, mangled, or amputated proximal extremity Paralysis (partial or complete) Burns with anatomical factors	Falls from a height greater than 10 feet or more than three times the child's height High-risk motor vehicle crash, including: Passenger compartment intrusion >18 inches (or >12 inches on the occupant side) Ejection (partial or complete) from the vehicle Fatality in the same passenger compartment Auto-pedestrian or auto-bicyclist collision where the child is thrown, run over, or impacted at >20 mph Motorcycle or bicycle crash with the child thrown and impact speed >20 mph Burn injuries associated with significant mechanism-of-injury factors

Primary Assessment/Primary Survey

The primary survey in pediatric trauma follows the ABCDE approach, ensuring that life-threatening injuries are managed immediately:

1. *Airway*: Ensure that the airway is open and clear. Use interventions like suctioning or inserting an airway adjunct (e.g., oropharyngeal airway) if necessary.

For traumatic injuries, it is also important to exclude and identify cervical trauma, with the help of doctor on duty. Prior to exclusion of the same, manual in-line stabilization needs to be done, and log rolling needs to be done to turn the child, in order to move the child or examine the back.

2. *Breathing*: Evaluate the rate, depth, and quality of breathing. Administer oxygen or support ventilation if the child is in respiratory distress. If the child is in respiratory failure, airway may need to be secured.

3. *Circulation*: Check for adequate blood flow by evaluating pulse, skin perfusion, and blood pressure. Manage any external bleeding and initiate fluid resuscitation if needed.
4. *Disability*: Assess the child's neurological status using the Pediatric Glasgow Coma Scale and monitor for signs of head injury or spinal cord damage. Serial neurological examination is imperative due to possibility of progression of injury (as ongoing occult intracranial bleed). Neurological status can be serially assessed using standardized scales as Pediatric Glasgow Coma Scale.
5. *Exposure*: Fully expose the child to check for hidden injuries while taking care to prevent hypothermia by covering them appropriately after examination. Monitoring blood glucose and temperature is important. It is important to examine the back of the child as well after logrolling.

Figure 2.2 elucidates in detail triage of patients as per initial assessment and primary assessment.

Secondary Survey and Adjuncts

A secondary survey is a more detailed examination after stabilizing the child. It includes:

- A head-to-toe assessment to identify any missed injuries
- Diagnostic adjuncts like X-rays, ultrasound, or CT scans to clarify the extent of injuries

Adjuncts to the secondary survey provide a more accurate picture of the child's condition and guide further treatment or disposition.

PCPs also assess the patient continuously during transport and manage any complications.

Safe Patient Transfer and Transport

PCPs are an indispensable part of the transporting team, which together coordinates preparation of the patient for transfer (e.g., securing the airway, ensuring IV lines and monitoring are in place), coordinating with the trauma transport team, monitoring and maintaining the record of events and procedures performed, and communicating with the receiving facility to ensure continuity of care.

PCPs' responsibilities in transport include the following:

1. *Patient Stabilization:* PCPs must ensure that the patient's airway is clear, breathing is adequate, and circulation is maintained. Any life-threatening issues such as hemorrhage or respiratory failure should be addressed immediately.
2. *Monitoring Vital Signs:* Continuous monitoring of the patient's heart rate, respiratory rate, oxygen levels, and blood pressure is crucial to detect any signs of deterioration during transport.

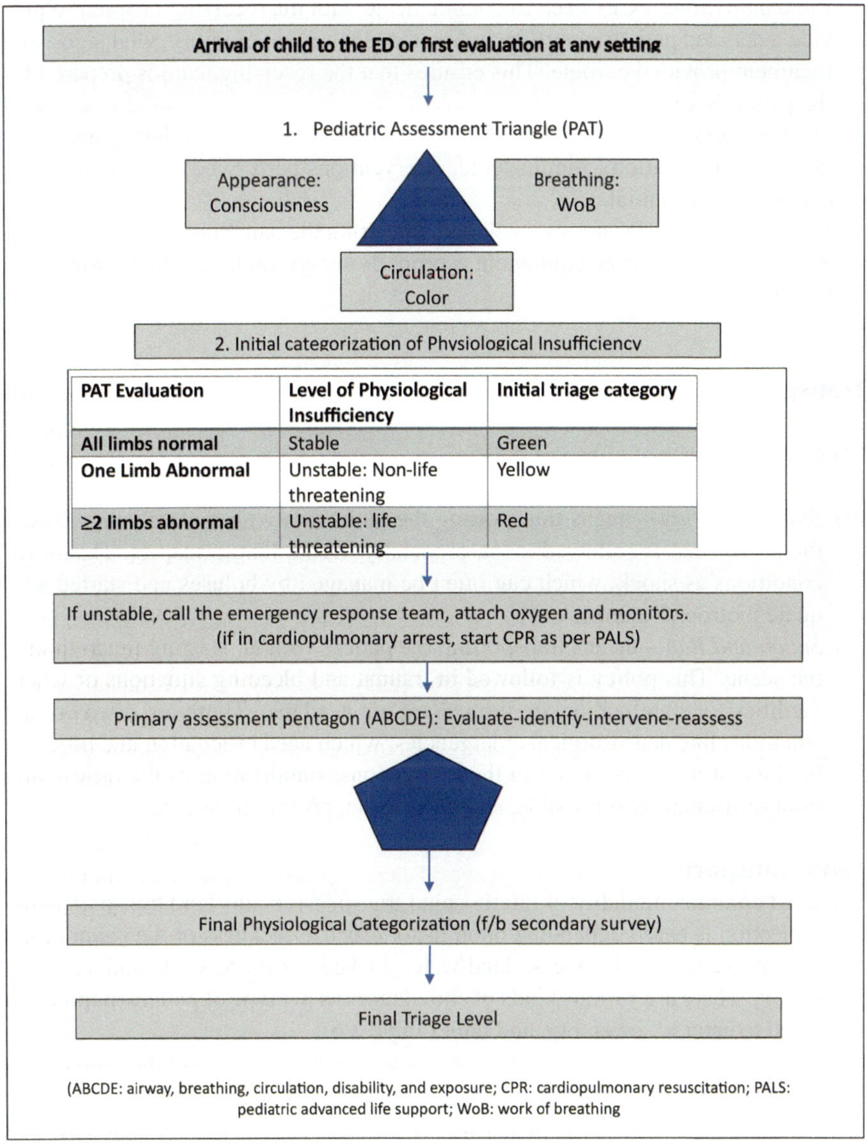

Fig. 2.2 Triage of patients as per initial assessment and primary assessment

3. *Communication:* PCPs need to communicate with the receiving hospital to provide a detailed patient report, including the mechanism of injury, vital signs, and treatment provided enroute. This ensures that the receiving team is prepared for the patient's arrival.
4. *Documentation:* Accurate documentation of the care provided during transport, including medications administered, interventions performed, and the patient's condition, is essential.
5. *Patient Safety:* PCPs are responsible for securing the patient on the stretcher and ensuring all monitoring equipment is properly set up and functioning throughout the journey.

Transport Policies

There are two types of transport policies

(a) *Stand and Play*—means transporting the patient only after stabilizing. This is the policy that is followed most, especially during long transport. This is for conditions as shock, which can often be managed by boluses and started adequate inotropic support.
(b) *Scoop and Run*—means transporting the patient without wasting much time at the scene. This policy is followed in trauma and bleeding situations or where facilities for stabilization are limited/are not available. These are often critical situations like neurosurgical emergencies, which need evacuation and little can be done at the scene. Even in these situations, stabilization of the airway and fluid resuscitation, if possible, should be done, prior to transport.

Land Transport

The most common modality of interhospital transport remains land transport; however, selection is based depending upon factors such as sickness of the patient/time critical interventions, distances, land/water locked location, cost, and resource availability. There are various kinds of ambulances as per type of patient, population they need to cater to, inventory, and built (Table 2.6).

Handover

This is one of the most important parts of transport. It is the exchange between health professionals of information about a patient, accompanying either a transfer of control over, or of responsibility for, the patient. Until the handover takes place, it is often assumed that the responsibility is with the previous team. Handover needs to be structured since repetitive and relevant narrative often hampers the communication process and wastes precious time. It is also important to determine context of handover. For example, a call made by the referring hospital to find out availability of ICU beds may not need detailed history as compared to handover bedside upon completion of transfer from the referring to the referred hospital and tailor the conversation accordingly (Table 2.7).

Table 2.6 Elements of transport

"The right patient is taken at the right time, by the right people to the right hospital and receives the right care throughout"		
The Critical Care Transport Team must consist of at least a doctor and a nurse with a minimum of Basic Life Support (BLS) and Pediatric Advanced Life Support (PALS) or equivalent qualifications. They must have the ability to provide acute medical interventions, pharmacology, and technological life support systems consistent with tertiary level care		
Transporting team	*Team leader*	Responsible for staffing, training, guidelines, and for liaison with other referring hospitals Responsibilities of team leader: (a) Communication with the referring hospital/parents, (b) stabilizing and monitoring the child during transport, (c) filling transport checklist and consent form, (d) well trained in obtaining vascular access, including intraosseous access and securing airway, (e) prescribe/administer necessary medications during transfer This role is to be taken by the senior most and most experienced personnel such as doctor or advanced nurse practitioner.
	Transport nurse	(a) Should be skilled in the nursing care of critically ill child (securing vascular access, tubes, etc.). (b) Should ensure all transport drugs are available and in a usable condition before and during the transport. (c) Should be familiar with all the required paperwork and ensure that they are filled appropriately. (d) Monitor and document vitals. (e) Familiar with equipments and ensure that they are in working condition. (f) Pre-transport checklist must be filled (transport doctor and nurse should be trained in PALS).
	Paramedic	(a) Ensure all equipment is available and in a usable condition. (b) They should be trained in assisting the team. (c) Help in bag and tube ventilation during transport if ventilator not available. (d) Help in moving the stretcher and oxygen cylinder.
	Transport driver	(a) Ensure vehicles are in good condition for transport. (b) Familiar with alternate routes and time taken to reach the destination. (c) Helps in moving the stretcher, when mobilizing the patient.

(continued)

Table 2.6 (continued)

Transport equipment	*Mode of transport*	Ambulance—Emergency ambulance designated for ACLS and BLS transfers must be appropriately equipped. Each retrieval should be triaged based on severity of illness, risk to patient, and experience and competence of staff.
	Monitoring equipment	Should be appropriate for age and weight. Checklist of equipment and drugs must be maintained and checked regularly.
Transport bag	This includes equipment needed for airway management, breathing-related equipment, cardiovascular-related drugs, and equipment.	
	Airway bag	Laryngoscope handles and blades (appropriate size), laryngoscope blades, Yankauer suction, Dynaplast, uncuffed ETTs, cuffed ETTs, 10 ml syringe, laryngeal masks, Guedel airway, face masks, suction tubing, bougie, intubation stylet, and suction catheter
	Similarly, the transport bag should have subsections or smaller bags each containing material for different aspects of physiology: breathing bag, circulation bag, monitoring bag, drug bag, emergency drug bag, PPE kit, etc.	
	Trauma and burns kit	This may include sand bags, spine board (included separately in ambulance), adjustable neck collar, splint for immobilization as Thomas splint, sling for immobilization, sterile gauze, bandages, sterile dressings, and tourniquet.
	For specialized transfers such as ECMO, iNO, and air transfers, specialized bags need to be developed.	
Checklists	Pre-transport checklist includes separate checklists for communication, equipment, ambulance, staffing, drugs, and infection control. Disease-specific checklists which may be necessitated. Separate checklists for patient monitoring en route, fire safety, and emergency plan are also needed. Checklists for handover and post-transport checklists to get all the equipment back are also a useful concept.	

(continued)

Table 2.6 (continued)

Types of Road Ambulances
Road ambulances are categorized according to the level of care they are equipped to provide:
1. *Type A—Medical First Responder Ambulance:*
2. Intended to deliver emergency medical care at the scene while the vehicle remains stationary. It may be any CMVR-approved Category M or L vehicle, equipped for basic stabilization and first response prior to transport.
3. *Type B—Patient Transport Vehicle (PTV):*
4. Designed for transporting stable patients who are not anticipated to require active emergency interventions during transit. Commonly used for interfacility transfers or noncritical patient movement.
5. *Type C—Basic Life Support (BLS) Ambulance:*
6. A purpose-built, ergonomically designed vehicle, staffed with trained personnel and equipped for basic patient monitoring and noninvasive airway management. Suitable for patients requiring ongoing observation and basic support en route.
7. *Type D—Advanced Life Support (ALS) Ambulance:*
8. Configured for the transport and intensive management of critically ill or injured patients, this vehicle carries advanced medical equipment and highly trained personnel capable of invasive airway management, advanced resuscitation, and continuous intensive monitoring.

Table 2.7 Handover tools that can be used by PCPs

Tools (acronym)	Details
SBAR	Situation, Background, Assessment, Recommendation (SBAR) model
ISBAR	*I*dentification, *S*ituation, *B*ackground, *A*ssessment, and *R*ecommendation
I-PASS:	I—illness severity, P—patient summary, A—action list, S—situational awareness and contingency planning, and S—synthesis by receiver
SIGNOUT:	S—Sick, I—Identifying data (name, age, gender, diagnosis), G—General hospital course, N—New events of day, O—Overall health status/clinical condition, U—Upcoming possibilities with plan, rationale, T—Tasks to complete overnight with plan, rationale, Any questions?
ANTICipate (written handouts)	A—administrative data, N—new information (clinical update), T—tasks (what needs to be done), I—illness, and C—contingency planning/code status

Intrahospital Transport

Transport is as relevant inside the hospital, be it shifting a sick traumatic brain injury child to CT room for imaging or shifting him to operation theater for surgery, and the concept involving pre-transport preparedness using checklists, handover between the transferring locations, and continuous monitoring with watchful expectancy remains the same. The modalities of intrahospital transport are elucidated in Table 2.8.

Table 2.8 Various modalities of intrahospital transport

Sl. no	Method	Uses	PCP responsibility
1.	*Manual bed/stretcher transport* This is the most common method of intrahospital transport, where the patient is transferred from one location to another on a hospital bed or stretcher.	It is often used for: Noncritical patients who are stable but need diagnostic tests (e.g., CT scans, MRIs, or X-rays) or treatment in another department (e.g., operating room) Patients under anesthesia or sedation following surgical procedures	Ensure all patient equipment (e.g., IV lines, monitors) are safely secured. Monitor vital signs, especially in postoperative patients. Coordinate with the receiving unit, informing them of the patient's condition and care requirements. Ensure the bed or stretcher has side rails up to prevent falls.
2.	*Wheelchair transport* This method is used for ambulatory patients who can sit up but may have limitations due to injury or illness.	It is suitable for patients undergoing noninvasive or diagnostic procedures like ultrasounds or consultations in other departments.	Ensure the patient is comfortable and properly positioned in the wheelchair. Assist with movement if the patient has limited mobility or strength. Monitor the patient for signs of discomfort or dizziness, particularly in postsurgical or weakened patients.
3.	*Specialized beds or transfer chairs* For patients with specific medical conditions, specialized beds or transfer chairs may be used.	These can be reclined or adjusted based on the patient's requirements, making them ideal for: Orthopedic patients who need specific support for injured limbs Cardiac or respiratory patients who may need to be positioned upright during transport for better oxygenation	Adjust the bed or chair to the patient's medical condition (e.g., elevated head for respiratory patients). Monitor the patient's vital signs and comfort level during the transport.

(continued)

Table 2.8 (continued)

Sl. no	Method	Uses	PCP responsibility
4.	*Portable ventilator or life support equipment transport* This method is used for critically ill patients who require continuous life support, including mechanical ventilation or complex monitoring.	These patients are typically being transferred to the ICU, operating room, or for diagnostic imaging that requires advanced care.	Ensure all life support equipment (ventilators, infusion pumps, monitors) is portable and properly functioning during transport. Monitor vital signs continuously and be prepared to intervene if the patient's condition deteriorates. Work closely with the transport team, which may include respiratory therapists or critical care nurses, to ensure safe transfer.
5.	*Transport with accompanying medical personnel* For critically ill or unstable patients, intrahospital transport may require a team of medical personnel, including nurses, respiratory therapists, or physicians, to accompany the patient.	In need of immediate interventions or whose condition may deteriorate during transport Needing specialized care (e.g., neonates, trauma patients, or those on ventilators)	Coordinate with the transport team to ensure seamless handovers between departments. Continuously assess the patient's status and provide life-saving interventions if necessary. Ensure the availability of emergency medications and equipment during transport.
6.	*Automated or robotic transport* Some hospitals use automated transport systems, such as robotic carriers, to move noncritical patients, samples, or supplies between departments.	This system is typically used for: Stable patients who do not require close monitoring Efficient handling of nonurgent transfers, such as transporting a patient for routine tests	Ensure the patient is stable and capable of undergoing automated transport. Communicate with receiving departments to coordinate care once the patient arrives.

Case Resolution

Let us now return to the case scenario and integrate the key concepts discussed above through a reflective case-based analysis (Table 2.9).

Prompt triage, early recognition of severity, and PCP-led stabilization enabled safe transport and timely surgical intervention. The child underwent emergency craniotomy and was later discharged with full neurological recovery. This case

Table 2.9 Reflective case-based analysis

Brief case history	An 11-year-old male child was struck by an electric pole while riding a bicycle without wearing a helmet. He was found unresponsive at the scene by bystanders, and emergency medical services (EMS) were called. The child's condition deteriorated en route to the hospital.	
Scene assessment (by EMS)	The child is found lying on the roadside near the bicycle. There is a visible head injury with swelling and minor abrasions on the face and arms. The child is unresponsive, breathing irregularly, and has no helmet.	
Initial rapid (PAT) assessment	*Appearance*: The child is unresponsive. Limp body tone, no purposeful movement. No eye contact or interaction with surroundings *Work of Breathing*: Irregular breathing. Shallow breaths and labored respirations. Audible gasping, indicating possible airway compromise *Circulation to Skin*: Pale skin, with cool extremities. Capillary refill is delayed (>3 s), suggesting poor perfusion.	
Initial assessment from PAT:	*The child appears to be in respiratory failure and shock, requiring immediate lifesaving interventions.*	
Primary survey (ABCDE approach)		
Primary assessment		
Airway	The child's airway appears compromised due to the unresponsive state. There are no obvious obstructions, but the child's head injury may compromise airway patency.	Open the airway using the jaw-thrust maneuver (avoid head tilt due to possible cervical spine injury). Consider placing an oral airway adjunct if needed.
Breathing	The child's breathing is shallow and irregular, with poor chest rise. Oxygen saturation is dropping (measured at 85%).	Administer high-flow oxygen via a non-rebreather mask. If breathing does not improve, consider bag-valve-mask (BVM) ventilation.
Circulation	The pulse is weak and rapid (tachycardia). Skin is pale and cool with delayed capillary refill (>3 seconds).	Establish intravenous (IV) access and begin fluid resuscitation with normal saline boluses (20 mL/kg), while continuously monitoring for signs of shock.
Disability	The child is unresponsive to verbal commands and painful stimuli (Glasgow Coma Scale = 7: eye response = 1, verbal response = 2, motor response = 4).	Reassess for any signs of improvement following resuscitation. Protect the cervical spine by immobilizing the neck with a cervical collar.
Exposure	Expose the child to assess additional injuries, including chest, abdomen, pelvis, and extremities. No visible signs of major trauma besides the head injury and abrasions	Cover the child with a warming blanket to prevent hypothermia.

(continued)

Table 2.9 (continued)

Secondary survey	
Head and neck:	There is significant swelling on the forehead, with possible skull fractures. Pupils are unequal, suggesting increased intracranial pressure (ICP) due to head trauma.
Chest:	Breath sounds are equal bilaterally. No rib fractures or deformities noted.
Abdomen:	The abdomen is soft, with no signs of tenderness or distention. No major abdominal injury is suspected at this stage.
Pelvis:	The pelvis is stable upon examination, with no signs of trauma.
Extremities:	No obvious deformities, but multiple abrasions on the arms and legs are noted. Distal pulses are weak.
Neurological exam:	As noted during the primary survey, the child has a Glasgow Coma Scale (GCS) of 7, indicating severe brain injury or impairment.
Intervention:	Perform a head CT scan (if possible) to assess for intracranial hemorrhage or skull fractures. Administer mannitol or hypertonic saline to reduce increased intracranial pressure, as indicated. Continued fluid resuscitation and close monitoring of vital signs are essential.
Transport and nursing responsibilities	
Preparation for transport:	*Stabilization before transport:* Ensure airway is maintained (consider intubation if necessary, due to neurological decline). Oxygen support via a non-rebreather mask or bag-valve-mask as required. Secure IV access for fluid and medication administration. Immobilize the cervical spine with a collar and use a backboard if spinal injury is suspected. Monitor vital signs continuously (heart rate, respiratory rate, oxygen saturation, blood pressure).
	Communication with the receiving facility: Communicate with the receiving trauma center, providing information on the child's condition, treatments provided, and the need for immediate neurosurgical evaluation due to suspected traumatic brain injury (TBI).
	PCP responsibilities: The PCP should continue monitoring the child's airway, breathing, and circulation during transport. Ensure that emergency medications and resuscitation equipment are readily available during transit. Administer IV fluids and medications as prescribed to prevent further deterioration. Document all interventions performed during transport, including changes in the child's condition and treatments administered.
Interhospital transport:	Due to the severe head injury, the child is transferred to a pediatric trauma center with neurosurgical capabilities. Air transport may be considered to reduce transport time if the trauma center is located far away.

(continued)

Table 2.9 (continued)

Post-transport care at trauma center	Upon arrival at the trauma center: The child will undergo a rapid neurological evaluation and head CT scan. Trauma and neurosurgical teams will assess the child for surgical intervention if there is an intracranial hemorrhage. Critical care in the Pediatric Intensive Care Unit (PICU) will follow, with close monitoring of neurological function, ICP, and overall condition.
Role of the PCP	Throughout the scenario, the PCPs' role includes: Rapid assessment using the Pediatric Assessment Triangle (PAT) and the ABCDE approach during the primary survey. Stabilization of the child before and during transport. Ongoing monitoring of vital signs, neurological status, and hemodynamic stability. Effective communication with the transport team and receiving facility to ensure seamless transfer of care.

highlights the vital role of structured triage, vigilant PCP-led care, and coordinated transport in optimizing outcomes for pediatric trauma victims.

Key Messages

- Pediatric trauma care is distinct from adult trauma management due to unique anatomical, physiological, and developmental characteristics, which require tailored triage, assessment, and stabilization protocols.
- The Pediatric Assessment Triangle (PAT) offers a rapid, visual, and noninvasive method to identify critically ill or injured children by assessing appearance, work of breathing, and circulation to skin.
- Early and accurate triage in the emergency department (ED) is crucial to prioritize care, prevent deterioration, and guide timely transfer decisions, using tools like IMNCI, ETAT, PREM, ESI, and IAP ALS.
- Primary survey (ABCDE approach) ensures systematic identification and immediate management of life-threatening issues. Airway protection, ventilation, circulation assessment, neurological evaluation, and exposure are core components.
- High-risk indicators (e.g., altered mental status, hypotension, abnormal respiratory rate) and specific mechanisms of injury (e.g., high-velocity accidents, falls >10 ft) warrant *up-triaging* to avoid missed critical injuries.
- Triage categorization (red-yellow-green-blue-black) facilitates resource prioritization, allowing PCPs to deliver lifesaving interventions to the most critically ill patients first.
- PCPs play a vital role in both interhospital and intrahospital transport, being responsible for stabilization, continuous monitoring, communication with receiving centers, and accurate documentation.
- Transport policies—"scoop and run" vs. "stand and play"—must be adapted based on patient condition and available resources. Even in rapid transfer scenarios, minimal stabilization (airway, fluids) is essential.

- Structured handover using tools like SBAR, ISBAR, and I-PASS enhances continuity of care during patient transfer by improving communication, reducing errors, and streamlining transitions between teams.
- Preparedness with transport equipment and checklists, along with trained personnel (doctor, nurse, paramedic, driver), ensures safe and efficient transfer, minimizing morbidity during critical windows of pediatric trauma care.

Bibliography

1. Advanced Trauma Life Support (ATLS®). (2018). Student course manual (10th ed.). American College of Surgeons.
2. American Academy of Pediatrics Committee on Pediatric Emergency Medicine. (2019). The role of emergency medical services in children's access to emergency care. Pediatrics, 144(5), e20192750.
3. American Heart Association. (2020). Pediatric advanced life support provider manual. American Heart Association.
4. Automotive Industry Standards Committee Under Central Motor Vehicle Rules – Technical Standing Committee Ministry Of Road Transport And Highways (Department Of Road Transport And Highways) Government Of India. Constructional and Functional Requirements for Road Ambulances (National Ambulance Code) [Internet]. Automotive Research Association Of India; 2013. Available from: http://www.nisc.gov.in/PDF/AIS_125.pdf
5. Bledsoe, B. E., Porter, R. S., Cherry, R. A., & Snyder, S. R. (2020). Paramedic care: Principles & practice (Vol. 5: Special considerations) (5th ed.). Pearson Education
6. Breaux J, McLendon R, Stedman RB, Amedee RG, Piazza J, Wolterman R. Developing a Standardized and Sustainable Resident Sign-Out Process: An AIAMC National Initiative IV Project. Ochsner J. 2014;14(4):563–8.
7. Burgess A, van Diggele C, Roberts C, Mellis C. Teaching clinical handover with ISBAR. BMC Medical Education. 2020 Dec 3;20(2):459.
8. Committee of Health and Family Welfare department, Government of National Capital Territory of Delhi. Registration of Ambulances [Internet]. Available from: http://health.delhigovt.nic.in/wps/wcm/connect/1c884d00406954a5b44dbc34262e20fd/cat.pdf?MOD=AJPERES&lmod=-288077341
9. D'Empaire PP, Amaral ACKB. What every intensivist should know about handovers in the intensive care unit. Rev Bras Ter Intensiva. 2017;29(2):121–3.
10. Dieckmann RA, Brownstein D, Gausche-Hill M. The pediatric assessment triangle: a novel approach for the rapid evaluation of children. Pediatr Emerg Care. 2010 Apr;26(4):312–5.
11. Dieckmann, R. A., Brownstein, D. R., & Gausche-Hill, M. (2010). Pediatric assessment triangle: A novel approach for the rapid assessment of children. Pediatric Emergency Care, 26(1), 74–78.
12. Emergency Triage Assessment and Treatment (ETAT) course [Internet]. World Health Organisation; [cited 2025 Apr 23]. Available from: https://www.who.int/publications/i/item/9241546875
13. Facility based integrated management of neonatal and childhood illness (F-IMNCI) IMNCI chart booklet [Internet]. Ministry of Health & Family Welfare, Govt. of India; Available from: https://nhm.gov.in/images/pdf/programmes/child-health/guidelines/imnci_chart_booklet.pdf
14. Figaji AA. Anatomical and Physiological Differences between Children and Adults Relevant to Traumatic Brain Injury and the Implications for Clinical Assessment and Care. Front Neurol. 2017 Dec 14;8:685.

15. Fitzgerald, M., Cameron, P., Mackenzie, C., Farrow, N., Scicluna, P., & Gocentas, R. (2012). Trauma resuscitation errors and computer-assisted decision support. Archives of Surgery, 147(3), 256–262.
16. Ghosh S, Ramamoorthy L, Pottakat B. Impact of Structured Clinical Handover Protocol on Communication and Patient Satisfaction. J Patient Exp. 2021 Mar 3;8:2374373521997733.
17. Horwitz LI, Moin T, Green ML. Development and Implementation of an Oral Sign-out Skills Curriculum. J Gen Intern Med. 2007 Oct;22(10):1470–4.
18. IAP ALS-BLS [Internet]. [cited 2025 Apr 23]. Available from: https://www.iapalsbls.com/
19. Jhamb, U, Saxena, R. Transport of sick kids: TaSK Module. IAP Presidential plan. Indian Academy of Pediatrics. 2021. Ed. 1. 1-368.
20. James H. E. (1986). Neurologic evaluation and support in the child with an acute brain insult. *Pediatric annals, 15*(1), 16–22.
21. Khilnani P, Chhabra R. Transport of critically ill children: how to utilize resources in the developing world. Indian J Pediatr. 2008 Jun;75(6):591–8.
22. Liu TT, Cheng CT, Hsu CP, Chaou CH, Ng CJ, Jeng MJ, et al. Validation of a five-level triage system in pediatric trauma and the effectiveness of triage nurse modification: A multi-center cohort analysis. Front Med (Lausanne). 2022 Nov 1;9:947501.
23. Maconochie, I. K., Aickin, R., Hazinski, M. F., & Atkins, D. L. (2015). Pediatric basic and advanced life support: 2015 international consensus. Circulation, 132(16_suppl_1), S177–S203.
24. Mowafi, H., & Dworkis, D. (2020). Prehospital trauma care systems: A global review. BMJ Global Health
25. National Highway Accident Relief service scheme (NHARSS). Specifications of Advance Life Support ambulance for Procurement [Internet]. Available from: https://morth.gov.in/sites/default/files/circulars_document/Specifications_of_Advance.pdf
26. Neha Thakur, Samir Misra. Pediatric Trauma Resuscitation Module (PTRM). First edition. New Delhi: Jaypee Brothers Medical Publishers (P) Ltd; 2024.
27. Paneitz DC, Ahmad S. Pediatric Trauma Update. Mo Med. 2018;115(5):438–42.
28. Reilly PL, Simpson DA, Sprod R, Thomas L. Assessing the conscious level in infants and young children: a paediatric version of the Glasgow Coma Scale. Childs Nerv Syst. 1988 Feb;4(1):30–3.
29. Srinivas, M., & Basavarajappa, K. G. (2021). Pediatric trauma care: An Indian perspective. Indian Pediatrics, 58(6), 523–529.
30. Subbarao, I., & Lyznicki, J. M. (2021). Pediatric emergency preparedness and response. In J. L. Ligon (Ed.), Disaster medicine (pp. 185–194). Springer.
31. The Canadian Triage and Acuity Scale.
32. Theodorou CM, Galganski LA, Jurkovich GJ, Farmer DL, Hirose S, Stephenson JT, et al. Causes of Early Mortality in Pediatric Trauma Patients. J Trauma Acute Care Surg. 2021 Mar 1;90(3):574–81.
33. Topjian AA, Raymond TT, Atkins D, Chan M, Duff JP, Joyner BL, et al. Part 4: Pediatric Basic and Advanced Life Support: 2020 American Heart Association Guidelines for Cardiopulmonary Resuscitation and Emergency Cardiovascular Care. Circulation. 2020 Oct 20;142(16_suppl_2):S469–523.
34. Wiebe, D. J., & Carr, B. G. (2020). Pediatric trauma systems: Where we are and where we need to go. Journal of Trauma and Acute Care Surgery, 89(6), 1197–1204.
35. World Health Organization. (2016). Guidelines for essential trauma care (2nd ed.). World Health Organization. https://apps.who.int/iris/handle/10665/42565

Crisis Resource Management and Disaster Preparedness in Pediatric Trauma Care

3

Anil Raj Assariparambil and Vimal Krishnan S

Learning Objectives

By the end of this chapter, the reader should be able to:

- Understand the core principles of Crisis Resource Management (CRM) and how they apply to pediatric trauma care in high-stress, resource-limited settings.
- Recognize the unique challenges of pediatric trauma during a mass casualty incident (MCI) and initiate appropriate triage and stabilization measures.
- Maintain situational awareness and make timely decisions, effectively allocating limited resources during dynamic trauma scenarios.
- Demonstrate leadership skills and coordinate team roles, ensuring efficient task distribution and clear communication during pediatric emergencies.
- Collaborate effectively within a multidisciplinary team, contributing to disaster preparedness and improving outcomes in pediatric trauma response.

A. R. Assariparambil
Department of Medical-Surgical Nursing, Manipal College of Nursing, Manipal Academy of Higher Education, Manipal, Karnataka, India
e-mail: anil.raj@manipal.edu

V. Krishnan S (✉)
Department of Emergency Medicine, Kasturba Medical College, Manipal, Manipal Academy of Higher Education (MAHE), Manipal, Karnataka, India

Centre for Resuscitation, Acute Care and Simulation Training (CReST), Manipal Academy of Higher Education (MAHE), Manipal, Karnataka, India
e-mail: vimal.krishnan@manipal.edu

N. T. Rai (ed.), *Pediatric Trauma Resuscitation Manual (PTRM) for Primary Care Providers*, https://doi.org/10.1007/978-981-95-4979-5_3

Introduction

Pediatric trauma care in crisis situations requires a coordinated, systematic approach to ensure optimal patient outcomes. Crisis Resource Management (CRM) focuses on enhancing teamwork, communication, leadership, and critical decision-making under high-pressure conditions. At the same time, disaster preparedness ensures efficient resource allocation and response during mass casualty incidents (MCI). PCPs play a critical role in managing pediatric trauma by rapidly assessing and stabilizing patients, collaborating with multidisciplinary teams, and adapting to evolving challenges. This chapter equips PCPs with essential skills to navigate high-stakes emergencies, minimize errors, and deliver effective, lifesaving care in pediatric trauma scenarios.

Disaster planning at all levels—national, state, tribal, local, and regional—must prioritize the unique needs of children, including their physical, mental, behavioral, and developmental requirements. PCPs should play a key role in disaster planning, response, and recovery, leveraging their expertise in patient care and public health. Healthcare facilities must create preparedness plans to ensure continuous care for children during and after disasters. Collaboration among PCPs, local hospitals, public health agencies, emergency management teams, educators, and nongovernmental organizations is essential to address children's needs in crisis situations effectively. Access to appropriate equipment, medications, and supplies for children must be ensured. Research and best practices for pediatric disaster care should be supported, with a call for federal backing. Disaster drills should include children as victims and responders, tailored to their capabilities. PCPs should educate families on emergency preparedness and resilience while seeking ongoing training in pediatric disaster response. It is also vital for all PCPs and first responders to understand the specific needs of children during disasters.

Case Scenario

A 6-year-old child is brought to the emergency unit of a district hospital following a mass casualty incident (MCI) involving a school bus crash during morning rush hour. Multiple pediatric patients are expected, and an MCI alert has already been activated.

The child arrives via ambulance, secured on a spinal board with a cervical collar in place. Emergency Medical Services (EMS) report that he was unresponsive at the scene but began responding to painful stimuli during transport. His identity remains unknown, and his parents have not yet been located, making consent and communication difficult.

The emergency bay is crowded, with teams managing a surge of critical cases. Two PCPs—Meena, a nurse practitioner, and Arjun, an emergency technician—are assigned to receive the child amid the chaos.

On initial assessment, the child has multiple traumatic injuries, including a suspected head injury, a deformed and bleeding right femur, and signs of respiratory distress. Vital signs are concerning:

- Heart rate: 140 bpm
- Respiratory rate: 35 breaths/min
- Blood pressure: 90/60 mmHg
- Oxygen saturation: 88% on room air

On auscultation, air entry is reduced on the right side of the chest, raising concern for a possible pneumothorax. The child remains on spinal precautions, and the care area continues to receive additional casualties.

Reflective Questions

1. What are the core principles of Crisis Resource Management (CRM), and how do they enhance patient safety in pediatric trauma care?
2. How does effective triage in a Mass Casualty Incident (MCI) help prioritize pediatric trauma patients, and what system is commonly used?
3. Why is situational awareness critical in a crisis, and how can fixation errors impact decision-making in pediatric emergencies?
4. How do leadership, teamwork, and closed-loop communication contribute to effective pediatric trauma management?
5. What are the key components of disaster preparedness for pediatric trauma, and why is ongoing training essential for PCPs?

Crisis Resource Management (CRM)

A crisis is a time-sensitive event where the outcome determines whether adverse consequences will follow. It is a complex situation involving the environment, the patient, and the healthcare workers. Effective crisis resolution requires managing the problem rather than focusing solely on the patient's physiological changes.

Crises present significant challenges for several reasons. The underlying problems or triggers may be poorly defined or ambiguous. Crises often appear to arise suddenly, leaving little time for information gathering and analysis. The data collected may be incomplete, contain errors, or conflict with other information. Proper filtering and analysis of this data are crucial to making accurate decisions.

Crises evolve rapidly, often leading to a swift deterioration in the patient's condition that demands immediate action. The treatment goals may be unclear or conflicting, further complicating decision-making. The situation's urgency places considerable time pressure especially on PCPs to respond effectively.

The nature of a crisis triggers stress responses in PCPs. These responses may include fear, anxiety, tachycardia, and tachypnea. Mental reactions can manifest as cognitive blockages, fixation on specific ideas, tunnel vision, and a sense of panic.

The heightened cognitive workload may lead to "load shedding," where certain information or tasks are relegated to the background and overlooked.

Managing critical events effectively requires adherence to fundamental principles. Seven key points of Crisis Resource Management (CRM) provide a structured approach to handling crises. These principles emphasize teamwork, communication, resource utilization, situational awareness, and decision-making under pressure, ultimately improving patient outcomes in high-stakes situations (Table 3.1).

I. *Understanding and being familiar with your environment*

Familiarity with your work environment is crucial in a crisis, impacting decision-making and resource utilization. Being unprepared can increase stress and hinder response effectiveness. Key aspects to know include:

Table 3.1 Crisis Resource Management (CRM) principles in pediatric trauma care

CRM principle	Key actions
1. Situational Awareness	Identify key ED zones: resuscitation bay, trauma cart, imaging suites, and exits. Ensure critical equipment is accessible (airway kits, IV tools, blood). Recognize crowding and equipment shortages; adapt accordingly.
2. Anticipation and Strategic Planning	Prepare airway tools: BVM, suction, and intubation kit. Anticipate shock due to fractures/head injury. Plan for oxygen, IV access, fluids (20 mL/kg), and analgesia. Coordinate with radiology, surgery, and ICU.
3. Timely Escalation	Activate trauma team early. Request support from senior clinicians, respiratory therapists, and blood bank. Involve social work and law enforcement for ID and consent.
4. Leadership and Role Assignment	Assign a team leader to direct care. Allocate roles: airway, IV, vitals, and documentation. Monitor task flow and correct delays, overlaps, or missed steps.
5. Effective Communication	Use SBAR to structure updates. Apply closed-loop communication (e.g., confirm task completion). Share updates regularly as patient status evolves.
6. Focused Attention and Decision-Making	Reassess ABCDE frequently. Monitor vitals and escalate as needed. Use POCUS for pneumothorax or bleeding. Watch for neuro/respiratory decline.
7. Task Delegation and Resource Use	Match tasks to skill level (e.g., experienced provider manages airway). Reassign roles as priorities shift. Prioritize limited resources. Document all actions in real time.

- Team capabilities
- Local operational protocols
- Location of equipment, drugs, and supplies
- Proper use and limitations of emergency equipment

II. *Anticipating potential issues and planning ahead*

Understanding patient care now and in the future helps predict and prevent critical events. When prevention isn't possible, planning minimizes risks and improves outcomes.

Key strategies include:

- Using checklists and established crisis procedures (e.g., DRSABCD, *Danger, Response, Send for help, Airway, Breathing, CPR, Defibrillation*)
- Practicing for likely emergencies
- Training in crisis management to reduce stress

Effective planning involves:

- Seeking help when needed
- Recognizing when senior support is required
- Identifying the crisis endpoint early and prioritizing necessary steps

III. *Seeking help at an early stage*

Early calls for help ensure optimal patient care by gathering necessary staff and resources. Effective help includes:

- Cognitive: Second opinions or alternative management approaches
- Physical: Extra hands for procedures
- Organizational: Resource coordination
- Sub-team Support: Handling specific tasks like transfusion or surgery

Barriers to seeking help may be personal, interpersonal, or cultural. To overcome this, many facilities promote help-seeking through staff assist buttons, MEWS, and mandatory reporting criteria.

IV. *Taking charge and assuming leadership responsibilities*

Effective leadership in crisis requires a clear, designated leader with technical expertise, composure, and organizational skills. A strong leader:

- Provides clear direction while overseeing the situation
- Uses audible, direct communication with names/roles and eye contact

- Summarizes the treatment plan to ensure shared understanding
- Engages the team respectfully and confidently
- Adapts to team dynamics for maximum effectiveness

Leadership may shift, but the new leader should clearly state, *"I am now the team leader."* Encouraging team input enhances overall effectiveness.

V. *Communicating clearly and effectively*

Clear communication is crucial in emergencies, requiring team members to listen, share information, and act accordingly. Stress can hinder communication, so extra effort is needed.

Key elements of effective communication:

- Clear, calm verbal exchanges using simple, standardized language
- Positive nonverbal cues like eye contact and gestures
- Closed-loop communication to confirm and clarify instructions
- Assigning a team member to manage interactions with family/carers

Communication Techniques:
Closed-loop communication ensures accuracy by having the receiver repeat back information.
Graded assertiveness (PACE) escalates concerns in a structured manner: Probe, Alert, Challenge, Emergency.

Standardized reporting tools:
- SBAR (Situation, Background, Assessment, Recommendation) for concise patient updates
- SEGUE for structured, safe team communication (Seek attention, Elicit information, Give information, Understand others, and End of the interchange)

Effective two-way communication improves situational awareness and patient safety.

VI. *Allocating attention wisely by utilizing all available information*

The situation can change rapidly as new details emerge. Staying aware of your surroundings, including available resources, team actions, and evolving conditions, is essential. Situational awareness is maintaining a big-picture view while integrating new information and managing available resources. In emergencies, clinicians must continuously assess the changing situation and team actions.

A key challenge is *fixation errors*, where focus on one detail causes critical oversights. Task fixation occurs when a team member becomes absorbed in a single task, neglecting broader responsibilities, such as a leader fixating on a procedure instead of directing the team.

Diagnosis fixation happens when a clinician commits to an initial diagnosis without considering alternatives, potentially missing life-threatening conditions. Maintaining awareness and adaptability is crucial for effective crisis management.

VII. *Distributing tasks efficiently and leveraging all available resources*

Effective workload distribution ensures tasks are completed efficiently based on urgency and skill level. To prevent overdependence on one team member, individuals should communicate when they feel overwhelmed or unable to complete a task. Tasks should be reallocated quickly to appropriate team members, and if staffing is limited, the team must optimize the existing skill mix. Understanding and appreciating each other's workload fosters teamwork and efficiency. Roles should be assigned at the start of an emergency but may need adjustments as the situation evolves. Team members must voice concerns if given a role beyond their capabilities to ensure safe and effective care.

Disaster Preparedness in Pediatric Trauma Care

The pediatric population is highly vulnerable and disproportionately impacted during disasters and needs special attention. The following factors make it challenging to manage children during disaster situations:

- *Anatomy and Physiology:* Children have unique anatomical and physiological traits that make them more vulnerable to trauma and environmental hazards. Their smaller blood volume, thinner skin, and lower body fat increase their fluid and heat loss risk. Children absorb more force per unit area due to their smaller mass, resulting in distinct injury patterns. Their skeletal immaturity and ligamentous laxity further influence trauma outcomes. Additionally, their higher surface area-to-mass ratio increases the risks of toxin absorption and harmful gas inhalation. High metabolic rates and rapid heart and respiratory rates complicate shock assessment. PCPs inexperienced in pediatric care must have quick access to pediatric vital signs and medication dosages, as children are also more susceptible to hypothermia and toxin inhalation. Regulating their temperature early is particularly important, especially for younger children.
- *Development and Psychology:* Children's developmental and emotional differences pose significant challenges for PCPs, particularly those with limited pediatric experience. Infants and young children rely on their caregivers for communication and emotional support. During disasters, separation from caregivers can occur due to injury, death, or chaos, complicating medical care and emotional stability. Without caregivers, young children need constant supervision, which adds strain to already overwhelmed PCPs. Additionally, children often struggle to understand the reality of a disaster, leading to emotional distress such as confusion, fear, or withdrawal, which can hinder effective assessments and care.

- *Educational Vulnerability:* Disasters significantly disrupt children's academic performance, with some changing schools up to 11 times in just 3 months. Infants and young children, unable to care for themselves, require safe housing, protection, and age-appropriate supplies. These unique needs must be prioritized in disaster response and preparedness planning.

Systematic changes in disaster preparedness are essential for effective pediatric trauma care. Integrating disaster planning into schools and institutions, along with pediatric-focused drills and training, benefits families and communities. Emergency plans at the state, regional, and local levels must address the legal and operational systems needed for large-scale disasters. These plans should include pre-disaster strategies, management, assessment, multidisciplinary collaboration, and data-driven approaches to identify and address the specific needs of the pediatric population (Table 3.2).

Table 3.2 Core domains and action points for pediatric trauma management in mass casualty incidents (MCI)

Equipment readiness	Conduct regular checks and drills to ensure availability of pediatric-specific supplies and equipment.
Simulation and drills	Participate in pediatric trauma simulations regularly to improve real-time readiness during MCI scenarios.
Effective triage	Apply pediatric triage systems like JumpSTART to categorize based on injury severity; the child in this case is red (immediate).
Role assignment	Delegate tasks clearly based on urgency and skill—airway management, bleeding control, fracture support, and vitals.
Team coordination	Use structured communication tools like SBAR to ensure clarity and prioritization of care tasks.
Age-appropriate assessment	Recognize pediatric-specific physiology; early signs like tachypnea and hypoxia may indicate serious compromise despite stable vitals.
Airway and breathing	Manage airway immediately; provide oxygen and prepare for chest decompression if pneumothorax is suspected.
Fluid resuscitation	Administer isotonic fluids (e.g., normal saline) at 20 mL/kg for suspected hypovolemic shock.
Efficient use of resources	Allocate limited supplies (equipment, medications, blood products) to the most critically injured pediatric patients.
Psychological support	Use calm, age-appropriate language to comfort the child, even if unresponsive, to reduce psychological stress.
Family support	Follow protocols for treating unaccompanied minors; continue efforts to identify and inform family members.
Post-disaster debriefing	Use after-action reviews to identify strengths and areas for improvement in disaster response.

Pre-disaster Planning and Preparedness

Training and Protocol Development

Effective pediatric disaster response starts with comprehensive training and well-structured protocol development. PCPs, particularly nurses, must be equipped with pediatric-specific knowledge and skills through regular simulations, drills, and continuing education programs. Training should focus on trauma assessment, pediatric triage systems (such as JumpSTART), communication strategies, and psychological first aid. Protocols need to be clearly outlined and standardized to ensure a coordinated response during emergencies. These protocols should include guidelines for triage, transport, reunification with caregivers, and age-appropriate care. By incorporating pediatric-focused protocols into hospital and community emergency plans, we enhance readiness and minimize confusion during actual events, ultimately improving outcomes for children in disaster situations.

- Participate in disaster drills and simulation exercises (e.g., mass casualty incidents, bioterrorism, natural disasters).
- Develop triage protocols tailored to pediatrics (e.g., JumpSTART triage for children).
- Familiarize with hospital disaster plans and regional emergency response systems.
- Ensure knowledge of evacuation procedures for neonatal and pediatric units.

Stockpile and Equipment Readiness

Ensuring the readiness of stockpiles and equipment is a crucial aspect of pediatric disaster preparedness. Emergency supplies should include child-sized medical equipment, such as airway tools, IV kits, splints, and personal protective gear, along with age-appropriate medications and nutritional supplies. Pediatric trauma kits must be easily accessible and regularly updated to meet the specific needs of children during mass casualty events. In addition to medical supplies, it is essential to have items like diapers, formula, comfort objects, and safe sleeping arrangements for infants and young children. Facilities should perform regular inventory checks and maintain emergency stockpiles to ensure functionality and availability during crises. By prioritizing pediatric equipment readiness, we enhance the efficiency and effectiveness of disaster response, ensuring that children receive timely and appropriate care.

- Ensure pediatric-sized medical supplies (e.g., endotracheal tubes, IV catheters, resuscitation equipment) are available.
- Maintain adequate stocks of medications, including pediatric analgesics, antibiotics, and sedation drugs.
- Use Broselow tapes for weight-based dosing in emergency settings.

Communication and Coordination

Effective communication and coordination are crucial for managing pediatric care during disasters. Establishing clear and reliable communication channels among hospitals, emergency services, public health agencies, and community organizations is essential to ensure a swift and organized response. Pediatric-specific protocols should be integrated into emergency communication systems to convey vital information, such as child identification, triage status, and caregiver reunification. Coordination also requires assigning roles, streamlining the flow of information, and ensuring that all stakeholders, including schools, childcare centers, and pediatric care units, understand their responsibilities. Building pre-established partnerships and conducting regular joint exercises can enhance interagency collaboration, minimize delays, and improve overall disaster readiness. This approach ensures that children's needs are prioritized and addressed efficiently during emergencies.

- Establish clear communication protocols within the hospital and with external agencies (EMS, public health, FEMA).
- Educate families on personal emergency plans, including emergency contacts and evacuation procedures.

Triage and Emergency Response in Pediatric Trauma Disasters

Triage and emergency response during pediatric trauma disasters require specialized approaches due to the unique physiological and emotional needs of children. Standard adult triage systems may not be suitable, making pediatric-specific tools like the JumpSTART triage system essential for accurately assessing and prioritizing young patients. Rapid identification of life-threatening injuries, age-appropriate resuscitation, and immediate stabilization are critical for improving survival rates. Emergency response teams must be trained to recognize subtle signs of shock or distress in children, as these manifestations may differ from those seen in adults. In addition to providing physical care, offering emotional support and maintaining calm environments are crucial during pediatric emergencies. Efficient triage and well-coordinated emergency protocols help ensure that children receive timely and appropriate care in the chaotic aftermath of a disaster.

Pediatric-Specific Triage Systems

- Use the *JumpSTART triage system* for rapid assessment of pediatric casualties:

  1. *Green*—Minor (walking wounded)
  2. *Yellow*—Delayed (stable but needs medical attention)
  3. *Red*—Immediate (life-threatening but survivable with intervention)
  4. *Black*—Expectant (unlikely to survive)

- Consider age-specific physiology (e.g., children compensate well for shock initially but can deteriorate rapidly).

Airway and Breathing Management

- Prioritize airway stabilization (higher risk of airway obstruction in children due to anatomy).
- Use bag-mask ventilation before intubation in younger children.

Circulation and Fluid Resuscitation

- Early recognition of shock (pediatric patients show late hypotension)
- Rapid IV or IO (intraosseous) access for fluid resuscitation (20 mL/kg isotonic fluids)

Psychological and Family Support

- Assign child-life specialists or social workers to help with emotional trauma.
- Keep families together when possible to reduce stress and anxiety.
- Provide age-appropriate explanations of the situation to pediatric patients.

Post-disaster Recovery and Ongoing Support

Post-disaster recovery and ongoing support are essential for addressing the long-term physical, emotional, and psychological effects of trauma in children. Many children may experience lasting distress, anxiety, or post-traumatic stress disorder (PTSD), necessitating age-appropriate mental health interventions, counselling, and social support systems. Key priorities are reuniting children with their families and restoring a sense of normalcy through stable housing, education, and community programs. Healthcare facilities should provide follow-up medical care for injuries and monitor for any delayed complications. Ongoing training for PCPs, schools, and caregivers is crucial to ensure continued preparedness and resilience in affected communities. A well-structured recovery plan helps children regain stability, heal from trauma, and rebuild their lives after a disaster.

Debriefing and Mental Health Support

- Conduct team debriefings to discuss response effectiveness and emotional well-being.
- Provide psychosocial support for both patients and staff to manage post-traumatic stress.

Infection Control and Long-Term Care

- Monitor for outbreaks or post-disaster infections (especially in displaced populations).
- Address nutritional and hydration needs, especially in prolonged disaster scenarios.

Community and Policy Involvement

- Advocate for pediatric disaster policies at hospital and government levels.
- Engage in public health initiatives for better pediatric disaster preparedness.

Case Resolution

As the 6-year-old boy was wheeled into the emergency unit, Meena, the nurse practitioner, and Arjun, the emergency technician, sprang into action. Despite the surrounding chaos and the arrival of multiple injured children, they immediately applied the principles of Crisis Resource Management (CRM)—maintaining composure, assigning roles, and focusing on safety and resource prioritization. Meena took leadership of the case, while Arjun prepared resuscitation equipment and monitored vital signs.

Using the JumpSTART triage system, designed specifically for pediatric mass casualty incidents, Meena rapidly categorized the child as immediate (red) based on his altered consciousness, respiratory distress, and perfusion abnormalities. This ensured he would be prioritized for early intervention and resource allocation, even as more casualties arrived at the hospital.

They noted the child's respiratory rate was elevated, oxygen saturation was low, and air entry was diminished on the right, raising suspicion of a pneumothorax. Arjun provided high-flow oxygen, while Meena contacted the on-call trauma coordinator for guidance on preparing for possible needle decompression. With the child still on spinal precautions and a deformed, bleeding femur, they applied direct pressure and improvised limb stabilization.

Throughout the intervention, Meena and Arjun demonstrated situational awareness, constantly scanning for changes in the child's status, the environment, and the flow of patients. They avoided fixation errors by not focusing solely on the suspected head injury and ensured other life-threatening conditions—such as tension pneumothorax and hemorrhagic shock—were addressed in parallel. This broader awareness helped them prioritize actions appropriately in a rapidly evolving environment.

Leadership and teamwork were critical. Meena communicated all instructions using closed-loop communication, confirming that tasks were understood and completed, such as "Arjun, apply pressure to the femur bleed. Let me know once it's done." This structured, clear communication reduced the risk of errors and maintained focus.

With no family available and consent still pending, Meena documented the child's status under a temporary identifier and ensured all critical actions were recorded. The team coordinated with EMS to prepare the child for transfer to a higher center once stabilized.

In the background, the hospital's disaster preparedness protocol had kicked in—supplies were being restocked, emergency tags distributed, and space for triage cleared. Meena reflected on how ongoing simulation training and drills helped her and Arjun remain calm and efficient. Regular updates in CRM, MCI triage, pediatric trauma care, and simulation-based preparedness had prepared them to operate under pressure, despite being nonphysician providers in a high-stakes scenario.

Key Messages

- PCPs must develop pediatric-specific knowledge and skills through regular training, simulations, and continuing education to respond confidently and effectively during disasters.
- Knowing the work environment, including the location of pediatric equipment, emergency exits, and protocols, helps PCPs act swiftly and efficiently under pressure.
- Familiarity with pediatric triage systems such as JumpSTART allows PCPs to assess and prioritize injured children appropriately based on their unique physiological responses.
- Communication should be clear, concise, and structured using tools like SBAR and closed-loop communication to ensure safe handovers and reduce errors during emergencies.
- PCPs must understand their role within a multidisciplinary team and be prepared to lead, assign tasks, and support team coordination in high-pressure situations.
- Seeking help early and coordinating with other staff and services ensures timely interventions and better outcomes for critically injured children.
- Providing emotional support using age-appropriate language and reassurance is essential to reduce psychological distress for both children and their families.
- PCPs play a key role in checking and maintaining readiness of pediatric-specific equipment and supplies to ensure rapid availability when disasters strike.
- Post-disaster responsibilities include monitoring for complications, offering psychological support, and facilitating reunification of children with their families.
- Continued learning through refresher courses and updated training modules helps PCPs stay current with best practices in pediatric disaster response.

Bibliography

1. Bagwell, H. B., Liggin, R., Thompson, T., Lyle, K., Anthony, A., Baltz, M., Melguizo-Castro, M., Nick, T., & Kuo, D. Z. (2016). Disaster Preparedness in Families With Children With Special Health Care Needs. Clinical Pediatrics, 55(11), 1036–1043. https://doi.org/10.1177/0009922816665087
2. Baker, A. H., Lee, L. K., Sard, B. E., & Chung, S. (2024). The 4 S's of Disaster Management Framework: A Case Study of the 2022 Pediatric Tripledemic Response in a Community Hospital. Annals of Emergency Medicine, 83(6), 568–575. https://doi.org/10.1016/J.ANNEMERGMED.2024.01.020
3. Burke, R. V., Iverson, E., Goodhue, C. J., Neches, R., & Upperman, J. S. (2010). Disaster and mass casualty events in the pediatric population. Seminars in Pediatric Surgery, 19(4), 265–270. https://doi.org/10.1053/J.SEMPEDSURG.2010.06.003
4. Chiu, M., Goodman, L., Palacios, C. H., & Dingeldein, M. (2022). Children in disasters. Seminars in Pediatric Surgery, 31(5), 151219. https://doi.org/10.1016/J.SEMPEDSURG.2022.151219
5. Dahl-Grove, D., Chung, S., Ruffing, R., Fallat, M. E., Dingeldein, M., Aldrink, J. H., & Escobar, M. A. (2025). How Pediatric Readiness can Impact Pediatric Trauma From

Every Day to Mass Events. Journal of Pediatric Surgery, 162135. https://doi.org/10.1016/J.JPEDSURG.2024.162135
6. Drayna, P. C., Hansen, A., Boggs, R., & Locklair, M. R. (2012). Disaster Management and Emergency Preparedness for Children and Youth With Special Health Care Needs. Clinical Pediatric Emergency Medicine, 13(2), 125–132. https://doi.org/10.1016/J.CPEM.2012.04.002
7. Mace, S. E., Doyle, C., Fuchs, S., Gausche-Hill, M., Koenig, K. L., Sorrentino, A., & Johnson, R. W. (2012). Pediatric patients in a disaster: part of the all-hazard, comprehensive approach to disaster management. American Journal of Disaster Medicine, 7(2), 111–125. https://doi.org/10.5055/AJDM.2012.0087
8. Nursing Management of Pediatric Disaster. (2020). Nursing Management of Pediatric Disaster. 10.1007/978-3-030-43428-1

Emergency Room (ER) Evaluation of a Child with Trauma

4

Chandu Raj B and Nisha Toteja

Learning Objectives

By the end of this chapter, the reader should be able to:

- Understand the key anatomical and physiological differences in children that influence injury patterns and emergency care in pediatric trauma.
- Apply a structured and prioritized approach to the initial assessment of injured children, using age-appropriate strategies.
- Perform the essential steps of the primary survey, including the use of appropriate tools and interventions for airway, breathing, circulation, disability, and exposure.
- Identify the components of a thorough secondary survey in pediatric trauma and recognize when to escalate care or seek advanced support.
- Emphasize the importance of continuous monitoring and re-evaluation following initial stabilization to detect deterioration early.
- Recognize the value of effective teamwork, role clarity, and communication in delivering safe and coordinated pediatric trauma care.

Introduction

Pediatric trauma is a major global health challenge and remains one of the leading causes of death and disability in children under the age of 18. Road traffic accidents, falls, drowning, burns, and non-accidental trauma continue to contribute to high

C. Raj B
Trauma Centre, AIIMS Rishikesh, Rishikesh, Uttarakhand, India

N. Toteja (✉)
Pediatrics, AIIMS Guwahati, Guwahati, Assam, India

N. T. Rai (ed.), *Pediatric Trauma Resuscitation Manual (PTRM) for Primary Care Providers*, https://doi.org/10.1007/978-981-95-4979-5_4

pediatric injury rates, particularly in low- and middle-income countries (LMICs) like India, where resources, infrastructure, and access to timely care remain limited. What makes pediatric trauma even more complex is the fact that children are not merely smaller versions of adults. Their unique anatomical, physiological, developmental, and psychological characteristics demand tailored approaches to assessment, stabilization, and treatment. For example, subtle signs of shock or head injury may be overlooked unless age-specific responses are well understood.

In many primary care and prehospital settings, primary care providers (PCPs)—including nurses, emergency technicians, paramedics, and undergraduate medical trainees—are often the first responders to pediatric trauma. They play a vital role in triage, airway management, basic life support, family engagement, and safe referral. The initial few minutes of care can be decisive in a child's survival and recovery. Yet, these frontline providers frequently operate under significant constraints: lack of equipment, absence of senior physicians, overwhelming patient load, and emotional stress.

This chapter explores the unique challenges of pediatric trauma care through the lens of PCPs, emphasizing practical, context-sensitive strategies for initial assessment and decision-making. A structured approach using tools like the Pediatric Assessment Triangle (PAT), age-based vital sign interpretation, and trauma-informed communication is essential. Special attention is given to common injury patterns in children, teamwork in resource-limited environments, and the importance of timely re-evaluation. By equipping PCPs with the right knowledge and tools, we can close the gaps in early trauma care and improve outcomes for children across diverse clinical settings.

Case Scenario

You are on duty in the emergency unit of a rural Primary Health Center (PHC) during the evening shift. A 6-year-old boy named Raghav is brought in by the local ambulance service after falling from a tamarind tree, estimated to be around 20 feet high. The incident occurred in a village about 10 km away, and transport to the PHC took nearly 50 min. He was initially unresponsive and is now showing partial responsiveness.

Raghav arrives immobilized on a long spine board, with his head secured using lateral blocks, and is receiving supplemental oxygen via face mask. He is unaccompanied by family members, and a neighbor who witnessed the fall is the only person available to provide information. On examination, gurgling breath sounds are heard, suggesting airway compromise.

His vital signs on arrival are:

- Heart rate: 180 bpm
- Blood pressure: 70/38 mmHg
- Respiratory rate: 40 breaths per min
- SpO_2: 84% on oxygen

Raghav opens his eyes to painful stimuli, makes incomprehensible sounds, and withdraws to pain—indicating a GCS score of 8 (E2V2M4).

Managing the emergency unit are Anita, a mid-level nurse practitioner with basic pediatric trauma training, and Faizal, an EMT posted recently under rural outreach services along with junior doctors. With no senior doctor present, limited airway equipment, and no imaging facilities, Anita and Faizal must act quickly to stabilize Raghav and prepare him for urgent referral to a pediatric trauma center.

Reflective Questions

1. What immediate steps should be prioritized by PCPs in a resource-limited setting when managing a child with suspected polytrauma?

Anatomical and Physiological Considerations

Children are not scaled-down adults, and the approach to pediatric trauma patients needs to be tailored to their physiological and anatomical uniqueness and responses. Table 4.1 highlights these considerations. Tables 4.2 and 4.3 give the age-specific vitals and various quick calculations commonly used by children.

Table 4.1 Unique anatomical and physiological considerations in children

	Features	Implications
Primary survey		
Airway	*Infants have a relatively more prominent occiput.*	A large occiput tends to flex the head forward in infants. Placement of shoulder roll in younger infants may be required to achieve sniffing position for optimal visualization of vocal cords during intubation.
	Smaller airway	Greater risk of obstruction from foreign bodies Loose teeth may dislodge into the airway. Airway resistance significantly increased with minimal airway edema.
	Larger tongue and smaller oral cavity	A larger tongue and a smaller oral cavity increase obstruction risk. Correct head and jaw positioning is essential for visualization during endotracheal tube placement.
	Short trachea	Increased risk of endotracheal tube dislodgement and right main stem intubation
	The larynx is cephalad and more anterior.	The larynx is anatomically located at C2–C3 cervical vertebrae. Visualization is difficult in untrained hands.
	The shape of the epiglottis	Epiglottis are floppy and horseshoe-shaped, making intubation difficult.

(continued)

Table 4.1 (continued)

	Features	Implications
Breathing	*Ribs positioned more horizontally*	Limited rib expansion thereby reducing tidal volume
	Diaphragmatic breathing	The diaphragm is the primary muscle of respiration. A higher position of the diaphragm also restricts chest expansion.
	Lower number of fatigue-resistant type 1 fibers	Diaphragm muscles lack type 1 muscle fibers and hence easily fatigue.
	Respiratory rate	A higher metabolic rate results in a higher respiratory rate, which is also age-dependent.
Circulation	*Blood volume proportion relative to body weight is higher.*	Smaller blood losses may lead to more significant circulatory compromise.
	Hypotension is a late sign.	Due to compensatory tachycardia and increased vascular resistance in response to hypovolemia, children can tolerate significant volume loss (>30%) before becoming hypotensive.
	Fixed-stroke volume	Tachycardia is the most predominant compensatory response in infants and younger children.
	Smaller vessels/more subcutaneous tissue	Difficulty obtaining vascular access due to small veins and increased subcutaneous tissue Intraosseous access may be required if intravenous access attempts fail in a child with critical injuries.
Disability—CNS	*Open sutures, presence of fontanelle*	Fontanelles may indicate intracranial pressure changes in infants with open fontanelles. Bulging fontanelles suggest increased intracranial pressure; sunken fontanelles suggest fluid loss.
	Thinner cranial bones	Thinner bones provide less protection to brain tissue. The chances of intracranial hemorrhage are higher.
	Head relatively larger	Higher center of gravity Prone to falls with toppling over and impact to the cranium The chances of traumatic brain injuries are higher.
	Cognitive and psychological development vary with age	Nonverbal developmental stage makes interpretations of sensorium challenging.
	Hypoglycemia	Higher consumption due to higher metabolic rate Lesser glycogen stores Predisposed to hypoglycemia Hypoglycemia may also cause altered sensorium. Dextrose must be assessed in all critically injured children. Dextrose-containing maintenance fluids should be administered in children <25 kg.

(continued)

Table 4.1 (continued)

	Features	Implications
Exposure	*Relatively small size*	A single impact may injure multiple organ systems.
	Higher BMR and surface area	A larger surface-area-to-body-mass ratio increases heat loss and insensible fluid losses. Hypothermia and hypovolemia are significant concerns in children.
Secondary survey		
Chest	*The chest wall is more compliant.*	Deeper injuries, such as pulmonary contusions, are more common than rib fractures.
	Increased mobility of the mediastinal structure	Higher risk of tension pneumothorax or large vessel transection due to mediastinal movement.
Abdomen	*Relatively thin abdominal wall*	Visceral injuries are common due to a poorly protective musculoskeletal system.
	Abdominal organ proportions and placement	Viscera are more anteriorly exposed, unprotected by the thoracic cage, and closely packed. Solid organ injury is common in blunt trauma to the abdomen. The bladder in infants is intra-abdominal, thus prone to injury.
	The diaphragm is more horizontal	The flatter diaphragm pushes the liver and spleen below the rib cage.
Musculoskeletal	*Growth plates are not fused.*	Fractures through growth plates affect future growth.
	Cartilaginous bones	More flexible bones result in greenstick/atypical fracture patterns.

Table 4.2 Age-specific vital signs for children

Normal pediatric vital signs by age group			
Age group	Respiratory rate	Heart rate	Min systolic BP
Term baby	40–60	100–170	50
3 months	30–50	100–170	50
6 months	30–50	100–170	60
1 year old	30–40	110–160	70–90
1–2 years	25–35	100–150	80–95
2–5 years	25–30	95–140	80–100
5–12	20–25	80–120	90–110
>12 years	15–20	60–100	100–120

Source: Harriet Lane Handbook 21st edition

Table 4.3 Calculations used in the pediatric population

Calculations in pediatric populations	
Calculations of weight based on age	
Age	*Expected weight*
3–12 months	(Age in months +9)/2
1–6 years	(Age in years × 2) + 8
7–12 years	(Age in years × 7–5)/2
Systolic blood pressure based on age	
Age	*SBP*
Neonate (0–28 days)	Hypotension if SBP < 60 mmHg
Infant (1–12 months)	Hypotension if SBP < 70 mmHg
Child 1–10 years	SBP- 90 + (age × 2) mmHg
	Lower limit of SBP- 70 + (age × 2) mmHg
Child >10 years	Hypotension if SBP < 90 mmHg
ET calculations based on age	
ET tube size	(Age/4) + 4
ET tube depth	Age/2 + 12 or ET tube size × 3

*Adapted from Neha Thakur, Samir Misra. Pediatric Trauma Resuscitation Module (PTRM). First edition. New Delhi: Jaypee Brothers Medical Publishers (P) Ltd.; 2024

Initial Approach

The emergency room (ER) evaluation for children mirrors that of adults in its rapid and systematic structure but with adaptations to meet the unique physiological needs of pediatric patients. The process is designed to prioritize the recognition and management of life-threatening conditions to prevent death or severe disability. Time is of the essence in such scenarios, and immediate, straightforward interventions are initiated in a carefully prioritized manner to stabilize the child as quickly as possible.

In pediatric trauma care, the initial assessment and resuscitation of the patient is carried out by a multidisciplinary trauma team, whose size and specific composition may vary depending on the institutional setting. This team-based approach ensures that all critical aspects of patient care are addressed simultaneously and efficiently. Typically, the trauma team includes a designated team leader, an airway manager, trauma nurses, trauma technicians, residents, and occasionally medical students. Additional support may come from specialists in anesthesiology, surgery, internal medicine, pediatrics, and other allied healthcare personnel.

The role of the team leader is pivotal. Rather than becoming directly involved in hands-on tasks, the leader oversees the entire process, coordinating efforts, ensuring proper sequence of assessment and interventions, and maintaining situational awareness throughout the resuscitation. Each member of the team is assigned a specific role, contributing their expertise in real-time to create a cohesive and streamlined response.

This model of simultaneous assessment and intervention—often referred to as a *horizontal approach*—is designed to reduce delays in identifying and managing life-threatening injuries. It ensures that critical actions such as securing the airway, controlling hemorrhage, and initiating fluid resuscitation occur without unnecessary delays. Ultimately, the goal is to resuscitate and stabilize the pediatric trauma patient rapidly, prioritize injuries appropriately, and prepare for definitive treatment, all while minimizing preventable morbidity and mortality.

The overarching goals of the emergency department evaluation in pediatric trauma are threefold: First, to rapidly identify any life-threatening conditions that require urgent intervention; second, to stabilize the child's condition through immediate and often simple treatments; and third, to determine the next appropriate steps—whether that involves initiating definitive treatment within the facility or organizing safe and timely transfer to a higher-level pediatric trauma center.

This structured yet flexible approach helps ensure that no critical step is missed and that pediatric trauma patients receive effective, lifesaving care from the moment they arrive (Fig. 4.1).

Preparation

Patient assessment begins immediately at the scene of the accident. Effective communication with the receiving facility is essential. Proper coordination allows the trauma team to stay alert, anticipate needs, and make necessary preparations.

- Preparation occurs in two main phases:
  1. Prehospital phase
  2. Hospital phase

PCPs' responsibilities in preparation

1. *Prehospital phase*
   - Control life-threatening external bleeding.
   - Maintain a patent airway with immobilization of the cervical spine.

1. Preparation
2. Triage
3. Primary survey (A, B, C, D, E - Assessment)& interventions
4. Adjuncts to the primary survey
5. Consideration of transfer
6. Secondary survey
7. Adjuncts to the secondary survey
8. Post-resuscitation monitoring and re-evaluation
9. Definitive care

Fig. 4.1 Structured approach to pediatric trauma

- Immobilize the patient for transfer.
- Gather and communicate essential information (time of insult, age, mechanism of injury, patient history) to the receiving facility.
- Immediate transport to the closest appropriate facility, preferably a trauma center.

2. *Hospital phase*
   - Assemble the trauma team, following standard precautions.
   - Assign roles and responsibilities.
   - Prepare the resuscitation area; control the room temperature.
   - Test and organize equipment for airway, breathing, and circulation.
   - Make sure to have prewarmed isotonic crystalloids and blankets or warming devices readily available.
   - Ensure prompt blood bank, laboratory, radiology, and operation theater (OT) backup.

Triage

Sorting/prioritizing based on injury severity, prognosis, and available resources. Triage is done to assign patients to designated care areas with appropriate and timely resource allocation. There are various validated triaging tools available based on setting and nationality.

Purpose of Triage:

1. Identify life-threatening injuries.
2. Prioritize patient care.

Most triaging systems categorize patients into 3–5 levels based on severity. These include specialized pediatric triaging systems, such as JUMPStart, pediatric trauma triage, the field triage scheme, Canadian triage and acuity score (CTAS), Pediatric Assessment Triangle (PAT), and pediatric early warning scores (PEWS). A simplified color-coded 4-level triage system based on the severity of injury is as depicted in Fig. 4.2. Triage categories based on situations are shown in Table 4.4.

PCPs' responsibilities in triaging

- *Sort/prioritize patients:* Assess injury severity and urgency.
- *Assign to triage zones*: Red, yellow, green, or black areas based on injury severity
- *Prioritize treatment*: Adjust priorities based on severity and resource availability

Primary Survey (A B C D E Assessment)

The overarching aim of primary survey in a polytrauma pediatric patient is to rapidly identify and addressing lifethreatening injuries using a structured ABCDE approach. It also prioritizes further assessment, resuscitation, and transportation.

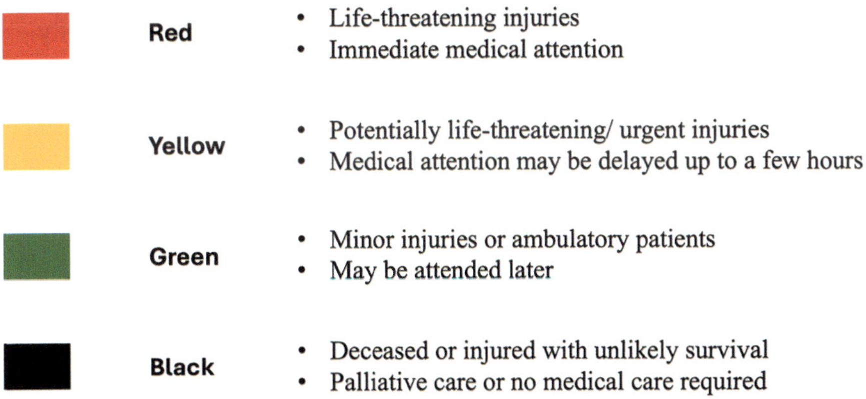

Fig. 4.2 Simplified color-coded 4-level triage system

Table 4.4 Triage categories based on the situation

The categories based on the situation are:		
1	*Multiple casualty*	The number and gravity of injuries do not exceed the facility's capabilities to render care.
2	*Mass casualty*	The no. of patients and severity of injuries exceed the treatment facility's capability. Priority is given to patients with the highest chance of survival using minimal resources.

The process is not always linear and varies with the number of victims and available team members. Focus on immediate airway, breathing, and circulation threats and treat any life-threatening injuries before proceeding to further assessments.

The sequences of assessments and interventions in the primary survey are given in Fig. 4.3.

A PCP can quickly assess the general condition of the child by asking:

- "What is your name?"
- "What happened to you?"

A clear response indicates a patent airway, good breathing, adequate brain function, and no immediate life threats. Inadequate/inappropriate responses require immediate and thorough assessment and management.

Airway Management with Cervical Spine Protection

The top priorities in trauma care are:

- Ensure effective airway management and adequate ventilation.
- Simultaneously restrict cervical spine movement throughout the ER evaluation.

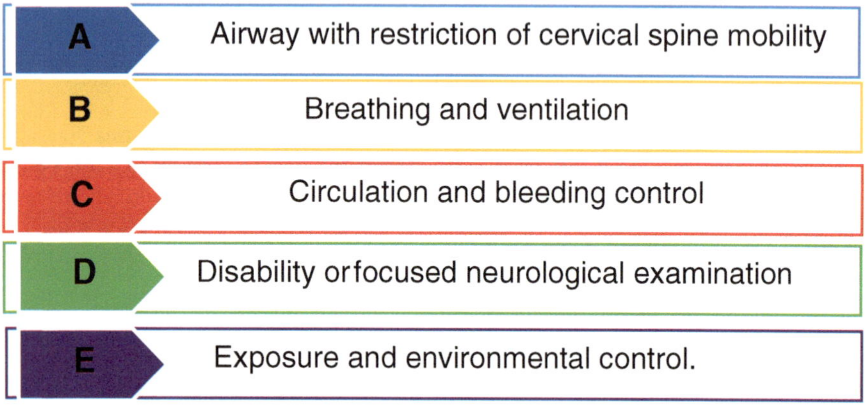

Fig. 4.3 Order of assessments and interventions in the primary survey [6]

Pediatric considerations:

- Airway is assessed by "look," "listen," and "feel" for airflow during breathing.
- Positioning measures such as chin lift and jaw thrust may be required to align the airway and prevent the tongue from falling back. If cervical injury is suspected, jaw thrust alone is preferred to avoid undue mobility of the head.
- Cervical immobilization must be maintained manually by manual inline stabilization (MILS) (Fig. 4.4) or using an appropriate-sized cervical collar or head blocks.
- The "sniffing position" is optimal for visualization during intubation and may require padding under the shoulder and back in younger children.

- *Airway categorization:*
  - *Stable/open airway:* No obstruction; provide supplemental oxygen
  - *Unstable but maintainable airway:* Obstructed by factors like tongue falls, bleeding, vomitus, or fractures, this airway can be managed by positioning, suctioning, or placing adjuncts such as an oropharyngeal airway (OPA) or nasopharyngeal airway (NPA). Airway adjuncts such as OPA can only be used in an unconscious patient without a gag reflex as a temporizing measure to maintain airway patency.
  - *Unstable and not maintainable:* If the patient is at a high risk of obstruction over time due to factors like inhalation injury, strangulation, or tracheal fracture, the presence of stridor, or airway patency that cannot be established by simple measures listed above, definitive airway should be placed. Figure 4.5 gives steps to airway assessment and management.

Definitive airway: A definitive airway may be required in cases of severe airway compromise or requirement of prolonged ventilation or an inability to protect the airway due to impaired Glasgow Coma Scale (GCS). A definitive airway is one with a tube placed in the trachea and cuff inflated below the level of the vocal cords. Most commonly, oral

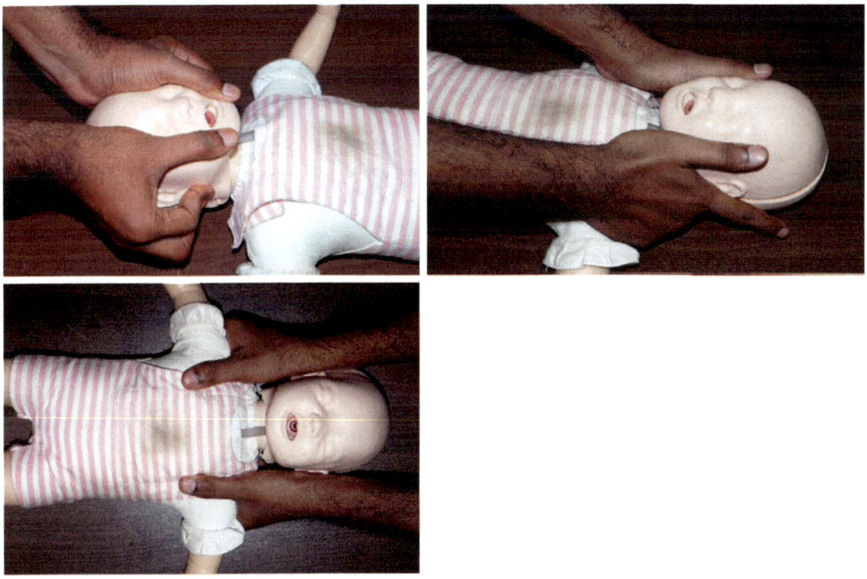

Fig. 4.4 Different approaches to manual in-line stabilization of cervical spine in children (MILS)

endotracheal intubation is used as a definitive airway. In difficult intubations, a definitive airway may be secured surgically with needle cricothyrotomy in children younger than 12 years or surgical cricothyrotomy in those older than 12 years.

Airway management with cervical spine movement restriction is crucial to prevent secondary neurological damage in trauma patients. Practitioners must be skilled in airway adjuncts, understand the impact of airway maneuvers, and know how to manage the cervical spine.

Manual in-line stabilization (MILS):
- MILS may worsen the laryngoscopic view, making intubation difficult.
- When using MILS, consider alternative devices like video laryngoscopes, supraglottic airway devices (SADs), or optical stylets.

Cervical spine protection:
- After airway management, protect the cervical spine with a hard cervical collar (Philadelphia Collar).
- During airway assessment, reopen the cervical collar and have a team member manually restrict cervical spine motion.

Rapid sequence intubation/drug-assisted intubation: To facilitate orotracheal intubation, children require special positioning, age-appropriate equipment sizes, and weight-based doses of drugs for sedation-paralysis. These can be determined by using the length-based tapes (Fig. 4.6).

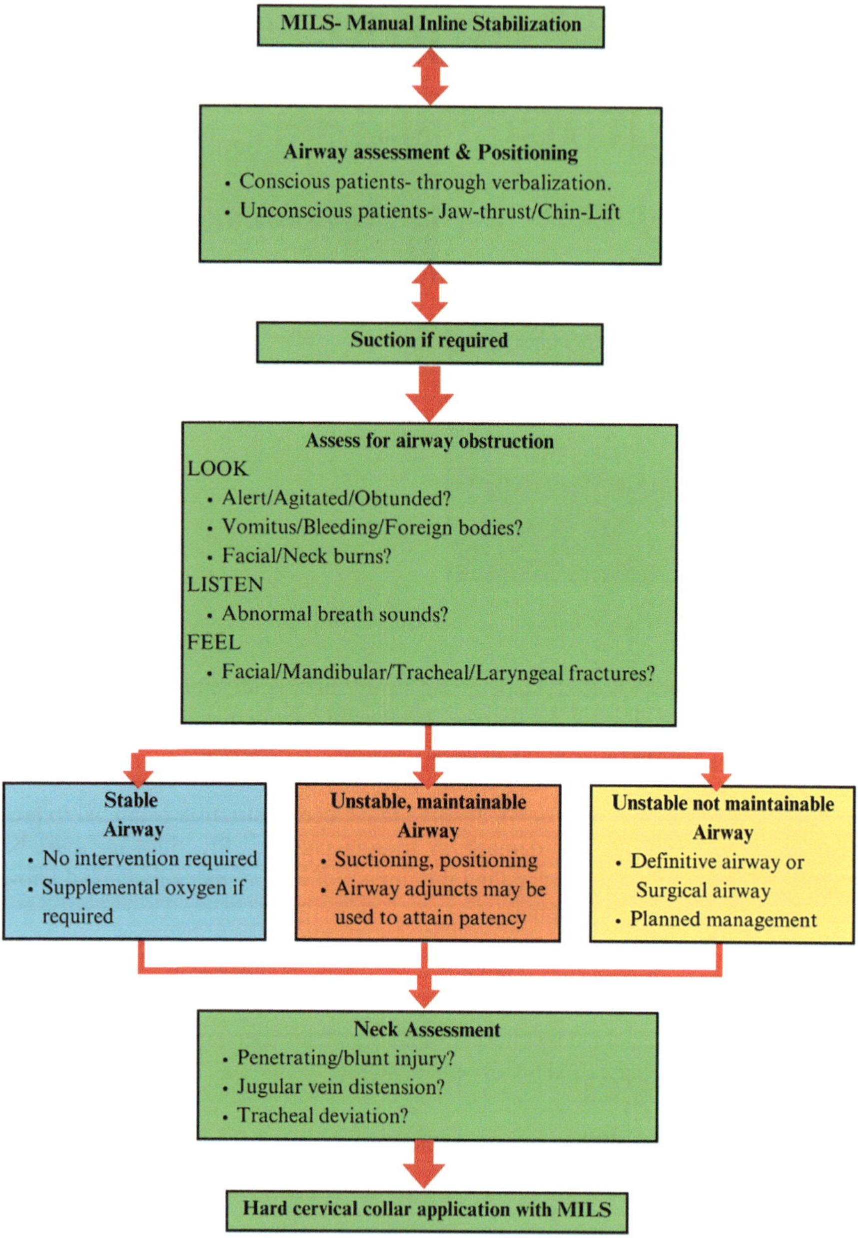

Note: - *Maintain MILS for cervical spine mobility restriction throughout the airway assessment and management.*

Fig. 4.5 Algorithm of airway assessment and management

The assessment indicates that Raghav's airway may be compromised. There are abnormal gurgling sounds that do not respond to suctioning and positioning measures, and his GCS is 8 with SpO2 of 90% on a non-rebreathing mask.

Endotracheal intubation was planned to secure the airway given a low GCS.

A rigid cervical collar was applied.

Broselow pediatric emergency tape/Broselow tape [BT]

- *Purpose*: Broselow tape estimates weight and guides medication dosages, equipment sizes, etc., in pediatric emergencies (Fig. 4.6).
- *Age Group*: For children up to 12 years old or under 36 kg
- *Usage*: Align the tape with the child's head and measure to heel.
- *Indication*: Used in emergency settings to quickly determine the correct medication dosages, equipment sizes, and other medical interventions based on the child's length

Surgical airway: In situations such as severe maxillofacial trauma or inhalational burns, orotracheal intubation or supraglottic devices may not be feasible as definitive airways, and these patients may require an emergent placement of a surgical airway, such as needle cricothyrotomy or surgical cricothyrotomy. Table 4.5 gives the salient features of the two common surgical airways.

PCPs' responsibilities in airway

- *Stabilize cervical spine:* Use padding and manually restrict motion (MILS) throughout ER evaluation and apply a hard cervical collar after airway management.

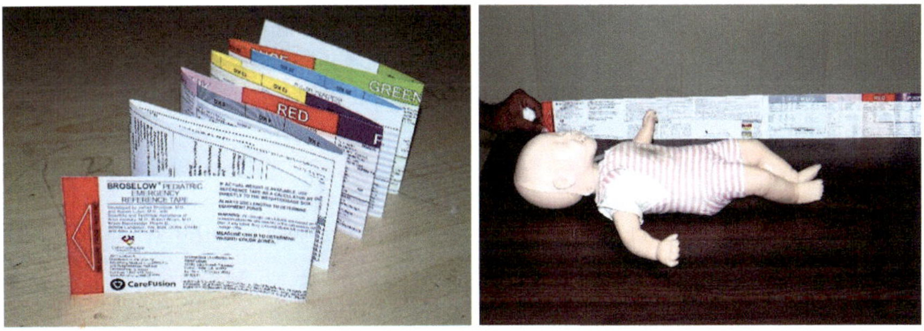

Fig. 4.6 Broselow tape (length-based estimation of weight)

Table 4.5 Needle cricothyrotomy versus surgical cricothyrotomy in children

	Needle cricothyrotomy	Surgical cricothyrotomy
Indication	Cannot intubate, cannot ventilate (CICV) scenario in children aged <12 years requiring emergent airway	Cannot intubate, cannot ventilate (CICV) scenario in children or adolescents aged >12 years requiring emergent airway
Procedure	A needle and catheter are inserted percutaneously through the cricothyroid membrane to create an airway.	Through an incision made in the cricothyroid membrane, a tube (e.g., tracheostomy tube or endotracheal tube) is inserted directly into the trachea.
Equipment	A large-bore intravenous catheter, syringe, and a high-pressure oxygen source or jet ventilator are typically used.	Scalpel and endotracheal or tracheostomy tube
Advantages	Faster to perform Less invasive Easier to learn	May provide more sustained and reliable ventilation, especially in severe upper airway obstruction cases
Disadvantages	(a) Only a temporary solution (b) Cannot be maintained for extended periods (less than 1 h) (c) Can lead to CO2 retention and pneumothorax	(a) More invasive (b) Bleeding, injury to surrounding structures, perforation (c) Requires time and technical expertise

- *Airway assessment:* Talk to the child and check for obstructions (tongue, foreign bodies, fractures).
- *Categorize and manage airway*
  - *Patent airway:* Provide supplemental oxygen.
  - *Compromised airway:* Immediate management with the trauma team
  - *Threatened airway:* Plan and manage with the team.
- *Establish airway:* If the airway is uncertain, establish a definitive airway or temporarily use an oropharyngeal airway for unconscious patients. And prepare and assist with a surgical airway if needed.
- *Alternative airway devices:* Prepare devices like video laryngoscopes, supraglottic airway devices (SADs), bougie, or optical stylets for use if needed.

Breathing and Ventilation

Effective gas exchange is essential for optimal oxygenation and carbon dioxide elimination.

All injured patients should receive supplemental oxygen to optimize oxygenation.

Breathing assessment technique:

- Use the "LOOK, LISTEN, and FEEL" method to assess breathing.
- Inspect the neck and thorax for key signs:
  - Jugular vein distension
  - Tracheal deviation
  - Chest wall movement
  - Visible chest injuries

- Crepitus on palpation
- Subcutaneous emphysema
- Decreased or absent air entry during auscultation
- Abnormal sounds on percussion

Life-threatening chest injuries: Identify and address these injuries during the primary survey:

- Tension pneumothorax
- Massive hemothorax
- Open pneumothorax
- Cardiac tamponade
- Tracheal-bronchial injury

Pneumothorax:

- A simple pneumothorax can become a life-threatening tension pneumothorax if a patient is intubated and given positive pressure ventilation before chest tube decompression. Table 4.6 depicts the assessment and management of life-threatening chest injuries during primary survey.

PCPs' responsibilities in breathing and ventilation

- *Breathing assessment:* Use "LOOK, LISTEN, and FEEL" to assess the neck and thorax for life-threatening chest injuries.
- *Oxygen administration:* Provide supplemental oxygen to all injured patients.
- *Pneumothorax management:* Avoid positive pressure ventilation before chest tube decompression to prevent tension pneumothorax.
- *Tension pneumothorax:* Perform/assist with needle decompression; prepare and assist with chest tube placement.
- *Open pneumothorax:* Apply a sterile three-way occlusive dressing, followed by placing a chest tube at a distant site and surgically repairing the open wound.
- *Cardiac tamponade:* Assist with pericardiocentesis and prepare for thoracotomy.
- *Pain management:* Administer analgesics to improve ventilation.

While preparing for endotracheal intubation, a quick assessment of the vital signs revealed a heart rate of 160 beats per min, blood pressure of 70/50 mmHg, and an SpO2 level of 89% on a non-rebreather mask. The patient exhibited labored breathing with asymmetrical chest movement on the right side. Distended neck veins were observed, and the percussion note was hyperresonant on the right, indicating a right-sided tension pneumothorax. The trauma team performed needle decompression, followed by the placement of a chest tube. After the insertion of the right ICD and drainage of tension pneumothorax, respiratory parameters have improved, with SpO2 96% on mechanical ventilator after endotracheal intubation. A quick look at the monitor shows that Child C has a heart rate of 170 per min, BP of 72/40 mmHg, weak peripheral pulses, and delayed CFT.

Table 4.6 Assessment and management of life-threatening chest injuries during the primary survey

S. no.	Chest injuries	Assessment	Management
1	Tension pneumothorax	Neck vein distension Tracheal deviation +/– Asymmetrical chest rise U/L decreased air entry Hyperresonant sound on percussion Subcutaneous emphysema +/– Signs of shock	Needle decompression Followed with chest tube placement Oxygen support Analgesics
2	Massive hemothorax	Collapsed neck vein Asymmetrical chest rise U/L decreased air entry Dull sound on percussion Signs of shock	Chest tube placement Fluid replacement Oxygen support Analgesics
3	Open pneumothorax	Sucking chest wound Asymmetrical chest rise U/L absent or decreased air entry Signs of tension pneumothorax +/–	Sterile three-way occlusive dressing Chest tube placement Oxygen support Analgesics
4	Cardiac tamponade	Neck vein distension Symmetrical B/L chest rise B/L air entry present Muffled heart sound Signs of shock	Pericardiocentesis Early evacuation for thoracotomy
5	Tracheal or bronchial injury	Hemoptysis +/– Cyanosis +/– B/L absent or decreased air entry Tracheal crepitation +/– Subcutaneous emphysema +/– Signs of tension pneumothorax +/–	Endotracheal tube placement below the injury or surgical airway Oxygen support Analgesics

Circulation and Hemorrhage Control

- The primary cause of shock in traumatic injuries is hypovolemia due to blood loss unless proven otherwise. Children can maintain normal systolic pressure even with a 30% decrease in blood volume.

Key priorities:

- Recognize shock promptly.
- Control the hemorrhage.
- Administer fluid resuscitation.

Early signs: Tachycardia, cold extremities, delayed capillary refill time, weak peripheral pulses, narrow pulse pressure, mottled skin, decreased urine output.

Clinical observations for shock:

- Assess the level of consciousness, skin perfusion, and pulse.
- Assume shock in injured children who are cool to the touch with a rapid heart rate.

Categories of shock in trauma

- Hemorrhagic (due to blood loss)—Most common
- Nonhemorrhagic
  - Obstructive (tension pneumothorax/cardiac tamponade)
  - Cardiogenic (direct myocardial injury)
  - Neurogenic (high cervical cord injuries)

Management

- *Hemorrhage control:*
  - Remember the mnemonic *"BLOOD ON THE FLOOR, LOOK FOR FOUR MORE."*
  - The most common site of hemorrhage is either external bleeding (on the floor) or in four internal compartments: thorax, abdomen, pelvis/retroperitoneum, and long bones.
- Stop external bleeding with direct pressure or a tourniquet in case of the limb. Mark the time of tourniquet application.
- Adjunct to primary survey includes point-of-care ultrasonography using eFAST to diagnose internal bleeding.
- In case of suspicion of pelvic fracture (pelvic compression test positive, leg length discrepancy, blood on the urinary meatus), a pelvic binder can be placed centered on the greater trochanter to splint the fracture and prevent blood loss in the pelvic cavity.
- If the cause of hemodynamic instability is not localized and the patient is not responding well to adequate fluid resuscitation, an urgent surgical laparotomy and/or CT angioembolization may be required (Fig. 4.7).

Venous access:

- Two large, wide-bore intravenous accesses must be secured in all critically injured children with shock.
  - Percutaneous peripheral (e.g., antecubital fossa, saphenous vein) are most commonly used.
  - Intraosseous (e.g., proximal tibia, distal femur) may have to be used in case of failed attempts to secure peripheral intravenous access.

Fluid resuscitation:

- Initial 20 ml/kg of prewarmed isotonic crystalloids bolus, repeated according to the child's physiological response.

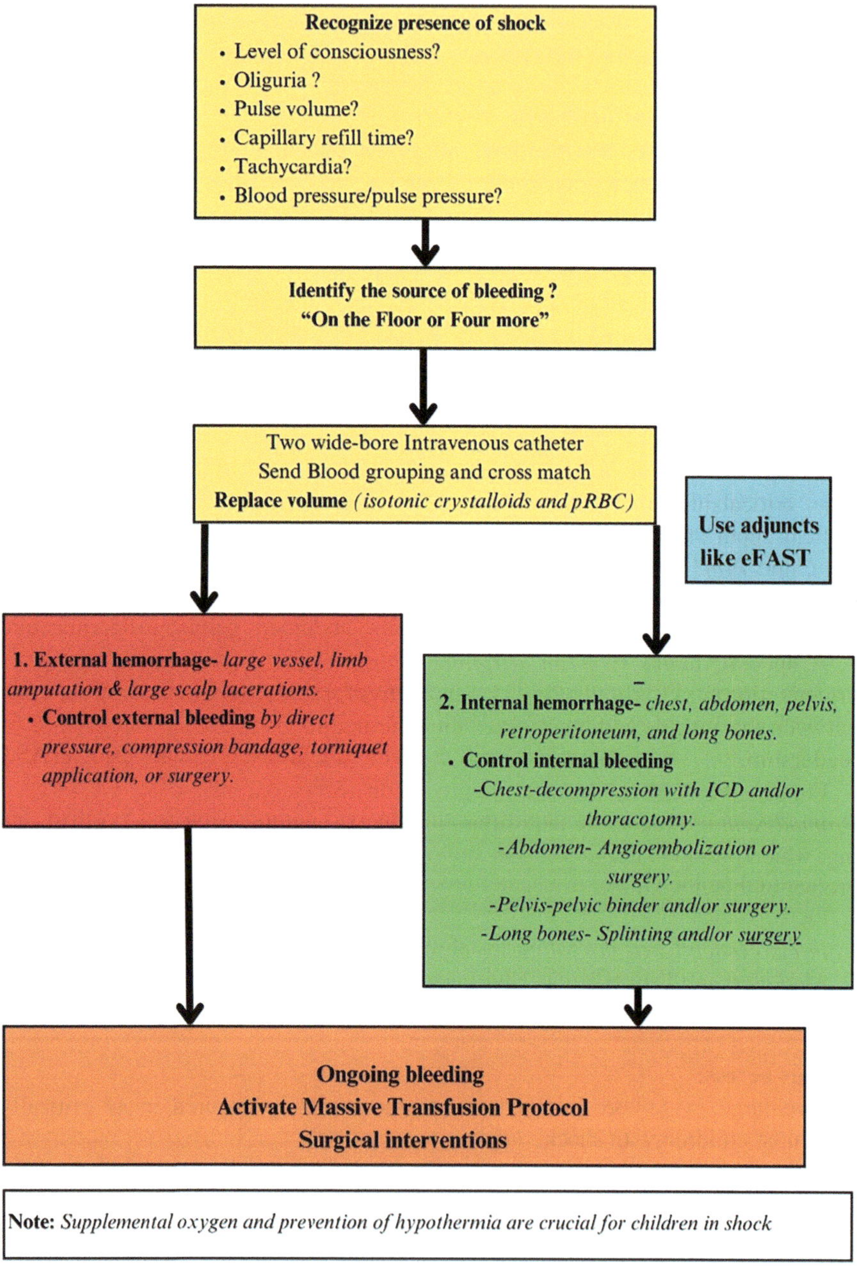

Fig. 4.7 Assessment and management of shock

  - Another 20 ml/kg of crystalloid bolus may be repeated.
  - Remember to estimate weight from length-based tapes (Broselow's tape) for calculating drug or fluid volume for resuscitation.
  - Further volume replacements may be done with the blood products.
- Continued hemodynamic instability after crystalloid resuscitation or after a certain volume of packed red blood cell transfusions (PRBC) may warrant massive transfusion protocol (MTP) activation.

Massive Transfusion Protocol (MTP)
MTP involves transfusion of PRBC: FFP: Platelets in ratios of 1:1:1 to prevent trauma-induced coagulopathy. Most studies advocate MTP activation if:

- 40 ml/kg PRBC requirement in 24 h
- Packed red blood cell (PRBC) transfusion of 50% of total blood volume (TBV) in 3 h
- PRBC transfusion of >10% of TBV/min

Please note that TBV for a preterm infant is 90–100 ml/kg, a term neonate/infant <3 months is 80–90 ml/kg, and for a child >3 months, 70 ml/kg.

Tranexamic acid: If given within the first 3 hours can potentially have a mortality benefit in pediatric trauma patients with ongoing bleeding. For children <12 years, a dose of 15 mg/kg is administered followed by infusion of 2 mg/kg/h for at least 8 h or until the bleeding stops whereas >12 years can be treated with adult dosages of 1 g loading dose over 10 min within the first 3 h post-injury, followed by a 1 g infusion over 8 h.

The lethal triad in trauma, hypothermia, acidosis, and coagulopathy must be prevented with the MTP protocol and due attention to the management of hypothermia.

Responses to fluid resuscitation:
- *Responders:* Stabilized by crystalloids and possibly blood
- *Transient responders:* Initial improvement, followed by deterioration
- *Nonresponders:* Require massive blood transfusion and possibly early surgery

Indicators of hemodynamic stability:
- Tachycardia resolving
- Normal sensorium
- Good peripheral pulses, normal skin color, and warm extremities
- Increased systolic blood pressure
- Urine output (1–2 ml/kg/h in case of infants and 0.5–1 ml/kg/h in older children)

PCPs' responsibilities in circulation and hemorrhage control

- *Recognize shock:* Assess the level of consciousness, skin perfusion, and pulse to detect shock early.
- *Hemorrhage control:* Manage bleeding using direct pressure, pressure bandages, tourniquets, pelvic binders, and splints.
- *Venous access:* Secure two large-bore IV cannulas, collect blood samples for grouping matching, and assist in intraosseous lines, or, less commonly, central line, and venous cutdowns.
- *Fluid replacement:* Assist with fluid resuscitation and blood replacement and activate the massive transfusion protocol.
- *OT preparation:* If a life-threatening hemorrhage cannot be controlled in the emergency department, prepare for surgery.
- *Thermoregulation:* Prevent hypothermia using prewarmed blankets, warm IV fluids, and blood products.

Following initial circulatory assessment shows that Child C was in shock with heart rate of 170 per min, BP of 72/40 mmHg, weak peripheral pulses, and delayed CFT. Two wide-bore intravenous accesses were established, and blood grouping for crossmatch was sent. Fluid bolus 20 ml/kg of warmed normal saline was rapidly infused, followed by another bolus of 20 ml/kg, and eFAST was performed, which was positive. A Foley catheter was inserted to document urine output and response to fluid resuscitation.

After receiving two boluses of crystalloids, the child's HR was 130/min, BP improved to 100/70 mmHg, skin perfusion improved, and pulses were well felt.

However, his GCS is still 8, and pupils are sluggishly reacting and unequal.

Disability or Neurological Status

Traumatic brain injury (TBI) is the leading cause of mortality in pediatric trauma patients. Any decrease in consciousness may indicate reduced cerebral oxygenation, perfusion, or traumatic brain injury.

The primary goal is to identify those that require immediate lifesaving surgical interventions and prevent secondary brain injury by maintaining adequate oxygenation and perfusion.

Table 4.7 Pediatric Glasgow Coma Scale (pGCS) and its modification in infants

Behavior	Response in children	Response in infants	Score
Eye opening (E)	Spontaneous	Spontaneous	4
	To sound	To sound	3
	To pressure	To pressure	2
	None	No response	1
	Non-testable		NT
Verbal response (V)	Appropriate words or social smile, fixes and follows	Coos and babbles	5
	Cries but consolable	Irritable cries	4
	Persistently irritable	Cries in response to pain	3
	Restless, agitated	Moans in response to pain	2
	None	No response	1
	Non-testable	Non-testable	NT
Best motor response (M)	Obeys commands	Spontaneous purposeful movements	6
	Localizing	Withdrawal to touch	5
	Normal flexion	Withdrawal to pain	4
	Abnormal flexion	Responds to pain with decorticate posturing (abnormal flexion)	3
	Extension	Responds to pain with decerebrate posturing (abnormal extension)	2
	None	None	1
	Non-testable	Non-testable	NT

Adapted from James H. E. (1986). Neurologic evaluation and support in the child with an acute brain insult. *Pediatric annals*, *15* (1), 16–22

Rapid neurological evaluation:

- Assess the patient's level of consciousness by GCS or modified GCS (nonverbal or younger children) (Table 4.7) or AVPU (Alert, Verbal, Pain, or Unresponsive) scale
- Check pupillary size and reaction.
- Look for any lateralizing signs.

Causes of altered consciousness:

- Consider hypoglycemia, alcohol, narcotics, or other drugs as potential causes.
- Assume changes in consciousness are due to TBI until proven otherwise.

Additional neurologic findings: Unequal, fixed, or dilated pupils and the presence of Cushing's triad (bradycardia, irregular respirations, and a widened pulse pressure) may indicate cerebral herniation, requiring immediate intervention.

Management of suspected TBI

1. Supportive measures
   Airway and Breathing:
   - Ensure a definitive airway.
   - Maintain normal PaCO2 levels (35–40 mmHg) and PaO2 > 60 mmHg to ensure proper oxygenation and ventilation.

   Circulation: Maintain normovolemia using crystalloids and/or blood products.
   - Head end elevation
   - Prevention of fever, seizures, and hypoglycemia
2. Medical management
   - Osmotic agents—Mannitol at a dose of 0.25–1 g/kg can be used in euvolemic patients for acute neurological deterioration, such as unequal pupils, focal deficits, and worsening sensorium.
   - Alternatively, hypertonic saline at a 3–5 ml/kg dose may be better tolerated in hypotensive patients.
   - Anticonvulsants—Levetiracetam can be given to treat seizures.
3. Surgical management
   All clinically *significant* TBIs must be managed in consultation with the neurosurgical team.

Indications of early neurosurgical referral/consultation:

1. Expanding skull hematoma
2. Depressed skull fractures
3. Penetrating head injuries
4. GCS < 8 despite initial resuscitation or worsening GCS particularly motor scores.
5. Cranial imaging is suggestive of intracranial bleeds, cerebral edema, or impending herniation.

PCPs' responsibilities in disability

- *Rapid neurological evaluation:* Assess the patient's consciousness level and pupillary size and reaction.
- *Consider causes of altered consciousness:* Assist in managing consciousness changes due to CNS injury but rule out hypoglycemia, alcohol, narcotics, or drugs.
- *Identify additional neurologic findings:* Detect cerebral herniation early and assist in immediate intervention.
- *Management techniques in primary survey:* Ensure proper oxygenation and ventilation to maintain normal PaCO2 levels and normovolemia using crystalloids or blood products.

The patient's low GCS and dilated, sluggish right pupil indicate a possible traumatic brain injury. Since we don't have a neurosurgeon, we have decided to transfer the patient to a trauma center for further evaluation.

Exposure and Environmental Control

Children are more susceptible to hypothermia due to their larger body surface area and immature body temperature regulation. Hypothermia contributes to the lethal triad of hypothermia, metabolic acidosis, and coagulopathy.

Primary evaluation steps:

- Undress the child: Completely remove garments by cutting them off for a thorough examination.
- Examination: Perform a proper examination, including a "log roll" to assess the child's back.
- Remove spine board: Immediately remove the spine board to prevent early pressure injuries.
- Preventing hypothermia
- Cover the patient: Use a prewarmed blanket or external warming device.
- Prewarmed fluids: Ensure intravenous fluids are prewarmed before infusing.
- Warm environment: Maintain a warm resuscitation area.

PCPs' responsibilities in exposure and environment

- *Primary evaluation:* Undress the child for a thorough examination and remove the spine board to prevent early development of pressure injuries.
- *Preventing hypothermia:* Cover the patient adequately, ensure intravenous fluids are prewarmed before infusion, and warm the resuscitation area.

Adjuncts to the Primary Survey

Table 4.8 depicts the adjuncts to primary survey.

Consideration of Transfer

Indications to transfer:

- Transfer the child if their condition exceeds the resources of the current facility.
- The decision should be made after completing the primary survey and resuscitation as needed.

Ensure effective communication between the referring and receiving facilities. Do not delay the transfer for in-depth diagnostic evaluations. Perform only the necessary evaluations to resuscitate, stabilize, and ensure the child's safe transfer.

Table 4.8 Adjuncts to the primary survey

S. no.	Adjuncts	Remarks
1	ECG	Diagnoses blunt cardiac injury and assesses heart function Dysrhythmias may indicate blunt cardiac injury.
2	Pulse oximetry	Monitors oxygen levels (SpO_2)
3	Capnography	A noninvasive method to evaluate respiratory adequacy by assessing end-tidal CO_2 levels
4	Arterial blood gases (ABG)	Assesses oxygenation, ventilation, and acid-base status Low pH, rising lactate, or base deficit levels may indicate worsening shock.
5	Urinary catheter	Monitors urinary output to assess volume status and renal perfusion Avoid transurethral catheterization if urethral injury is suspected (e.g., blood at the meatus or perineal bruising).
6	Gastric catheters	Decompresses the stomach Reduces the risk of aspiration Assesses upper GI tract bleeding
7	Chest X-ray	Identifies life-threatening chest injuries Verifies the placement of chest tubes
8	Pelvic X-ray	Identifies pelvic fractures Assesses the need for early blood transfusion
9	FAST/eFAST	Detects intra-abdominal bleeding, pneumothorax, and hemothorax

PCPs' responsibilities in patient transfer

- *Ensure patient stability:* Monitor and assess the patient's vital signs and condition for transport.
- *Prepare equipment:* Verify that all necessary medical equipment and supplies are packed and functional.
- *Secure the patient:* Properly secure the patient on the transport stretcher or bed to prevent movement.
- *Coordinate with the transport team:* Communicate with the transport team to plan and execute a safe transfer.
- *Maintain communication:* Keep open lines of communication with both the sending and receiving facilities.
- *Document information:* Accurately document the patient's condition before transport.

> *Properly communicate Raghav's condition to the trauma center in situation, background, assessment, and recommendation (SBAR) format* (Table 4.9).

Table 4.9 SBAR handover format for communication while transferring children with pediatric trauma

Situation: A 6-year-old boy Raghav fell from a 20-feet height. Currently intubated Right-side tension pneumothorax was treated with chest tube placement. Transferring to a trauma center for further care	*Assessment:* Airway secured. Circulation improving post-fluid bolus and transfusion (BP: 100/70 mmHg) GCS remains 8 and dilated right pupil; possible traumatic brain injury
Background: Raghav presented with abnormal breathing sounds and a compromised airway (GCS: 8, Spo2: 84%) Developed hypovolemic shock (BP: 72/40 mmHg, pulse: 180 bpm) Initial interventions: Intubation, needle decompression, chest tube insertion, fluid resuscitation, and blood transfusion	*Recommendation:* Immediate transfer to a trauma center for neurosurgical evaluation and intensive care

Accurately document the patient's condition and transfer the patient to the nearest trauma center via *ICU ambulance with a trained trauma nurse.*

Secondary Survey

- Begins after the primary survey is complete, resuscitation is initiated, and vital signs are normalized.
- If the child's condition deteriorates at any time, reassess ABCDE using the primary survey.

Components of the secondary survey:

- Medical history: Collect detailed history, including reassessment of all vital signs.
- *Head-to-toe examination:* Conduct a comprehensive physical examination to identify hidden injuries.
- History collection (AMPLE mnemonic):
  A: Allergies
  M: Medications
  P: Past illness/pregnancy
  L: Last meal
  E: Events/environment related to injury
- Physical examination: Perform a systematic and thorough review of the body (head to toe) to identify hidden injuries (Table 4.10).

Table 4.10 Head-to-toe examination in secondary survey

Head-to-toe evaluation	Assessment
Head and maxillofacial	Inspect and palpate the entire head and face for lacerations, contusions, or fractures. Reassess pupillary response and level of consciousness. Examine the eyes for hemorrhage, penetrating injuries, visual acuity, and the presence of contact lenses. Evaluate cranial nerve function. Inspect ears and nose for any cerebrospinal fluid (CSF) leakage. Inspect the oral cavity for bleeding, mucosal lacerations, and dental injuries.
Cervical spine and neck	Inspect for signs of blunt or penetrating trauma, tracheal deviation, and use of accessory muscles. Palpate for tenderness, deformity, swelling, subcutaneous emphysema, and symmetry of pulses. Auscultate the carotid arteries for bruits.
Chest	Inspect the chest wall for blunt or penetrating injuries and abnormal respiratory effort. Palpate the chest for tenderness, crepitus, subcutaneous emphysema, and evidence of trauma. Percuss for hyperresonance or dullness indicating underlying pathology. Auscultate for bilateral breath sounds and heart sounds.
Abdomen	Inspect the anterior and posterior abdomen for bruising, abrasions, or penetrating wounds. Palpate for tenderness, involuntary guarding, and rebound tenderness. Auscultate for the presence or absence of bowel sounds.
Genitourinary/ rectal	Inspect for contusions, hematomas, lacerations, and urethral bleeding. Perform rectal examination to assess for gross blood, anal sphincter tone, bowel wall integrity, and bony fragments.
Skin/extremities	Assess for bruising, abrasions, lacerations, swelling, and deformities. Evaluate skin color, temperature, and signs of cyanosis or pallor. Check for tenderness and restriction of joint movement.
Back and sacrum	Inspect the entire back and buttocks for injuries, bruises, or lacerations. Palpate the spine for tenderness or step-offs. Palpate scapulae and sacroiliac joints for tenderness.

Adapted from Neha Thakur, Samir Misra. Pediatric Trauma Resuscitation Module (PTRM). First edition. New Delhi: Jaypee Brothers Medical Publishers (P) Ltd.; 2024

PCPs' responsibilities in secondary survey

- *Review medical history:* Obtain and review the child's medical history and any relevant information from caregivers.
- *Perform a detailed assessment:* A comprehensive head-to-toe examination to identify any injuries.
- *Reassess vital signs:* Monitor and record vital signs, including heart rate, respiratory rate, and blood pressure.
- *Assess pain levels:* Evaluate and document and manage the child's pain accordingly.

- X-rays of the spine & extremities
- Computed Tomography (CT) scans of the head, chest, abdomen, and spine
- Magnetic Resonance Imaging (MRI) of the spine
- Contrast-enhanced urography
- Contrast angiography
- Transesophageal ultrasound
- Bronchoscopy
- Esophagoscopy

Fig. 4.8 Adjuncts of the secondary survey

- *Ensure comprehensive documentation:* Record all findings and interventions accurately in the patient's medical record.
- *Coordinate with trauma team:* Communicate findings and collaborate with the team for further treatment and care.

Adjuncts to the Secondary Survey

Perform specialized diagnostic tests once the patient is hemodynamically stabilized during the secondary survey. These tests help identify specific injuries that may not be apparent during the primary survey. Common adjuncts used in trauma patients are outlined in Fig. 4.8.

Post-resuscitation Monitoring and Re-evaluation

Constant re-evaluation of trauma patients is essential to detect new findings and any deterioration.

PCPs' responsibilities in re-evaluation

- Continuous monitoring of vital signs, oxygen saturation, and urinary output
- Periodic arterial blood gas (ABG) analysis and end-tidal CO_2 monitoring
- Provide effective pain relief with small, reasonable doses to ensure the child's comfort.

Definitive Care

- If the child's treatment needs exceed the facility's capabilities, consider transferring the child.
- The decision to transfer is based on a thorough assessment of the child's injuries and the institution's resources, including personnel, equipment, and capabilities.

Case Resolution

Recognizing that Raghav's condition was rapidly deteriorating, Anita, the mid-level nurse practitioner, and Faizal, the emergency medical technician, promptly initiated emergency care. They observed abnormal gurgling breath sounds, a Glasgow Coma Scale (GCS) of 8, and SpO_2 of 84% on high-flow oxygen—clear signs of airway compromise and altered mental status, pointing toward potential head injury and traumatic airway obstruction.

In a resource-limited setting, the immediate priorities for PCPs include securing the airway, supporting breathing and circulation, maintaining spinal precautions, and seeking timely medical assistance. Anita applied a rigid cervical collar, ensured manual stabilization of the spine, provided supplemental oxygen, and elevated the child's head slightly to optimize breathing. Faizal monitored vital signs and began preparing IV equipment, recognizing the need for rapid circulatory support.

Simultaneously, Anita activated the on-call junior physician stationed at the PHC.

Upon arrival, the physician confirmed the need for endotracheal intubation due to a low GCS and gurgling breath sounds. During airway preparation, the team identified asymmetric chest movement, distended neck veins, and hyperresonance on the right—hallmarks of a right-sided tension pneumothorax. The physician promptly performed needle decompression, followed by intercostal chest drain (ICD) insertion, significantly improving the child's respiratory status and SpO_2.

Despite respiratory improvement, Raghav's circulation remained unstable: heart rate 170 bpm, BP 72/40 mmHg, delayed capillary refill. Two wide-bore IV lines were established, and the team administered two boluses of 20 mL/kg warmed normal saline. An eFAST scan was performed and found to be positive for intra-abdominal fluid. A Foley catheter was inserted to monitor urine output.

Following fluid resuscitation, the child's heart rate reduced to 130 bpm, BP improved to 100/70 mmHg, and skin perfusion normalized. However, the GCS remained at 8, and pupils were unequal and sluggish, suggesting traumatic brain injury.

Given the limitations of the PHC—including absence of imaging and neurosurgical support—the team prepared for urgent referral to a pediatric trauma center. Critical information documented and communicated during the handover included the mechanism of injury (fall from 20 feet), initial vital signs and GCS, airway interventions (intubation), ICD placement, volume resuscitation given, response to treatment, eFAST findings, and the patient's current neurological status. Clear documentation and advance communication were done in structured SBAR format

(Situation, Background, Assessment, Recommendation) over the phone to coordinate with the receiving center, facilitating a seamless handover to ensure continuity of care and minimized delays at the receiving facility.

Through their actions, Anita and Faizal exemplified the core competencies of PCPs in trauma care—prioritizing stabilization, utilizing structured assessment tools like the PAT, and ensuring effective documentation and communication during referral.

Key Messages

- Children's unique anatomy and physiology makes them more vulnerable to airway obstruction, internal injuries, and rapid deterioration, necessitating tailored approaches to trauma care.
- The ABCDE primary survey remains the cornerstone of initial assessment, focusing on Airway protection (with cervical spine control), Breathing, Circulation, Disability (neurological status), and Exposure/environmental control (e.g., preventing hypothermia).
- Pediatric airway management requires early identification of obstruction; a child tolerating an oral airway typically needs definitive airway support. Note that surgical cricothyroidotomy is not recommended for children under 12 years.
- In trauma, shock is considered hypovolemic until proven otherwise. Immediate control of hemorrhage and fluid resuscitation with isotonic crystalloids are essential.
- Chest injuries such as a simple pneumothorax can rapidly progress to tension pneumothorax, especially if positive pressure ventilation is applied before chest decompression.
- Proper ventilation and oxygenation are essential to prevent secondary brain injury, along with maintaining adequate perfusion and conducting a focused neurological evaluation.
- The Broselow tape is a useful tool in emergency settings to estimate weight and guide drug dosing and equipment sizing in pediatric patients.
- Triage strategies, including color-coded systems like JumpSTART, help prioritize care based on injury severity, especially during mass casualty events.
- Hypothermia is a common and dangerous complication in pediatric trauma. Warm the child actively and monitor temperature as part of the exposure assessment.
- Bleeding control, including pressure dressings and tourniquets (used only when necessary), is vital. Always document the time when a tourniquet is applied.
- Begin the secondary survey only after completing the primary survey and stabilizing the child, focusing on a thorough head-to-toe examination and history (AMPLE).
- Transfer the child promptly if the necessary level of care exceeds the facility's capabilities. Do not delay for imaging or tests that won't change immediate management.

- A coordinated multidisciplinary trauma team, led by a designated team leader, ensures efficient resuscitation and reduces preventable deaths through clear communication and role assignment.

Bibliography

1. Advanced Trauma Life Support (ATLS) Student Course Manual. 10th ed. Chicago: American College of Surgeons; 2018. p. 4–21.
2. Cook SC, Thomas M, Nolan J, Parr M. Trauma Secondary Survey. Key Clinical Topics in Critical Care [Internet]. 2023 Jul 25 [cited 2024 Aug 15];385–385. Available from: https://www.ncbi.nlm.nih.gov/books/NBK441902
3. DeBoer S, Seaver M, Broselow J. Color Coding to Reduce Errors: The Broselow–Luten system streamlines pediatric emergency treatment. AJN The American Journal of Nursing. 2005 Aug 1;105(8):68–71.
4. Evangelista ME, Gaffley M, Neff LP. Massive transfusion protocols for pediatric patients: current perspectives. Journal of blood medicine. 2020 May 21:163–72.
5. Flavin MP, Dostaler SM, Simpson K, Brison RJ, Pickett W. Stages of development and injury patterns in the early years: a population-based analysis. BMC public health. 2006 Dec;6:1–0.
6. Georgiou A, Lockey DJ. The performance and assessment of hospital trauma teams. Scandinavian journal of trauma, resuscitation and emergency medicine. 2010 Dec;18:1–7.
7. Greene N, Bhananker S, Ramaiah R. Vascular access, fluid resuscitation, and blood transfusion in pediatric trauma. International journal of critical illness and injury science. 2012 Jan 1;2(3):135–42.
8. Holm-Knudsen RJ, Rasmussen LS. Paediatric airway management: basic aspects. Acta Anaesthesiologica Scandinavica. 2009 Jan;53(1):1–9.
9. James H. E. (1986). Neurologic evaluation and support in the child with an acute brain insult. *Pediatric annals*, *15*(1), 16–22.
10. Kahl L, Hughes HK. The Harriet Lane Handbook E-Book. Elsevier Health Sciences; 2017 Apr 2
11. Karki SB, Kale S, Saigal D. Laryngoscopic View after Application of Manual In-Line Stabilization–A Comparison with Early Morning Sniffing Position in the Same Patient. Anesthesia Essays and Researches. 2022 Jan 1;16(1):115–20.
12. Li C, Jiao J, Hua G, Yundendorj G, Liu S, Yu H, Zhang L, Yang X, Liu L. Global burden of all cause-specific injuries among children and adolescents from 1990 to 2019: a prospective cohort study. International Journal of Surgery. 2024 Apr 1;110(4):2092–103.
13. Lui A, Kumar KK, Grant GA. Management of severe traumatic brain injury in pediatric patients. Frontiers in toxicology. 2022 Jun 24;4:910972.
14. Neha Thakur, Samir Misra. Pediatric Trauma Resuscitation Module (PTRM). First edition. New Delhi: Jaypee Brothers Medical Publishers (P) Ltd; 2024. p. 23–39
15. Romig LE. Pediatric triage. A system to JumpSTART your triage of young patients at MCIs. JEMS: a journal of emergency medical services. 2002 Jul 1;27(7):52–8.
16. Ruhomauly Z, Betts K, Jayne-Coupe K, Karanfilian L, Szekely M, Relwani A, McCay J, Jaffry Z. Improving the quality of handover: Implementing SBAR. Future healthcare journal. 2019 Jun;6(Suppl 2):54.
17. Simon Junior H, Schvartsman C, Sukys GD, Farhat SC. Pediatric emergency triage systems. Revista Paulista de Pediatria. 2022 Jul 15;41:e2021038.
18. Theodorou CM, Galganski LA, Jurkovich GJ, Farmer DL, Hirose S, Stephenson JT, Trappey AF. Causes of early mortality in pediatric trauma patients. Journal of Trauma and Acute Care Surgery. 2021 Mar 1;90(3):574–81.
19. Tintinalli JE, Stapczynski JS, Ma OJ, Yealy DM, Meckler GD, Cline DM. Tintinalli's Emergency Medicine: A Comprehensive Study Guide, 8e. New York, NY, USA: McGraw Hill Education; 2016.

Airway and Breathing Management in Pediatric Trauma

5

Arun Varghese, Aneeqa Tahir, and Muhammed Elhady Muhammed Elgasim

Learning Objectives

By the end of this chapter, the reader should be able to:

- Understand key anatomical and physiological differences in the pediatric airway and thorax that make children more susceptible to airway obstruction and respiratory compromise during trauma.
- Apply the ABCDE framework effectively to assess and manage airway and breathing in pediatric trauma patients, with specific attention to signs of deterioration.
- Recognize clinical indicators of upper and lower airway compromise, such as stridor, hoarseness, gurgling, and abnormal chest movement, and interpret their significance in acute trauma care.
- Implement essential airway interventions, including positioning, suctioning, use of adjuncts (OPA/NPA), and bag-valve-mask ventilation, with an understanding of when to escalate to intubation.
- Support and assist in team-based airway management, understanding the roles and limitations of primary care providers (PCPs), nurses, and junior doctors in resource-limited settings.

A. Varghese
College of Nursing, AIIMS Gorakhpur, Gorakhpur, Uttar Pradesh, India

A. Tahir
Dumfries & Galloway Royal Infirmary, Dumfries, UK

M. E. M. Elgasim (✉)
Cork University Hospital, Cork, Ireland

N. T. Rai (ed.), *Pediatric Trauma Resuscitation Manual (PTRM) for Primary Care Providers*, https://doi.org/10.1007/978-981-95-4979-5_5

- Initiate and coordinate breathing support strategies, including oxygen delivery, positive pressure ventilation, and identification of thoracic injuries such as pneumothorax or flail chest.
- Demonstrate effective communication with families during high-risk airway scenarios, providing reassurance and information in a clear and compassionate manner.
- Document and communicate critical findings and interventions accurately during referral or transfer to higher centers, ensuring continuity and safety of care.

Introduction

In the critical moments following pediatric trauma, ensuring a patent airway and adequate breathing is paramount. Unlike adults, children present unique anatomical and physiological challenges that require careful consideration and timely intervention. For primary care providers (PCPs), especially those working in resource-limited or prehospital settings, understanding these nuances can significantly impact patient outcomes.

Children have proportionally larger heads, smaller airways, and more compliant chest walls, making them more susceptible to rapid airway obstruction and respiratory compromise. A swollen tongue, blood or vomitus, or even poor positioning can cause obstruction. Additionally, their higher metabolic rate and lower oxygen reserves mean that even brief periods of hypoventilation or apnea can lead to severe hypoxia.

This chapter focuses on equipping PCPs with the knowledge and practical strategies needed to effectively assess and manage airway and breathing issues in pediatric trauma. It explores the differences in pediatric airway anatomy, common mechanisms of obstruction, and structured approaches like the ABCDE framework to perform systematic assessments. The importance of early recognition of signs such as stridor, hoarseness, and altered breath sounds is emphasized, along with appropriate use of suction, airway adjuncts, oxygen delivery systems, and preparation for intubation when necessary.

We also highlight the importance of multidisciplinary teamwork and clear communication during high-risk airway management scenarios. In many instances, PCPs are the first to respond, often without immediate access to pediatric specialists. This chapter aims to empower frontline providers with actionable skills, ensuring they are prepared to stabilize the airway and support breathing until definitive care is reached.

Ultimately, safeguarding the pediatric airway is not just about techniques—it's about anticipation, vigilance, and confidence in applying basic principles under pressure. Through this, PCPs can play a lifesaving role in the golden hour of trauma care.

Case Scenario

You are working a day shift at a remote hill dispensary in Uttarakhand, functioning as a Primary Health Outpost with no in-house doctor on site but connected to the district hospital via teleconsultation. Midafternoon, a 5-year-old boy named *Kabir* is rushed in by a forest ranger and two locals. Kabir had been playing near a narrow hillside road when he was struck by a reversing jeep. The vehicle reportedly bumped him forcefully onto a rock outcrop, causing facial injuries and possible head trauma.

Kabir arrives wrapped in a blanket with no formal prehospital care. His neighbor had attempted basic first aid. There is no spinal immobilization. His father, visibly distressed, accompanies him but has limited understanding of the injury timeline. You, *Anuradha*, a nurse practitioner trained in pediatric triage, and *Paramjeet*, a community health officer (CHO), quickly begin the primary assessment while contacting *Dr. Shaan*, a junior medical officer on rotation from the district hospital who is arriving shortly by motorbike.

Kabir is semiconscious and making gurgling noises with each breath. There are bruises across his chin and neck, dried blood in the mouth, and visible swelling over the right side of the jaw. He is unable to speak and has significant respiratory distress.

Initial Vital Signs:

- Heart rate: 152 bpm.
- Respiratory rate: 54 breaths/min.
- SpO_2: 86% on room air.
- GCS: 10 (E3 V3 M4).
- Capillary refill time: >3 seconds.

Dr. Shaan arrives within minutes. Under guidance from the nurse team, he performs suctioning and applies a jaw thrust. Suspecting impending airway obstruction and potential cervical spine injury, he initiates airway management with manual in-line stabilization and prepares for definitive airway support while the team arranges emergency transfer by ambulance.

Reflective Questions

1. What early signs should alert PCPs to impending airway compromise in pediatric trauma patients?
2. How can PCPs use the Pediatric Assessment Triangle (PAT) to guide rapid decision-making when advanced diagnostics are unavailable?
3. What are the responsibilities of the trauma nurse or primary triage nurse in preparing for airway and breathing interventions in resource-limited settings?
4. What immediate stabilization steps should PCPs prioritize when managing suspected facial or airway trauma in children?
5. What key clinical information must PCPs document and communicate during interfacility transfer to ensure safe and timely escalation of care?

How Are Children Different?

Understanding children's unique anatomical and physiological features is essential to adequate airway and breathing management in pediatric trauma. These differences increase the risk of obstruction, injury, fatigue, and rapid deterioration (Table 5.1).

Table 5.1 Key anatomical and physiological differences in pediatric airway and breathing: implications for trauma management

	Feature	Anatomical/ physiological feature	Clinical implication
Airway	*Narrow diameter*	Smaller airway lumen compared to adults	Prone to rapid airway obstruction from secretions or swelling; increases resistance significantly
	Larger tongue and adenoids	Proportionally larger tongue and lymphoid tissue	Risk of upper airway blockage during sedation or unconscious states; complicates mask ventilation and intubation
	Floppy, long epiglottis	Epiglottis is U-shaped and more flexible.	Difficult laryngoscopic view; often necessitates straight blade use for better glottic exposure
	Higher, anterior larynx	Larynx is located higher and more anterior (C2–C3 level)	Increases complexity of intubation due to angle and depth
	Shorter trachea	Trachea is short and narrow in diameter	Greater risk of right main bronchus intubation; must verify ETT position with imaging or auscultation
	Larger occiput	Relatively larger occiput in infants	Neck flexion in supine position may obstruct airway; requires towel rolls to maintain neutral alignment
	Soft tissues	Delicate and compressible airway mucosa	Higher risk of airway trauma and bleeding during suction or intubation
	High metabolic rate, low FRC	Increased oxygen demand and low FRC due to body metabolism	Rapid desaturation during apnea or hypoventilation; requires efficient preoxygenation
Breathing	*Smaller airways*	Narrower bronchi and smaller diameter	Elevated work of breathing; higher risk of airway collapse and wheezing in reactive airway diseases
	Compliant chest wall	Cartilaginous, flexible rib cage and sternum	Injuries like pulmonary contusions may not manifest as fractures; silent hypoxia risk
	Diaphragm dependency	Respiration largely dependent on diaphragm movement	Fatigue sets in quicker during respiratory distress; inadequate accessory muscle support
	High respiratory rate and O_2 consumption	Rapid respiratory rate with limited oxygen storage	Quicker onset of hypoxia during respiratory compromise; must monitor closely
	Low functional residual capacity (FRC)	Low lung volume left after passive expiration	Reduced oxygen reserve limits apnea time; early intervention essential

Airway

Assess the upper airway and the anterior neck; look for signs of airway obstruction.

Airway Assessment in Pediatric Trauma

Signs of Airway Obstruction (Table 5.2)

- *Respiratory distress*, which may present with:
  1. *Tachypnea* (increased respiratory rate).
  2. *Paradoxical chest and abdominal movements.*
  3. *Use of accessory muscles*, with *sternal*, *intercostal*, or *subcostal retractions.*
- *Intrathoracic obstruction* (tracheal or bronchial)—may manifest as *wheezing* or *prolonged expiration.*
- *Extrapulmonary obstruction*—may present with:
  1. *Stridor*, *hoarseness*, or *voice changes* (suggesting laryngeal or upper tracheal injury).
  2. *Gurgling sounds* (due to contamination of the oropharynx).
  3. *Snoring* (from loss of pharyngeal tone due to decreased consciousness causing airway occlusion).

Table 5.2 Red flag signs in pediatric trauma—ABCDE assessment

Category	Red flag signs	Clinical implication
Airway sounds	stridor, hoarseness, or voice change gurgling snoring	Suggests *upper airway obstruction* or *loss of tone*
Anatomical findings	facial, oral, mandibular, or neck trauma swelling of tongue, pharynx, or neck visible hematoma	High risk of *progressive airway obstruction*
Respiratory effort	tachypnea or irregular breathing paradoxical chest-abdominal movements use of accessory muscles (sternal, intercostal, subcostal retractions)	Indicates *increased work of breathing* and *partial obstruction*
Oxygenation	cyanosis low SpO_2 despite oxygen supplementation	Reflects *inadequate oxygen delivery*
Circulatory signs	tachycardia venous distension expanding neck hematoma	May indicate *obstructive shock* or *airway compression*
Neurological status	decreased consciousness restlessness or agitation	*Impaired airway protection* or *hypoxia*
Palpatory findings	subcutaneous emphysema laryngeal tenderness or crepitus tracheal deviation	Suggestive of *tracheal or laryngeal injury*, *tension pneumothorax*, or *pneumomediastinum*

- *Cyanosis* or *low* SpO_2.
- *Visible swelling* of the *tongue*, *pharynx*, or *neck*.
- *External evidence of trauma* to the *face*, *mouth*, *mandible*, or *neck*.
- *Nonspecific systemic manifestations* such as *tachycardia*, *restlessness*, or *altered mental status*.

Mechanisms of Airway Obstruction

- *Direct trauma* to the airway or adjacent structures (e.g., maxillofacial, laryngeal, or tracheal injuries, compression from anterior neck hematoma or burn-related edema of the mouth, pharynx, or larynx).
- *Airway contamination* by *vomitus*, *blood*, *teeth*, or other *foreign bodies*.
- *Loss of pharyngeal tone* secondary to *head injury* or *drug/alcohol intoxication*.
- *Improper positioning*, especially *neck hyperflexion* in infants due to a *prominent occiput*.

Examination of the Anterior Neck

A thorough *anterior neck examination* helps identify signs of *actual or impending airway obstruction* at the *laryngeal or tracheal level* and detect *thoracic life threats* such as *tension pneumothorax* or *cardiac tamponade*.

Use the mnemonic *TWELVE-C* to guide assessment:

- *T—Tracheal deviation*: May indicate *tension pneumothorax* or *massive hemothorax*.
- *W—Wounds*: Blunt or penetrating injuries can cause *airway damage* or *progressive swelling*.
- *E—Emphysema (subcutaneous)*: Suggests presence of *pneumothorax* or *pneumomediastinum*.
- *L—Laryngeal tenderness or crepitus*: May suggest *laryngeal fracture*, often seen in "clothesline" injuries.
- *V—Venous distension*: Associated with *obstructive shock* due to *tension pneumothorax* or *cardiac tamponade*.
- *E—Esophageal injury*: Though not immediately life-threatening, *perforation* carries a high *mortality risk*.
- *C—Carotid hematoma, bruits, or swelling*: A *rapidly expanding hematoma* may obstruct the airway; *carotid injury* increases *stroke risk*.

Airway Management in Pediatric Trauma

1. *Cervical Spine Precautions*
   - Always maintain manual in-line stabilization (MILS).
   - Keep the head in a *neutral position*:
     – *Infants (<1 year)*: Place 1–2 folded towels under the trunk (buttocks to shoulders).

   - *Older children*: Use a rolled towel under the shoulders.
   - *Goal*: Align the occiput slightly lower than the back to prevent neck flexion and airway compromise.
2. *Opening the Airway*
   - Always use a *jaw thrust* (not head tilt or chin lift).
     - Place fingers behind the angle of the mandible and lift anteriorly.
3. *Clearing the Airway*
   - If gurgling or fluid sounds are present:
     - *Infants*: Use a 10-FG soft suction catheter.
     - *Older children*: Use a Yankauer suction.
     - Perform under direct vision using a laryngoscope or tongue depressor.
     - Avoid contact with the mucosa to prevent bleeding or laryngospasm.
4. *If Obstruction Persists*
   - Reposition the head and repeat jaw thrust.
   - Examine the mouth under direct vision.
   - Remove foreign bodies using *Magill forceps* or *Yankauer suction.*
   - Insert an *oropharyngeal airway (OPA)* if the airway improves with laryngoscopy but is otherwise inadequate.
5. *Oropharyngeal Airway (OPA)*
   - Correct size = distance from *incisors to angle of mandible.*
   - Refer to the skills chapter for sizing and insertion technique.
6. *Indications for Endotracheal Intubation*
   - Persistent obstruction despite OPA.
   - Inadequate oxygenation with supplemental O_2.
   - Hypoventilation or GCS deterioration.
   - Anticipated airway compromise (e.g., inhalation burns).
   - Need for sedation or safe transport.
   - Severe agitation or distress requiring controlled ventilation.
7. *Preparation for Intubation*
   - *Preoxygenation*:
     - T-piece circuit with high-flow O_2.
     - Apply *PEEP* and gentle positive pressure ventilation.
     - Use a nasal cannula (if no basal skull fracture).
     - Insert a small-bore orogastric tube to decompress the stomach.
   - *ETT size calculation*:
     - Cuffed ETT (mm ID) = *Age/4 + 3.5.*
     - Prepare three tubes: calculated size, 0.5 mm smaller, 0.5 mm larger.
   - *Introducer*: Use a stiletto for ETT ≤4.5 mm ID.
   - *Intubation approach*:
     - Always use *oral*, not nasal, route (especially in head injury).
     - Have *two working laryngoscopes* ready.
     - Ensure *Yankauer suction* is available and functioning.
     - Drugs prepared and labeled:
       - *Ketamine*: 0.25–2 mg/kg.
       - *Rocuronium*: 1.2–1.6 mg/kg.
       - *Saline flush*, patent IV cannula, and 3-way tap attached.

8. *Induction of Anesthesia*
   (i) *Preoxygenate* for 5 mins if possible:
      (a) T-piece circuit + PEEP > bag-mask-valve device > NRBM + high-flow O_2.
      (b) Nasal cannula at 2 L/kg/min (max 15 L/min) during apnea.
   (ii) *Drugs*:
      (a) 1st: *Ketamine*
      (b) 2nd: *Rocuronium* (timing may vary based on oxygenation)
   (iii) *Laryngoscopy*:
      (a) Left-hand technique; avoid dental pressure or lip injury.
      (b) Blade choice:
         (i) *<1 year*: Straight blade (e.g., Miller)
         (ii) *>1 year*: Curved blade (e.g., Mac 2 or 3)
   (iv) *ETT Insertion*:
      (a) *Depth = (Age/2) + 12 cm* at teeth.
      (b) Confirm bilateral breath sounds and absence in the stomach.
      (c) Secure with *cotton tape* or *Elastoplast.*
   (v) *Orogastric tube* on free drainage (avoid NGT in head injury).
   (vi) *Confirm placement* with AP chest X-ray (tip at medial clavicles).
   (vii) *Suction* ETT every hour or as needed.
   (viii) *Humidify* gases using a condenser humidifier ("Swedish nose").
   (ix) *Splint arms* as needed for safety and sedation.

9. *Can't Intubate, Can't Oxygenate (CICO)*
   - Escalate immediately to:
     - *Needle cricothyroidotomy*: Any age (temporary measure).
     - *Surgical cricothyroidotomy*: Children *>12 years.*

Specific airway problems in trauma: Suspect airway injury if:

- Fall onto a sharp object.
- Collision with a hidden wire.
- Blunt trauma from dashboard/front seat.
- Penetrating neck injury.

Think of laryngeal/tracheal rupture—Look for subcutaneous emphysema.

- *Airway Burns:* Always prioritize airway in cases with thermal injury, inhalation (flames, steam), and hot liquid aspiration. Suspect inhalation injury if exposed to fire/smoke in an enclosed space, even without facial burns.

Warning Signs:
- Stridor, drooling, facial/neck burns.
- Edema, tachypnea, respiratory distress.
- Late signs (e.g., recession) = need for immediate intubation.

Breathing

Respiratory distress is a frequent and potentially serious manifestation in children who have sustained significant trauma. Early recognition and understanding of its underlying causes are crucial for timely intervention. Common contributors include:

- *Direct airway injury* from trauma.
- *Airway obstruction*, which may result from vomitus, blood, soft tissue swelling, or loss of pharyngeal tone due to a low Glasgow Coma Scale (GCS) score.
- *Chest injuries*, including life-threatening thoracic trauma as previously described.
- *Abdominal injuries*, such as peritonitis or a ruptured diaphragm, which can compromise breathing.
- *Aspiration* of gastric contents or foreign material.
- *Shock or metabolic acidosis*, which often triggers compensatory tachypnea.
- *Pain, anxiety, or fear*, which can also contribute to increased respiratory effort.

Breathing Assessment in Pediatric Trauma

During the primary survey, examine the thorax to identify immediate or impending life threats. Use a look, listen, feel approach.

1. *Look.*
   - Expose the chest fully.
   - Assess work of breathing:
     - Tachypnea: May indicate chest injury, pain, acidosis, or anxiety.
     - Bradypnea may suggest head injury or intoxication.
     - Grunting or nasal flaring: Signs of severe distress (consider pulmonary contusion, hemothorax, tension pneumothorax).
   - Assess breathing adequacy:
     - Chest symmetry: Asymmetry may suggest pneumothorax or hemothorax.
     - Paradoxical movement: Flail chest.
     - Oxygen saturation: Normal ≥95%; investigate persistent hypoxia.
   - Assess systemic effects:
     - Pallor, cyanosis (late and may be masked in anemia).
     - Tachycardia (early ***hypoxia***), bradycardia (late and ominous).
     - Agitation or drowsiness: May indicate hypoxia or hypercapnia.
   - Check for external signs of trauma:
     - Bruising, abrasions, seatbelt marks, or wounds—clues to internal injury patterns.
2. *Listen.*
   - Air entry: Compare bilaterally; listen in multiple lung zones despite environmental noise.
   - Heart sounds: Muffled or absent may suggest tamponade.

3. *Feel.*
    - Surgical emphysema: Suggests pneumothorax.
    - Tenderness: Over ribs, clavicle, or sternum may indicate fractures.
    - Percussion: Check for dullness (hemothorax) or hyperresonance (pneumothorax).

Don't Forget the Neck!
If not already examined:

- Provide manual in-line stabilization before removing the collar.
- Assess for:
  - Tracheal deviation.
  - Wounds.
  - Subcutaneous emphysema.
  - Laryngeal tenderness or crepitus.
  - Venous distension.
  - Carotid swelling or bruit.
  - Dysphagia (if absent, esophageal injury is unlikely).

Breathing Management in Pediatric Trauma

Ensure the airway is patent and protected: Breathing interventions rely on a secure airway. Reassess frequently and escalate support as needed.

Oxygen and Ventilation Support

- If the child is *spontaneously breathing*: Administer 15 L/min oxygen via a non-rebreather mask (NRBM).
- If ventilatory support is needed:
  - Use positive pressure ventilation via anesthetic T-piece circuit (*preferred*).
  - Bag-valve-mask (BVM) with PEEP valve can be used but may not deliver consistent PEEP.
  - Avoid BVM in spontaneously breathing children with poor effort—some BVMs require negative pressure to open valves, which these children may not generate.

Monitoring and Reassessment

- Continuously monitor:
  - SpO_2, RR, HR, BP, and ECG.
- Observe response to oxygen/ventilation.
- Monitor trends and reassess regularly.

Bag-Valve-Mask (BVM) Ventilation

Use BVM if the airway is stable (with/without OPA) and the child requires assisted ventilation.

Steps:

- Select the correct mask and bag size:
- Bag sizes: 250 ml, 500 ml, or 1500 ml (based on age/size).
- Attach:
  - Mask to bag and bag to wall oxygen at 15 L/min.
- Deliver breaths:
  - Enough to cause visible chest rise.
  - Auscultate for bilateral air entry.
  - Allow passive expiration (I:E ratio ≈ 1:3).
  - Target rate: 20 breaths per minute.

Indications for Intubation

- Airway obstruction that persists despite use of an oropharyngeal airway (OPA).
- Inability to maintain adequate oxygenation even with supplemental oxygen.
- Hypoventilation or escalating work of breathing.
- Worsening level of consciousness (declining GCS).
- Requirement for prolonged mechanical ventilation.
- Anticipated airway compromise, such as in burn injuries.
- To control agitation, pain, or distress.
- To facilitate safe and secure transport.

Specific Management Considerations

The detailed management of specific thoracic injuries such as tension pneumothorax, open pneumothorax, massive hemothorax, flail chest, rib fractures, and pulmonary contusions require focused interventions that will be comprehensively addressed in the upcoming chapters. Primary care providers should be able to recognize the clinical signs suggestive of these injuries during the initial assessment and initiate basic stabilization while arranging for prompt transfer and definitive care.

Patient and Family Communication

Effective communication with families is vital in the care of injured children. In airway and breathing emergencies, caregivers should be reassured that interventions such as oxygen delivery, airway positioning, suctioning, or intubation are essential to support the child's breathing and prevent further complications. These procedures are often performed with medications to ensure the child's comfort and safety. PCPs must use clear, compassionate, and age-appropriate language when explaining the child's condition and the steps being taken. Families should be kept informed throughout the resuscitation and encouraged to share relevant medical history or comfort the child once stable. Their involvement not only enhances care coordination but also provides emotional reassurance during a distressing time.

Case Resolution

Upon initial assessment using the Pediatric Assessment Triangle (PAT), Anuradha and Paramjeet noted Kabir's abnormal appearance (reduced responsiveness), increased work of breathing (tachypnea, gurgling sounds, use of accessory muscles), and poor circulation (prolonged capillary refill). These findings prompted immediate prioritization of airway management and stabilization. The PAT framework proved invaluable in guiding urgent decision-making despite the absence of advanced diagnostic tools like X-rays or blood gases.

Signs of impending airway compromise—including gurgling respirations, facial swelling, hoarseness, and altered sensorium—were recognized early. Anuradha ensured airway suctioning equipment was ready, and a jaw thrust maneuver was used while maintaining cervical spine precautions. A rigid collar was improvised using a folded towel roll and tape, and supplemental oxygen was administered via non-rebreather mask. Despite this, SpO_2 remained below 90%, and stridor worsened, confirming the need for escalation.

Dr. Shaan, the junior physician, arrived and took clinical charge. Guided by the team, he performed a focused airway assessment and assisted with positioning and suctioning. Recognizing signs of progressive obstruction and low GCS, he prepared for endotracheal intubation. While definitive intubation was deferred until ambulance arrival due to lack of RSI medications and monitoring, bag-valve-mask ventilation was initiated with appropriate technique to prevent gastric insufflation and barotrauma.

The trauma nurse's role proved critical—Anuradha coordinated the preparation of airway equipment, ensured closed-loop communication among team members, and communicated vital signs and clinical changes to Dr. Shaan continuously. She also provided calm reassurance to Kabir's father and began documentation for referral.

Before transfer, key clinical data were documented, including injury mechanism, vitals, Glasgow Coma Scale, airway interventions attempted, oxygen delivery mode, and suspected cervical spine injury. A printed referral form was supplemented with a phone update to the receiving hospital to ensure continuity of care.

As the ambulance departed toward the tertiary trauma center with Dr. Shaan escorting the child, the team reflected on how a structured, team-based approach and early recognition of red flags helped prevent further deterioration. This case reinforces how even in limited-resource settings, well-trained PCPs can make life-saving decisions when guided by clinical acumen, teamwork, and prioritization principles.

Key Messages

1. *Always prioritize the airway first during primary survey:* In pediatric trauma, airway obstruction is a leading and reversible cause of death. Begin your assessment with airway patency. Use the jaw thrust technique, especially when cervi-

cal spine injury is suspected, and never delay airway interventions if compromise is evident.

2. *Recognize the anatomical vulnerabilities of the pediatric airway:* Pediatric airways are narrow, anterior, and highly collapsible. Children have larger tongues, a higher larynx, and a proportionally larger occiput, all of which increase the risk of obstruction. Even minor swelling or secretions can severely compromise airflow.
3. *Identify early signs of airway compromise:* Be vigilant for stridor, hoarseness, gurgling, snoring, or complete silence. Look for signs of respiratory distress such as intercostal retractions, tachypnea, use of accessory muscles, and altered mental status. These may precede sudden deterioration.
4. *Support the airway with positioning and adjuncts:* Ensure airway patency using manual positioning (neutral head alignment with in-line stabilization) and adjuncts like oropharyngeal (OPA) or nasopharyngeal (NPA) airways. Suction oral secretions or blood promptly to prevent aspiration.
5. *Prepare for intubation if non-definitive measures fail:* If airway obstruction persists or the child has a GCS ≤ 8, prepare for endotracheal intubation. Ensure that the most skilled clinician available performs the procedure. Preoxygenate with high-flow oxygen and confirm tube placement with capnography, chest rise, and bilateral air entry.
6. *Provide high-flow oxygen early and monitor continuously:* Administer 15 L/min oxygen via a non-rebreather mask at the first sign of respiratory distress. Continuously monitor SpO_2, respiratory rate, heart rate, and clinical response to ensure adequate tissue oxygenation and guide further interventions.
7. *Evaluate breathing with a systematic approach:* Use Look, Listen, and Feel:
   - Look for chest rise, symmetry, and signs of trauma.
   - Listen for breath sounds and air entry.
   - Feel for subcutaneous emphysema or tracheal deviation.
   - Assess for life-threatening conditions like tension pneumothorax, flail chest, or hemothorax.
8. *Manage life-threatening chest injuries promptly:* In cases of suspected tension pneumothorax, perform needle decompression followed by chest tube insertion. Do not delay if clinical signs are present—diagnostic tools like imaging may not be available in resource-limited settings.
9. *Avoid overventilation, especially in head injuries:* Overzealous ventilation can lower CO_2 levels excessively, reducing cerebral perfusion. In children with traumatic brain injury or hypovolemia, use gentle, controlled ventilation and aim to maintain normal CO_2 and oxygen levels.
10. *Reassess frequently and escalate when needed:* Airway and breathing status can change rapidly in pediatric trauma. Perform ongoing reassessment and be prepared to escalate support. Document all interventions and communicate clearly with receiving centers to ensure continuity of care during transfer.

Bibliography

1. American College of Surgeons. *Advanced Trauma Life Support® (ATLS®) Student Course Manual*. 10th ed. Chicago: ACS; 2018.
2. Emergency Nurses Association (ENA). *Trauma Nursing Core Course Provider Manual*. 8th ed. Des Plaines, IL: ENA; 2019.
3. International Liaison Committee on Resuscitation (ILCOR). *Pediatric Basic and Advanced Life Support Guidelines—2020 International Consensus on Cardiopulmonary Resuscitation and Emergency Cardiovascular Care Science With Treatment Recommendations*. Circulation. 2020;142(16_suppl_1):S140–S184.
4. Royal College of Paediatrics and Child Health (RCPCH). *Management of Seriously Ill or Injured Children: A Team Approach*. 4th ed. London: RCPCH Publications; 2016.
5. The Royal Children's Hospital Melbourne. *Trauma Manual—Airway Management* [Internet]. Melbourne: RCH; c2018 [cited 2025 Apr 25]. Available from: https://www.rch.org.au/trauma-service/manual/
6. The Royal Children's Hospital Melbourne. *Trauma Manual—Breathing Management* [Internet]. Melbourne: RCH; c2018 [cited 2025 Apr 25]. Available from: https://www.rch.org.au/trauma-service/manual/

Assessment and Management of Circulation: Shock and Fluid Management

6

Samuel Ravi and Sibabratta Patnaik

Learning Objectives

After reading this chapter, the reader will be able to:

- Recognize early clinical signs of hemorrhagic shock in children, including subtle indicators such as tachycardia, prolonged capillary refill time, altered sensorium, and cool extremities.
- Differentiate between the stages of hemorrhagic shock based on physiological parameters and severity of blood loss and understand their implications for urgent intervention.
- Apply the ABCDE approach systematically to assess and stabilize pediatric trauma patients, with an emphasis on airway protection, circulatory support, and neurologic assessment.
- Identify key anatomical and physiological differences in children that impact shock response, fluid needs, and resuscitation strategies.
- Implement initial emergency interventions, including airway management, oxygen delivery, intravenous access, and appropriate fluid resuscitation using crystalloids and blood products.
- Understand the indications for activating massive transfusion protocols in pediatric patients and the safe ratio-based administration of blood components.
- Support trauma-informed care by engaging with families, recognizing the emotional impact of pediatric trauma, and providing appropriate education and reassurance.

S. Ravi
Christian Medical College Vellore, Vellore, Tamil Nadu, India

S. Patnaik (✉)
Department of Pediatrics, AIIMS Bibinagar, Bibinagar, Telangana, India

N. T. Rai (ed.), *Pediatric Trauma Resuscitation Manual (PTRM) for Primary Care Providers*, https://doi.org/10.1007/978-981-95-4979-5_6

Introduction

Hemorrhagic shock remains a leading, yet preventable, cause of death in pediatric trauma patients. Unlike adults, children often maintain their blood pressure until significant blood volume is lost—typically 25–35%—which can mask the severity of their condition during early assessment. This unique physiological compensation underscores the importance of timely recognition and rapid intervention. Primary care providers (PCPs), especially in prehospital or resource-limited settings, play a crucial role in identifying signs of shock early, initiating lifesaving measures, and coordinating transfer to higher centers.

Pediatric patients differ significantly from adults in terms of anatomy, physiology, and injury patterns. Children have proportionally larger heads, thinner skin, higher metabolic rates, and less developed abdominal musculature, all of which influence how trauma affects them. In hemorrhagic shock, these differences can make both diagnosis and management more challenging. A seemingly minor injury may result in significant blood loss, and vital signs may remain deceptively stable until decompensation occurs.

This chapter provides a comprehensive guide to the early recognition and management of hemorrhagic shock in children. It emphasizes the use of a systematic ABCDE approach to identify life-threatening conditions, stabilize the child, and initiate appropriate resuscitative efforts. Key nursing interventions—including obtaining vascular access, initiating crystalloid infusion, monitoring perfusion parameters, and preparing for blood transfusion—are also highlighted.

Special attention is given to the emotional and psychological stress that pediatric trauma places on both the child and the family. The role of the healthcare team, especially the PCP, extends beyond physical care to include emotional support, family education, and multidisciplinary coordination.

By equipping frontline providers with practical, age-specific strategies, this chapter aims to improve outcomes and reduce preventable mortality in children presenting with hemorrhagic shock following trauma.

Case Scenario

You are on duty at a rural emergency unit in Eastern India with a basic pediatric setup, including limited monitoring and one oxygen cylinder. At 5:45 PM, a 9-year-old boy named Arnav is brought in by a bystander and his uncle after being hit by an auto-rickshaw while crossing a busy street. The incident occurred approximately 1 h ago. He was reportedly conscious immediately after the event but has become progressively drowsy.

On primary examination, Arnav is drowsy but withdraws to pain (AVPU: P). He has visible facial abrasions, contusions on his limbs, and a deep bruising injury across the upper abdomen. There is no obvious external bleeding. His vital signs are as follows:

- Heart rate: 110 bpm (feeble pulse)
- Blood pressure: 80/50 mmHg
- Respiratory rate: 32 per min
- SpO_2: 96% on room air
- Capillary refill time: 5 s
- Extremities: Cold and pale

A point-of-care arterial blood gas (ABG) reveals:

- pH: 7.24
- pCO_2: 37 mmHg
- HCO_3^-: 16 mmol/L
- Base excess: −7 mmol/L
- Lactate: 6 mmol/L

There is no pediatric specialist on site, and the next referral hospital is 2 h away. You initiate the ABCDE approach, provide high-flow oxygen, maintain spinal precautions, and begin fluid resuscitation while preparing for urgent transport.

Reflective Questions

1. What are the early signs of hemorrhagic shock in children, and how might they differ from adult presentations?
2. How can PCPs use bedside assessments to identify occult internal bleeding in pediatric trauma patients?
3. What immediate interventions should be prioritized when managing pediatric hemorrhagic shock in resource-limited settings?
4. How does blood gas interpretation support the diagnosis of hemorrhagic shock in this case?
5. What clinical parameters should be monitored closely during transport to ensure early detection of deterioration?

Anatomical and Physiological Considerations

Infants and children exhibit significant anatomical and physiological differences compared to adults, with these differences becoming more pronounced in younger children.

- Children have relatively larger body surface area and can lose a lot of fluid by evaporation; thus, they need comparatively more fluid to maintain their volume status.
- The cardiac output of infants and young children is heart rate dependent as their stroke volume is relatively constant. Contractility of infant's heart is less as compared to children and adults.

- Visibly smaller amount of blood loss in infants and children may be sufficient to produce poor perfusion and shock. For example, a 5 kg infant will have a blood volume of 400 ml and for it, 50–100 ml of blood loss is very significant.
- In children, cardiac output and oxygen delivery are higher on a per kilogram basis compared to adults. Therefore, any condition that increases oxygen demand or impairs oxygen delivery can rapidly lead to cardiovascular decompensation.
- IV access is difficult in children because of more subcutaneous fat and smaller veins.
- Metabolic rate is high in children, so the workload on heart is also more.
- Children have a proportionally larger total body water content compared to adults.
- Their renal tubules are immature, so the concentrating ability is less and sodium wastage is more.
- The pharmacokinetics and pharmacodynamics of drugs differ between children and adults and this may affect the dosing of many drugs.
- Children have a reduced ability to concentrate urine, which can lead to increased water loss.
- The expected urine output for an infant and child is 1–2 mL per kg body weight per hour. For older children, urine output is 0.5–1 mL/kg/h.

ABCDE Approach

When an injured child arrives in the ED, life-threatening injuries are to be ruled out as soon as possible and necessary treatment is to be started. The approach followed is the "ABCDE rule."

Use the *Pediatric Assessment Triangle* (CBC: consciousness, breathing, color) for the early recognition of a child in danger.

Then follow the ABCDE approach

- Once the child is evaluated systematically, problems are identified, and necessary interventions are initiated.
- Always re-evaluate after your intervention to see if it is working or not.
- Any life-threatening condition on evaluation, do the interventions immediately before going for further evaluation.

A is for airway – Establish and maintain airway patency.

B is for breathing

- Check the respiratory rate (consider age related).
- Check for signs of increased work of breathing like retractions, grunting, and nasal flaring, which indicate respiratory distress.
- Look for air entry clinically or by auscultation. Try to find abnormal sounds like grunting, stridor, crackles, etc.

- Oxygenation (color, pulse oximetry). *Be aware that hypoxemia can occur without other obvious clinical signs.*
- Use capnography if available.
- Consider doing chest ultrasound.

C is for circulation (age specific)

- Pulse rate, rhythm, and volume
- Capillary refill time (CRT) – *Be aware that CRT may not be reliable if the environment is very cold.*
- Assessment of end organ perfusions like urine output (kidney) and sensorium (brain)
- Preload evaluation: jugular veins, liver span, crepitation
- Blood pressure measurement with appropriate technique
- Lactate measurements and follow-up
- Consider point-of-care ultrasound to look for fluid status.

D is for disability check

- Level of consciousness is assessed by AVPU (Alert-Verbal-Pain-Unresponsive) score or by pediatric Glasgow Coma Scale (GCS). AVPU scoring is much easier in ED setups.
- Airway is not maintained at a GCS of 8 or less and these children will require endotracheal intubation.
- Look for pupillary size, symmetry, and reaction to light.
- Posturing or focal signs point to intracranial insult.
- Any seizure in trauma setting is a neurological emergency.
- Check blood glucose level.
- Neuroimaging may be considered urgently if no improvement in GCS after resuscitation, focal signs, or seizures.

E is for exposure

Child should be exposed completely to examine from head to toe.

- Look for any trauma or bruise in any hidden part; see for cyanosis or anemia.

Biomechanics of Injury Among Children

Children are especially vulnerable to severe injuries due to their anatomical characteristics—larger head-to-body ratio, weaker abdominal musculature, and limited protective reflexes. Falls from height or high-impact vehicular trauma can result in multisystem injuries, with the risk of head trauma and internal organ damage being particularly high. Recognizing common mechanisms of injury and their associated patterns helps primary care providers anticipate life-threatening conditions and prioritize interventions (Table 6.1).

Table 6.1. Common mechanisms of pediatric trauma and injury patterns

Mechanism of injury	Typical injury patterns
Child thrown from a vehicle during a crash	• Head injuries, multisystem injuries, possible hollow viscus injuries requiring urgent surgical intervention
Pedestrian-vehicle impact	• *Low-speed impact:* Lower limb fractures • *High-speed impact:* Polytrauma, head and cervical spine injuries, lower leg fractures
Motor vehicle occupant injury	• *Unrestrained child:* Multiple trauma, head and cervical spine injuries, scalp/facial lacerations • *Restrained child:* Thoracic and abdominal trauma, lower spine injuries
Height-related injuries	• *Low fall:* Upper limb fractures • *Medium fall:* Head and neck injuries, upper/lower limb fractures • *High fall:* Polytrauma involving head, neck, and extremities. Possible hollow viscus injuries requiring urgent surgical intervention
Bicycle fall injuries	• *Without helmet:* Head/neck lacerations, scalp and facial injuries, upper extremity fractures • *With helmet:* Predominantly upper limb fractures • *Handlebar injury:* Internal abdominal trauma (e.g., hollow viscus injury)

Pediatric Hemorrhagic Shock in Trauma

Hemorrhagic shock is a common cause of morbidity and mortality in pediatric trauma. Exsanguination at the scene and massive blood loss account for nearly 40% of trauma-related deaths. Polytrauma resulting from motor vehicle collisions, falls, blunt abdominal and pelvic injuries, open or multiple bone fractures, penetrating injuries, and vascular injuries comprises the majority of these cases. Children with multiple injuries often present in hypovolemic or hemorrhagic shock, which requires prompt recognition and intervention. In contrast to adults, children can maintain near-normal blood pressure until they have lost 25–35% of their circulating blood volume. This is attributed to their high sympathetic tone, which induces peripheral vasoconstriction to preserve blood pressure despite significant blood loss.

- Tachycardia is a very early sign of shock while hypotension is a late sign.
- Signs of poor peripheral perfusion include:
  - Prolonged capillary refill (>2 s)
  - Low volume or weak pulses
  - Mottling or paleness of the skin
  - Impaired sensorium

Pediatric traumatic hemorrhagic shock is a form of hypovolemic shock that arises due to significant blood loss, which may be either internal (such as from solid organ injury or pelvic fractures) or external (such as from open wounds or lacerations). This condition impairs oxygen delivery to vital tissues, leading to cellular

Table 6.2 Change in body parameters based on amount of blood loss

	Class I	Class II	Class III	Class IV
Category based on blood loss	Very mild	Mild	Moderate	Severe
Amount of blood loss (%)	<15%	16–25%	26–39%	40%
Heart rate	Normal	Increased	Progressive tachycardia	Progressive tachycardia
Pulse volume	Normal	Low volume	Weak peripheral pulse	Weak central pulse
Blood pressure	Normal	Narrow pulse pressure	Low BP	Significant hypotension
Peripheries	Warm and pink	Cold extremities	Cold and mottled	Cold, mottled, and cyanosed
Respiratory rate	Normal	Increased	More increased	More increased
Sensorium	Anxious	Irritable	Drowsy	Unresponsive
Urine output	Normal	Reduced	Oliguria with increased blood urea	Anuria
ABG	Normal pH	Normal pH	Metabolic acidosis	Severe acidosis with increased lactate

hypoxia and metabolic derangement. As blood volume declines, hypotension develops—often as a late and ominous sign in children especially when it becomes irreversible leading to high mortality. It is the duty of attending PCP to diagnose hemorrhagic shock before the blood pressure falls. Table 6.2 depicts the stages of shock and related clinical findings. Laboratory indicators, such as a rising base deficit and elevated serum lactate levels, further reflect tissue hypoperfusion. Although a late marker, a noticeable drop in hemoglobin concentration may also be observed, signifying the severity of blood loss. Early recognition and prompt resuscitative efforts are essential to improving outcomes.

Management of Pediatric Hemorrhagic Shock

Prehospital Priorities in Pediatric Trauma with Suspected Hemorrhagic Shock

- *Sensorium as a Red Flag*: In pediatric trauma, altered mental status (e.g., drowsiness, confusion, or reduced responsiveness) is a critical indicator of underlying physiological compromise—even in the absence of obvious external injuries. A declining sensorium may be the first sign of shock or brain injury and requires immediate intervention.
- *Initiate the ABCDE Approach*: On scene, begin the ABCDE (Airway, Breathing, Circulation, Disability, Exposure) assessment immediately, incorporating spinal precautions in all trauma patients, especially when there is a risk of cervical spine injury from mechanisms like vehicular impact or falls.

- *Oxygenation Support*: Provide high-flow oxygen using a non-rebreather mask to ensure adequate tissue oxygenation. This is especially important in hypovolemic states, where oxygen delivery is already compromised due to reduced perfusion.
- *Initiate Transport Without Delay*: Begin rapid but safe transport to the nearest appropriate facility while continuing assessment and interventions. Time-sensitive management can be lifesaving in hemorrhagic shock.

For a Child Showing Signs of Hypoperfusion Without Visible Bleeding

- *Presume Internal Hemorrhage*: In the absence of external bleeding, always suspect internal bleeding—particularly in mechanisms involving blunt trauma to the chest, abdomen, or pelvis. Children can compensate well initially, so subtle signs may precede obvious deterioration.
- *Ongoing Reassessment Is Crucial*: Continuously monitor vital signs (HR, BP, CRT, RR, SpO_2), level of consciousness (AVPU), and peripheral perfusion. Pediatric patients may decompensate quickly without clear warning.
- *Maintain Airway and Breathing*: Ensure a patent airway and support adequate ventilation. Avoid hypoxia at all costs as children have limited physiologic reserves.
- *Expedite Transfer to Definitive Care*: Rapid transport is essential. Ensure spinal stabilization during transfer, monitor continuously, and prepare for escalation of care en route, including fluid resuscitation or airway support if required.

Emergency Department Response in Pediatric Hemorrhagic Shock

Initial Assessment – Focus on Hemorrhage (ABCDE Framework)

Upon arrival to the emergency department, immediate resuscitation should follow the ABCDE approach with an emphasis on circulatory status and bleeding control:

- *Airway and Cervical Spine*: Ensure cervical spine immobilization is maintained throughout evaluation. Secure the airway, if necessary, using basic airway maneuvers or adjuncts.
- *Breathing*: Continue high-flow oxygen via a non-rebreather mask and monitor for signs of respiratory distress or compromise.
- *Circulation*:
  - Inspect for active external bleeding; apply direct pressure with sterile compresses.
  - Palpate central and peripheral pulses, noting their volume and regularity.
  - Evaluate capillary refill time (CRT) and skin temperature/color as indicators of perfusion.
  - Be alert to subtle signs of clinical deterioration: changes in mental status, tachypnea, or pallor.

Frequent reassessment is essential as children may compensate physiologically before rapidly decompensating.

Circulatory Interventions and Hemorrhage Control

- Initiate control of external bleeding with pressure dressings or tourniquets, if appropriate.
- Suspect internal bleeding in cases with poor perfusion but no visible hemorrhage.
- Establish two large-bore IV lines for fluid resuscitation and laboratory investigations.
- Begin infusion with crystalloids (e.g., 0.9% normal saline or Ringer's lactate) at 20 mL/kg while arranging blood products.
- Elevate the foot end of the spine board to improve venous return and preload in hypotensive children.
- Prepare for urgent operative management in cases of blunt abdominal trauma, pelvic fractures, or penetrating injuries.

Blood Transfusion and Massive Transfusion Protocol (MTP)

- Send urgent blood samples for type and crossmatch, complete metabolic panel (LFTs, KFTs, electrolytes including calcium), blood gas analysis, coagulation profile, and ROTEM (if available).
- If blood type is unknown and crossmatch is pending, O-negative PRBCs can be used.
- Administer tranexamic acid (TXA) at 15 mg/kg IV bolus (maximum 1 g), followed by an infusion at 2 mg/kg/h, especially in major trauma or ongoing hemorrhage.

Criteria for Pediatric Massive Transfusion Protocol

MTP activation, though rare in pediatric patients, may be indicated when:

- More than 50% of total blood volume is transfused within 24 h.
- Greater than 40 mL/kg of blood products are given in 24 h.
- Unlike adults, standardized scoring tools for pediatric MTP activation are lacking. However, the accepted transfusion ratio is:
- 1:1:1—fresh frozen plasma (FFP): platelets: packed red blood cells (PRBCs), adjusted to the child's body weight

Complications of MTP may include:

- Electrolyte disturbances (e.g., hypocalcemia, hyperkalemia)
- Coagulation abnormalities
- Immunologic reactions
- Volume overload

Family Support in Pediatric Trauma Care

A child's traumatic injury is not only a medical emergency but also an emotionally devastating event for the entire family. Parents and caregivers often undergo acute stress responses, which may range from anxiety, helplessness, guilt, and anger to sleep disturbances, emotional numbing, and social withdrawal. These reactions are natural in the aftermath of witnessing or being informed about a child's injury.

Primary care providers (PCPs) and emergency teams must recognize that emotional first aid for families is just as vital as medical intervention for the child. It is essential to create a calm, compassionate, and communicative environment, especially in the early hours of care. Keep families informed using clear, honest, and empathetic language without medical jargon. Providing consistent updates about the child's condition and interventions helps alleviate uncertainty and builds trust in the medical team.

Where available, involving a medical social worker or psychologist can be invaluable. These professionals assist in:

- Helping families process the trauma
- Providing coping strategies
- Facilitating access to mental health resources, financial aid, or hospital lodging if required
- Supporting siblings who may also be distressed or neglected in the chaos

Encourage family presence when medically safe as parental presence at the bedside can be comforting for both child and caregivers. For families from rural or resource-limited settings, practical concerns such as food, transportation, accommodation, and job security may further intensify their stress. Proactively connecting them with community support services, nongovernmental organizations, or hospital-based assistance programs can make a significant difference.

Lastly, follow-up care should include screening for post-traumatic stress in both the child and family members. Long-term psychosocial support may be necessary, especially in cases of prolonged hospitalization, disfigurement, or permanent disability.

In summary, a trauma-informed approach that includes robust family support not only aids emotional recovery but also enhances adherence to medical plans and improves overall outcomes for pediatric trauma patients.

Role and Responsibilities of a Primary Care Provider in Pediatric Hemorrhagic Shock

Primary care providers (PCPs) play a pivotal role in the early recognition, stabilization, and coordination of care for children presenting with traumatic hemorrhagic shock—especially in resource-limited or pre-referral settings. Their responsibilities encompass both clinical and supportive domains, ensuring holistic care for the pediatric patient and their family.

Key Responsibilities

- *Initial Assessment and Triage*: Rapidly evaluate the child's condition using established triage protocols to prioritize life-threatening conditions and allocate appropriate resources.
- *Emergency Interventions*: Initiate immediate, potentially lifesaving interventions such as airway management, fluid resuscitation, and hemorrhage control until advanced care is available.
- *Continuous Monitoring and Evaluation*: Conduct ongoing assessments of vital signs, neurological status, and perfusion markers to detect early signs of deterioration and guide further interventions.
- *Collaboration with the Multidisciplinary Team*: Work closely with pediatricians, emergency physicians, surgeons, anesthesiologists, and nursing staff to ensure timely escalation and coordination of care.
- *Family Support and Communication*: Provide clear, compassionate communication with caregivers. Offer emotional support, explain interventions, and involve families in decision-making where appropriate.

Critical Actions Checklist for the PCP

1. *Assign or Assume Team Roles* – Ensure clear task delegation within the healthcare team to streamline resuscitation.
2. *Obtain a Focused History* – Quickly gather relevant details from the caregiver regarding the mechanism of injury, time of incident, prior health conditions, and treatments already received.
3. *Perform Primary and Secondary Surveys* – Follow ATLS principles with the ABCDE approach to identify and address life-threatening conditions.
4. *Initiate Cardiac Monitoring* – Attach the patient to continuous ECG and pulse oximetry for real-time vital sign surveillance.
5. *Establish Vascular Access* – Secure one or two large-bore IV lines or intraosseous access if peripheral access is difficult.
6. *Administer High-Flow Oxygen* – Provide supplemental oxygen to optimize tissue perfusion and oxygenation.
7. *Assist Ventilation if Needed* – Use bag-valve-mask (BVM) ventilation for children with inadequate respiratory effort or altered consciousness.
8. *Begin Intravenous Fluid Resuscitation* – Administer appropriate isotonic crystalloids (e.g., 20 mL/kg bolus of NS or RL) while preparing for blood transfusion if required.
9. *Ensure Cervical Spine Immobilization* – Use a cervical collar or manual in-line stabilization during initial management and transfer.
10. *Prepare for Intubation Prior to Transfer* – In cases of severe shock, declining GCS, or compromised airway, consider early intubation to secure the airway before transport.

Case Resolution

Arnav, a 9-year-old boy, presented with clinical signs suggestive of hemorrhagic shock, a potentially fatal condition if not promptly recognized and managed. His cold extremities, prolonged capillary refill time (CRT) of 5 s, feeble pulse, and tachycardia are early indicators of hypovolemia, even though his blood pressure is only mildly low. In pediatric patients, hypotension is a late and often preterminal sign of shock due to their robust compensatory vasoconstriction. Hence, early warning signs such as altered mental status, cool skin, and poor peripheral perfusion must be diligently observed, especially in the absence of overt external bleeding.

In this case, bedside assessments proved essential. The presence of deep bruising over the upper abdomen raised suspicion for blunt abdominal trauma and possible internal hemorrhage, such as from liver or splenic injury. Without imaging support, the team relied on serial clinical examinations, including heart rate, CRT, skin temperature, and mental status, to monitor perfusion status.

The ABG findings further supported the diagnosis of hemorrhagic shock. The acidemia (pH 7.24), low bicarbonate (16 mmol/L), negative base excess (−7), and elevated lactate (6 mmol/L) indicated poor tissue perfusion and anaerobic metabolism—hallmarks of shock. These values served as biochemical confirmation of the clinical diagnosis and helped guide ongoing resuscitation.

Given the resource limitations (one oxygen cylinder, basic monitoring, no pediatric consultant), the PCP-led team prioritized lifesaving interventions: initiating high-flow oxygen, maintaining spinal precautions, starting 20 mL/kg crystalloid bolus, and preparing for early transport. Recognizing that delays could be fatal, they coordinated with the referral center for early surgical preparedness.

During transfer, the team closely monitored heart rate, CRT, sensorium, and urine output—simple but effective indicators of systemic perfusion in pediatric patients. They ensured the child remained warm, reassessed every 10–15 min, and were prepared to give additional fluid boluses if signs of shock persisted.

Arnav's case highlights the vital role of vigilant clinical observation, basic resuscitation skills, and early referral coordination in pediatric trauma care—even in the absence of advanced diagnostics. It reinforces that, for PCPs in rural or resource-constrained environments, early recognition and decisive action can save lives.

Key Messages

- Hemorrhagic shock is a critical and potentially fatal condition in pediatric trauma that requires immediate recognition and management.
- Primary care providers (PCPs) play a pivotal frontline role in the initial stabilization and ongoing care of children with hemorrhagic shock, especially in resource-limited settings.
- Timely identification of clinical deterioration through systematic assessment (e.g., ABCDE approach) and prompt initiation of resuscitative measures is essential for improving outcomes.

- Children have distinct anatomical and physiological characteristics that influence how they respond to trauma and shock, necessitating specialized pediatric-focused management.
- Following airway stabilization, early administration of isotonic crystalloids is critical while simultaneously preparing for blood transfusion in cases of ongoing hemorrhage.
- Effective hemorrhage control and early coordination with the trauma or surgical team are crucial to prevent ongoing blood loss and support definitive care.
- In cases of refractory shock, internal bleeding should be strongly suspected, and life-threatening conditions such as tension pneumothorax and cardiac tamponade must be ruled out.
- While pediatric massive transfusion protocols (MTPs) are not universally standardized, a balanced transfusion strategy with a 1:1:1 ratio of PRBCs, FFP, and platelets is generally recommended.
- Family-centered communication and emotional support are integral parts of trauma care and must be provided alongside medical management during critical illness.

Bibliography

1. Children's Health Queensland Hospital and Health Service. (2023, February 24). Clinical Assessment of the Pediatric Patient – Rapid Assessment / Primary and Secondary Survey / Vital Signs. Queensland Health Intranet. Retrieved December 4, 2023 from https://qheps.health.qld.gov.au/__data/assets/pdf_file/0019/724240/ns_00241.pdf
2. Holland AJ, Jackson AM, Joseph AP. Paediatric trauma at an adult trauma centre. ANZ J Surg. 2005;75:878–81. https://doi.org/10.1111/j.1445-2197.2005.03553.x. [DOI] [PubMed]
3. https://www.aliem.com/emrescupeds-em-resident-simulation-curriculum-pediatrics/case-7-multisystem-trauma/
4. Peden M, McGee K, Sharma G. The Injury Chart Book: A Graphical Overview of the Global Burden of Injuries. Geneva: World Health Organization; 2002.
5. Russell RT, Bembea MM, Borgman MA, Burd RS, Gaines BA, Jafri M, Josephson CD, Leeper CM, Leonard JC, Muszynski JA, Nicol KK, Nishijima DK, Stricker PA, Vogel AM, Wong TE, Spinella PC. Pediatric traumatic hemorrhagic shock consensus conference research priorities. J Trauma Acute Care Surg. 2023 Jan 1.

7 Pediatric Head and Maxillofacial Trauma

Manju Dhandapani, C. Vasantha Kalyani, Malar Kodi S, Asish Kishore, and Rachana Bhat

Learning Objectives

By the end of this chapter, the reader should be able to:

- Understand the anatomical and physiological differences in children that influence the assessment and management of head and facial trauma.
- Identify common mechanisms of pediatric traumatic brain injury (TBI) and maxillofacial fractures across different age groups.
- Perform systematic initial assessment using the Pediatric Assessment Triangle (PAT) and the ABCDE approach in head and facial trauma cases.
- Implement appropriate airway management strategies, including spinal motion restriction and suctioning techniques, in children with suspected facial injuries.
- Recognize signs of raised intracranial pressure (ICP) and neurological deterioration and respond with timely interventions and escalation.

M. Dhandapani
National Institute of Nursing Education, Post Graduate Institute of Medical Education & Research (PGIMER), Chandigarh, India

C. Vasantha Kalyani
College of Nursing, All India Institute of Medical Sciences (AIIMS), Deoghar, India
e-mail: Vasantha.nur@aiimsdeoghar.edu.in

M. K. S
College of Nursing, All India Institute of Medical Sciences (AIIMS), Rishikesh, India
e-mail: Malar.nur@aiimsrishikesh.edu.in

A. Kishore · R. Bhat (✉)
Department of Emergency Medicine, Kasturba Medical College, Manipal, India

Manipal Academy of Higher Education, Manipal, Karnataka, India
e-mail: Rachana.kmc@manipal.edu

N. T. Rai (ed.), *Pediatric Trauma Resuscitation Manual (PTRM) for Primary Care Providers*, https://doi.org/10.1007/978-981-95-4979-5_7

- Differentiate between various types of traumatic brain injuries (e.g., concussion, epidural hematoma, diffuse axonal injury) and facial fractures (e.g., mandibular, orbital, nasal) in pediatric patients.
- Stabilize and manage children with maxillofacial injuries, including soft tissue care, hemorrhage control, and supportive therapies.
- Prepare and execute safe referral and transfer of pediatric patients to higher centers with appropriate documentation and communication using SBAR framework.
- Educate caregivers on home care, warning signs, and rehabilitation needs following pediatric head and facial trauma.

Introduction

Head injury is one of the frequent presentations encountered in pediatric trauma cases within emergency departments. Its prevalence spans a broad spectrum of severity and causes, varying significantly with age and developmental stage. The epidemiology of pediatric head trauma reflects these variations—infants, for instance, are at particular risk for non-accidental trauma such as shaken baby syndrome, which demands high clinical suspicion and careful evaluation. In toddlers, head injuries commonly result from falls as they begin to walk and explore their surroundings. As children grow older, particularly in school-aged and adolescent groups, the leading causes shift toward motor vehicle collisions, bicycle accidents, sports-related injuries, and other high-energy mechanisms associated with recreational activities.

Fortunately, the majority of head injuries in children—approximately 80%—are categorized as mild, and in nearly 90% of these cases, neuroimaging reveals no structural abnormalities. Nonetheless, even seemingly minor head trauma requires thorough assessment due to the potential for subtle but significant neurological sequelae, such as those observed in concussions. On the more severe end of the spectrum, traumatic brain injuries (TBIs) can result in lasting cognitive and functional impairment, posing substantial challenges for the child's long-term development and quality of life.

An additional concern in pediatric head trauma is the risk of underlying child abuse, which is often under-recognized or inadequately reported. Recognizing red flags for non-accidental injuries—including inconsistent history, delay in seeking care, or signs of other physical harm—is critical before disposition from the emergency department. Furthermore, maxillofacial fractures—although uncommon in younger children—become more prevalent after the age of five due to bone ossification, and they often accompany high-impact trauma. A vigilant, age-sensitive approach by primary care providers (PCPs) is essential to ensure accurate diagnosis, timely intervention, and protection of the child's well-being.

Emergency management of pediatric traumatic brain injury (TBI) plays a pivotal role in determining patient outcomes, emphasizing the need for swift, coordinated, and evidence-based interventions. Early recognition; rapid stabilization of airway, breathing, and circulation; and timely neuroimaging are crucial steps in minimizing secondary injury and improving survival rates. The integration of advanced monitoring techniques and adherence to pediatric-specific protocols further enhances the quality of acute care. Equally important is the seamless transition from emergency treatment to definitive care, ensuring continuity and comprehensiveness in management. By prioritizing training for PCPs, investing in pediatric trauma systems, and fostering public awareness, we can improve emergency responses and optimize the prognosis for children affected by TBI.

Case Scenario

You are working an evening shift at a secondary care district hospital in Central India with a basic pediatric emergency setup. Your team includes you—a staff nurse experienced in pediatric triage—and a CHO (community health officer). The on-call junior resident doctor is stationed in the adjacent trauma room. Around 6:30 PM, a 6-year-old boy, Riyan, is rushed into your unit by his parents and neighbors.

According to the history, Riyan fell face-first from the second-floor balcony sill while playing unsupervised with friends. The fall occurred roughly 30 minutes before arrival. On examination, Riyan is bleeding from the nose and mouth, with noticeable facial swelling and distortion of midface contours. He is irritable and intermittently responsive—crying loudly at times, occasionally obeying commands but not making sustained verbal contact.

Initial Observations

- Consciousness: Semiconscious, responds to verbal stimulus (AVPU: V)
- RR: 24 breaths/min
- SpO_2: 95% on room air
- HR: 135 bpm
- BP: 100/70 mmHg
- Capillary refill time: 2 seconds

As a primary care provider (PCP), your immediate priority is to begin the ABCDE assessment, focusing first on airway patency. Given the facial injuries and altered sensorium, you check for gurgling, snoring, or signs of obstruction. You gently perform suctioning and assist with positioning to maintain a neutral head and neck posture, keeping spinal precautions in mind.

Reflective Questions

1. What key anatomical features should be considered when assessing head and facial trauma in children?
2. How can PCPs recognize the risk of associated cervical spine injury in pediatric head trauma, and what immediate precautions should they take?
3. Why is spinal motion restriction essential in children with suspected head injuries, and how can PCPs implement it in resource-limited settings?
4. What positioning techniques should be used to maintain airway patency in infants with suspected maxillofacial trauma?

Anatomical and Physiological Considerations

1. Children's skulls are thinner and more pliable, making them more prone to fractures. The brain is still developing, with ongoing synaptogenesis and myelination, which can influence injury outcomes.
2. A child's head is proportionally larger compared to their body, increasing the likelihood of head injuries in falls or accidents. The larger head in children causes a higher fulcrum leading to higher incidence of associated occipito-cervical spine injuries. Hence, taking appropriate spinal motion restriction precautions becomes an important and integral part of all pediatric head trauma management.
3. The presence of open fontanelles (Fig. 7.1) and sutures in infants can affect the dynamics of intracranial pressure (ICP) during trauma.
4. Children's craniofacial anatomy differs from that of adults, with softer bones and open sutures, which make them more prone to fractures from low-impact forces.
5. The management of airway is vital in pediatric maxillofacial trauma, as swelling and bleeding can quickly block smaller airways. Early assessment and stabilization of the airway are essential. The large occiput can cause challenges in appropriately positioning of the child for airway management in infants. Placement of a shoulder pad should aid in proper positioning in such situations as shown in Fig. 7.2.
6. While baseline ICP is lower in children, they are more susceptible to rapid increases due to swelling or bleeding. Signs of TBI in children may differ from adults, such as irritability, changes in feeding patterns, or altered activity patterns.
7. The developing brain exhibits plasticity, which can aid recovery but also means that injuries may disrupt critical developmental processes. Treatment strategies must consider the child's age, developmental stage, and unique physiological responses.

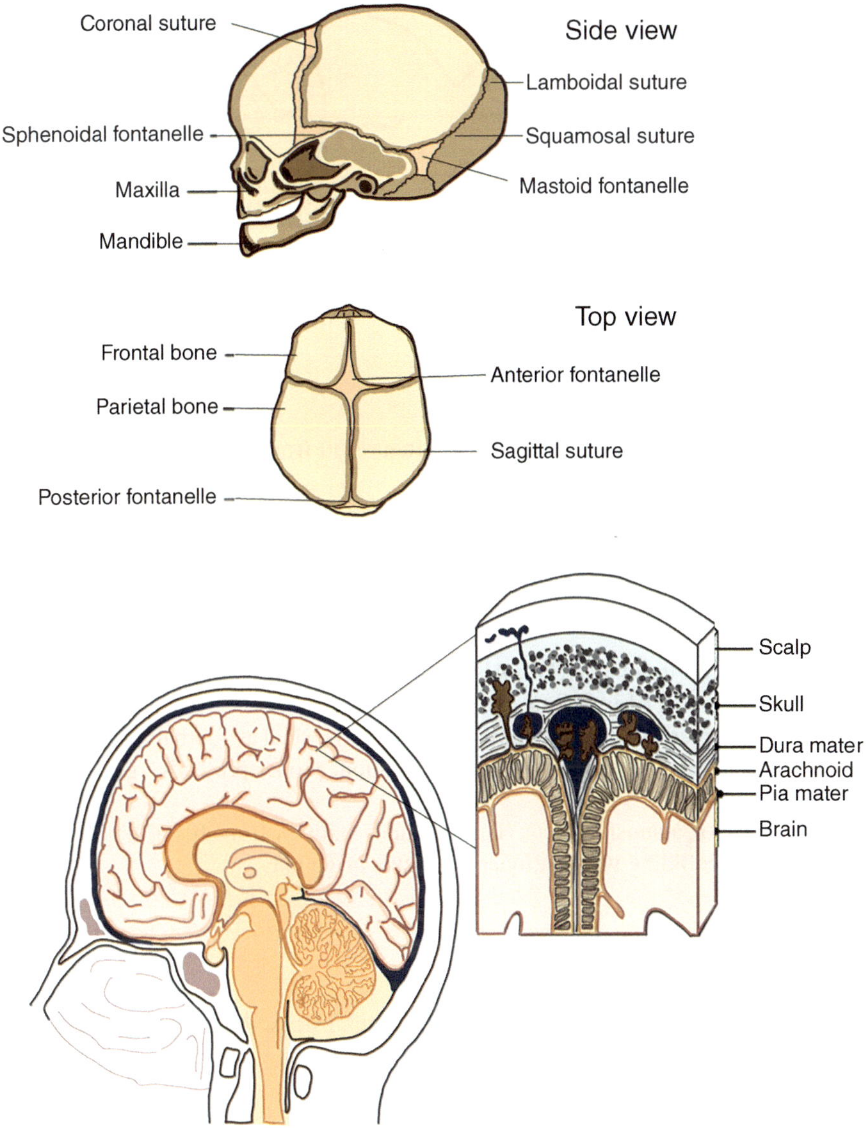

Fig. 7.1 Craniofacial anatomy in children and layers of the scalp

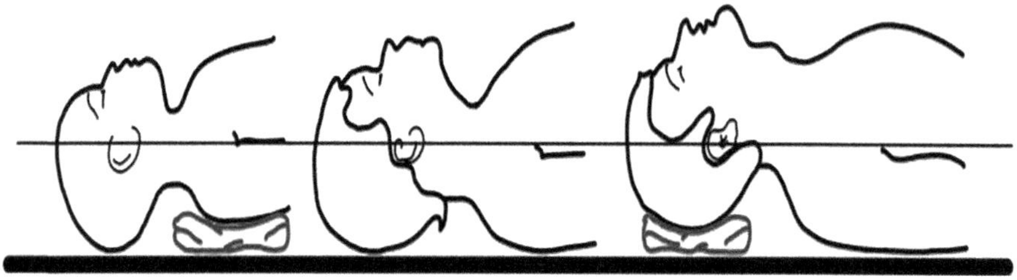

Fig. 7.2 Placement of a shoulder pad in proper positioning of airway depending on size of occiput

Common Mechanisms of Injury

Pediatric traumatic brain injuries (TBIs) often result from specific mechanisms that vary with age and developmental stage.

- Falls: The leading cause of TBI in children, especially those under 14 years old.
- Motor vehicle accidents (MVAs): A significant cause of TBIs in older children and adolescents. This includes injuries sustained as passengers, pedestrians, or cyclists.
- Abusive head trauma (AHT): Also known as shaken baby syndrome, this is a major cause of TBI in infants and young children.
- Sports and recreational activities: Contact sports, such as football or soccer, and activities like skateboarding or cycling without proper protective gear can lead to TBIs.
- Struck by or against objects: This includes injuries from being hit by falling objects or colliding with stationary objects during play.

Initial Assessment

The initial assessment of a child involves two main steps: the Pediatric Assessment Triangle (PAT) and the primary survey (ABCDE).

Pediatric Assessment Triangle (PAT)
The PAT is a quick way to assess the severity of a child's condition. It looks at three things:

1. *Appearance:* Check if the child is alert, responsive, and interacting normally. Look for signs of distress, such as crying or lethargy.
2. *Work of breathing:* Observe how the child is breathing, any periodic breathing, or any periods of apnea. Look for fast or slow breathing and abnormal sounds like wheezing or gurgling or stridor.
3. *Circulation to skin:* Check the skin color and temperature. Look for signs of poor blood flow, such as pallor (pale skin), mottling, or cyanosis (blue skin).

Primary Survey (ABCDE)
The primary survey is a more detailed assessment that focuses on identifying and managing life-threatening conditions. The *ABCDE approach* stands for Airway, Breathing, Circulation, Disability, and Exposure.

Airway (A)
- Ensure the airway is open and clear.
- Look for signs of obstruction, such as choking, high-pitched breathing sounds, or gurgling.
- Avoid hyperextension of the airway and position infant in neutral position. In high-velocity injuries/injuries with dangerous mechanisms, suspect associated cervical spine injuries and immobilize the C spine till further injuries are ruled out. If there is suspected cervical spine injury, the preferred method opening airway is a jaw thrust maneuver.
- The airway is susceptible to blockage from blood, vomit, tooth fragments, or foreign objects. Thus, prioritizing the removal of debris from the upper airway is crucial.
- If the noisy breathing persists after clearing the airway or child is unconscious and airway is not maintained, consider securing definitive airway/intubation. Anticipated difficult airways in children may necessitate fiber-optic intubation when indicated.

Breathing (B) Check the child's breathing.

- Look for rate, rhythm, depth, and effort.
- Listen for abnormal sounds (aspiration in maxillofacial injury or severe head injury) and check oxygen saturation.

Circulation (C)
- Assess circulation by checking the pulse, heart rate, capillary refill time, blood pressure, and skin condition. Look for signs of shock, such as rapid heart rate, weak pulse, or low blood pressure.
- Midface fractures as well as scalp injuries are notorious for heavy bleeding, where the source may at times be difficult to localize. Immediate measures such as applying local pressure, using sutures, and stabilizing the patient may be necessary.

Disability (D)
- Evaluate the child's neurological status. Check their level of consciousness using the AVPU scale (Alert, response to Voice, response to Pain, Unresponsive) or Glasgow Coma Scale (GCS) if familiar.
- Assess pupil size and reaction to light.
- Assess whether the child is moving all four limbs or if there is paucity of movement in any of the limbs.
- Check the blood glucose level.

Exposure (E)

- Fully expose the child to look for signs of trauma, bleeding, and other injuries while preventing hypothermia.
- The head and scalp form a significant proportion of body surface area of infants and preventing hypothermia by covering the same is crucial.
- Palpation of fontanelle may give crucial insights. Bulging fontanelle may indicate raised intracranial pressure. In children with fused fontanelle, the intracranial pressure may rise exponentially with worsening brain edema due to injury.

Role of Primary Care Provider

- *Quick Checkup:* Use the Pediatric Assessment Triangle (PAT) to see how serious the child's condition is quickly.
- *Detailed Checkup (ABCDE):* Check airway, breathing, circulation, disability (neurological status), and exposure (look for other injuries).
- *Airway:* Make sure the child's airway is open and clear while maintaining the in-line stabilization of cervical spine.
- *Breathing:* Support the child's breathing and give supplemental oxygen or prepare for necessary ventilator support.
- *Circulation:* Check pulse and blood pressure, and give IV fluids as ordered by the trauma team.
- *Disability/Neurological Check:* Check the child's level of consciousness using AVPU/GCS and pupillary reaction. Inform ED physician/neurosurgery team if there is a change in level of consciousness, unequal pupillary size, or sluggish or absent reaction or asymmetrical limb movements.
- *Exposure:* Look for other injuries and keep the child warm.

While assessing the child using ABCDE approach, the primary care provider should also emphasize on the following interventions.

- *Communication:* Talk with the team to share important information.
- *Recordkeeping:* Write down the child's condition and treatments given.
- *Family Support:* Help the child's family understand what's happening.
- *Procedure Preparation:* Help the trauma team to prepare for emergency procedures like intubation, X-rays, shifting for CT scan, etc., and provide assistance to trauma team as needed.
- *Ongoing Monitoring:* Keep checking the child's vital signs and be ready to act if something changes.

Specific Types of Traumatic Brain Injuries

Pediatric traumatic brain injuries (TBIs) can be classified into several types based on the nature and mechanism of the injury and neuroimaging. Here are the main categories:

1. *Concussion*:
   A mild TBI caused by a blow or jolt to the head. Symptoms may include confusion, headache, dizziness, and temporary loss of consciousness.
2. *Contusion*:
   A bruise on the brain tissue caused by direct impact. It may occur at the site of direct impact (coup contusions) or directly opposite to the site of impact (contrecoup contusions). It can lead to swelling and increased intracranial pressure.
3. *Epidural Hematoma:*
   Bleeding between the skull and the dura mater (outer brain membrane) due to the injury to the middle meningeal artery. May be associated with a skull fracture.
4. *Subdural Hematoma*:
   Bleeding between the dura mater and the brain due to the injury to bridging veins.
5. *Traumatic Subarachnoid Hemorrhage (SAH)*:
   Bleeding into the space between the brain and the thin tissues covering the brain. Can result from both mild and severe injuries.
6. *Diffuse Axonal Injury (DAI)*:
   Caused by rotational forces or severe shaking, leading to tearing of brain tissue. Often results in widespread damage and severe neurological deficits.
7. *Penetrating Brain Injury*:
   Caused by an object piercing the skull and brain tissue. Often leads to localized damage and high risk of infection.
8. *Second Impact Syndrome*:
   Occurs when a second TBI happens before the first one has fully healed. Can lead to rapid and severe brain swelling.

Each type of TBI has unique implications for diagnosis, treatment, and recovery.

Clinical Features of Traumatic Brain Injuries

1. *Neurological symptoms*:
   - Altered level of consciousness, ranging from irritability to confusion to coma
   - Seizures, which may occur immediately or later after the injury
   - Focal neurological deficits, such as weakness or numbness in specific areas

1. *Visible injury indicators*:
   - Scalp swelling or bruising, particularly in infants
   - Skull fractures or other visible head injuries
2. *Signs of increased intracranial pressure*:
   - Persistent vomiting
   - Pupillary changes, such as unequal pupil size or sluggish reaction to light
   - Cushing's triad: bradycardia, hypertension, and irregular breathing
3. *Physical symptoms*:
   - Headache, which may worsen over time
   - Nausea and vomiting, especially in the early stages
   - Dizziness or balance problems

4. *Visual and auditory changes*:
   - Blurred vision or sensitivity to light
   - Ringing in the ears (tinnitus) or hearing loss

Specific Types of Injuries in Pediatric Maxillofacial Trauma

Pediatric maxillofacial trauma encompasses a variety of injuries, primarily classified into fractures and soft tissue injuries as shown in Table 7.1.

Table 7.1 Pediatric maxillofacial trauma—specific injuries

Maxillofacial injury	Description and mechanism of injury	Clinical features
Mandibular fractures	Most common type of maxillofacial injury in pediatric patients (approximately 65% of cases) Can result from various mechanisms, including falls, motor vehicle accidents (MVAs), and sports injuries Unique anatomical features of children, such as greater flexibility of bones and the presence of developing teeth, influence the presentation and management of these fractures.	*Pain and swelling*: Localized swelling and tenderness in the jaw area *Trismus*: Difficulty in opening the mouth due to pain or muscle spasm *Malocclusion*: Misalignment of teeth or inability to properly close the mouth *Crepitus*: A grating sound or sensation when moving the jaw
Nasal fractures	Most common facial injuries in children (33.3% of pediatric maxillofacial trauma cases) Direct trauma such as falls, sports injuries, or physical altercations	*Nasal deformity:* This may include a visible deviation of the nasal bridge or tip, flattening of the nose, or asymmetry. Palpation may reveal crepitus or tenderness over the fractured area. Swelling, bruising, and pain around the nose and may extend to the periorbital region *Nasal obstruction:* Due to swelling of the mucosa or displacement of bone fragments *Epistaxis:* Due to damage to the nasal mucosa or blood vessels. Anterior (from the front part of the nose) or posterior (from deeper structures)

(continued)

Table 7.1 (continued)

Maxillofacial injury	Description and mechanism of injury	Clinical features
Zygomaticomaxillary complex (ZMC) fractures	Second most common type of maxillofacial fracture in children (approximately 27.5% of cases) Predominantly result from high-impact trauma, motor vehicle accidents (MVAs), and sports-related incidents	*Facial asymmetry:* Alterations in facial contour due to bone displacement *Periorbital ecchymosis:* Bruising around the eyes, commonly known as "raccoon eyes," indicative of orbital involvement *Limited eye movement:* Resulting from muscle entrapment or edema, potentially leading to diplopia *Nasal deformity:* Accompanying nasal injuries may cause visible deformities or obstruction.
Maxillary fractures	Account for approximately 17.5% of pediatric facial fractures Result from significant trauma, such as motor vehicle accidents (MVAs) or falls Frequently associated with other facial injuries	*Dental malocclusion:* Misalignment of teeth due to the displacement of the maxilla can lead to functional and aesthetic concerns. *Facial swelling and pain:* Localized swelling around the cheeks and upper jaw is common, often accompanied by tenderness on palpation. *Mobility of maxillary teeth:* Increased mobility or looseness of teeth in the maxilla may indicate associated dental injuries.
Orbital fractures	Usually occur following blunt trauma to the face Sports injuries: Contact sports like football or hockey Falls Motor vehicle accidents	*Orbital floor fractures (blowout fractures):* Occur when a forceful impact causes the orbital floor to break, often while the orbital rim remains intact. Commonly associated with entrapment of the inferior rectus muscle, leading to restricted eye movement and diplopia (double vision). *Orbital rim fractures:* Involve the bony edges of the orbit and are usually more extensive. Can lead to significant swelling and bruising around the eyes (periorbital ecchymosis). *Complications if not treated promptly:* Muscle entrapment leading to persistent strabismus (misalignment/squinting of the eyes) Vision loss due to optic nerve injury or severe hemorrhage

(continued)

Table 7.1 (continued)

Maxillofacial injury	Description and mechanism of injury	Clinical features
Frontal bone fractures	High-impact trauma such as falls from heights Direct blows to the forehead in sports or accidents *Types:* Linear fracture Depressed fracture Frontal sinus fracture	Patients may exhibit swelling, tenderness over the forehead, headache, or neurological symptoms. Injuries involving the frontal sinus cavity can lead to complications such as sinusitis or cerebrospinal fluid leaks (watery discharge through the nose) and pneumocephalus (air in the cranial cavity).
Soft tissue injuries	Lacerations and contusions Injuries to palate and tongue	In areas such as lips, cheeks, and oral mucosa due to blunt trauma Contusions lead to pain, swelling, and discoloration due to bleeding under the skin. Pain, swelling, and hematoma Secondary infection and scarring

Evaluation of TBI and Maxillofacial Injury

In the primary care or district emergency setting, early recognition and appropriate evaluation of traumatic brain injury (TBI) and maxillofacial trauma in children are critical for timely referral and stabilization. While advanced imaging and neurosurgical interventions may not be available on site, primary care providers (PCPs) play a pivotal role in initial assessment, stabilization and determining the need for urgent transfer.

1. *Clinical Assessment*

   A thorough clinical examination remains the cornerstone of evaluation in resource-limited settings:

   - *Neurological Status:*
     - Use the Pediatric Glasgow Coma Scale (PGCS) to assess consciousness and neurological function.
     - Monitor for changes in behavior, confusion, persistent crying, poor feeding (in infants), vomiting, or seizures—these may be subtle signs of evolving TBI.
     - Assess for pupillary size, symmetry, and reactivity to light.
   - *Head and Facial Examination:*
     - Look for scalp hematomas, lacerations, boggy swellings, or depressions that may indicate underlying skull fractures.
     - Inspect the nose, mouth, and periorbital region for signs of maxillofacial trauma (e.g., nasal bleeding, dental avulsion, malocclusion, periorbital bruising).

- Palpate the mandible, maxilla, and zygomatic arches for tenderness or crepitus.
- Assess for CSF leak from nose or ear (clear, watery discharge) suggesting basilar skull fracture.

- *Signs of Raised Intracranial Pressure (ICP):*
  - Observe for bradycardia, hypertension, irregular respirations, or altered mental status.
  - Watch for bulging fontanelle in infants or papilledema (if feasible).

2. *Imaging*

While many PCP settings may not have CT imaging, recognizing when imaging is indicated is essential:

- *CT Head* (Non-contrast):
  - Indicated in moderate to severe TBI (PGCS ≤13), suspected skull fracture, persistent vomiting, seizure, focal deficit, or altered mental status
  - Helps detect skull fractures, hematomas (epidural/subdural), brain contusions, or midline shift.
- *Facial Bone CT/3D Reconstruction:*
  - May be advised by the trauma team in referred centers for complex midface or orbital fractures.
  - 3D reconstructions assist in surgical planning.
- *FAST (Focused Assessment with Sonography for Trauma):*
  - Can be helpful in multi-trauma scenarios to rule out concurrent intra-abdominal injury.

3. *Laboratory Investigations*

Relevant in supporting diagnosis and preparing for referral or surgery:

- *Complete Blood Count (CBC):* Evaluate for bleeding or infection.
- *Electrolytes and Blood Glucose:* To identify metabolic causes of altered mental status.
- *Coagulation Profile:* Particularly if there are signs of bleeding or if the patient is on anticoagulants
- *Blood Grouping and Crossmatch:* If transfusion is likely
- *Toxicology Screening:* If substance ingestion, overdose, or poisoning is suspected (especially in adolescents)

4. *Monitoring and Documentation*

- *Vital Signs:* Document trends in heart rate, blood pressure, respiratory rate, temperature, and oxygen saturation.
- *Neurological Observations:*
  - Record GCS scores at regular intervals.
  - Note any new signs such as posturing, pupil changes, or vomiting.
- *Fluid Status and Input-Output Monitoring:* Especially important in children with vomiting, poor oral intake, or signs of shock

5. *Red Flags for Urgent Referral*

   PCPs should initiate urgent referral or call for higher-level trauma support in case of:
   - GCS ≤13 or deteriorating mental status
   - Suspected open or depressed skull fracture
   - Prolonged post ictal phase in post-traumatic seizure
   - Signs of basilar skull fracture (CSF leak, raccoon eyes, Battle's sign)
   - Facial deformity with suspected airway compromise or ocular involvement
   - Persistent vomiting, bradycardia, or hypertension

Management of TBI and Maxillofacial Injury

General Principles of Initial Management

In the primary care or district hospital setting, the role of the PCP is focused on early recognition, stabilization, and preparation for referral. Given the unique anatomy and physiology of pediatric patients, prompt and tailored interventions are critical.

1. *Airway Management*
   - Ensure a patent airway while assuming a cervical spine injury in all head trauma cases.
   - Use a jaw thrust maneuver to open the airway in a child with suspected spinal trauma.
   - Suction blood or secretions as needed and use airway adjuncts (OPA/NPA) if trained and indicated.
   - Be vigilant for signs of obstructed airway due to facial swelling, hematoma, broken teeth, or nasal bleeding.
   - Call for help early if airway compromise is suspected and advanced airway management is beyond PCP scope.

2. *Breathing and Oxygenation*
   - Provide high-flow oxygen via a non-rebreather mask.
   - Observe for signs of respiratory distress, hypoxia, or aspiration.
   - Elevate the head of the bed to 30° if not contraindicated to assist venous drainage and reduce intracranial pressure.

3. *Circulation and Hemorrhage Control*
   - Apply direct pressure to external bleeding from facial wounds.
   - Monitor vital signs and signs of shock (delayed capillary refill, tachycardia, hypotension).
   - Establish IV access and administer fluid bolus (20 mL/kg warm isotonic saline) if signs of hypovolemia are present.
   - Initiate blood grouping and crossmatching if available, especially if referral is delayed.

4. *Pain Management and Comfort Measures*
   - Administer age-appropriate analgesics (e.g., paracetamol or ibuprofen) as per weight.
   - Apply cold compresses to reduce swelling and provide comfort.
   - Provide gentle emotional reassurance to both child and caregiver.

5. *Wound Care and Tetanus Prophylaxis*
   - Clean visible wounds with sterile saline or antiseptic solution.
   - Dress wounds with sterile gauze.
   - Initiate tetanus prophylaxis as indicated for open injuries.

6. *Neurological Monitoring*
   - Assess and document GCS or AVPU scale at regular intervals:
     - Every 20 minutes for the first 2 hours
     - Every 30 minutes for the next 2 hours
     - Hourly thereafter till the child is stable or shifted out of ICU
     - Every 2 hours once the child is neurologically stable
     - Inform even a minor change to the physician or neurosurgeon.
   - Observe for new or worsening signs: pupil asymmetry, posturing, irritability, seizures, or vomiting.
   - Watch for CSF leak (clear discharge from nose/ears) and avoid nasal suction or NG tube insertion in such cases.
   - Don't suction nasally if anterior fossa fracture is present.
   - Avoid procedures that may increase ICP, such as forceful coughing or nose-blowing.
   - Administer antiepileptics as per institutional policy.

7. *Eye and Skin Care*
   - Monitor for corneal reflex; protect the eyes with lubricating drops or gentle taping if unconscious.
   - Keep the child warm to avoid hypothermia, especially during transfer preparation.

8. *Documentation and Communication*
   - Maintain a clear, timed record of all assessments, vitals, GCS trends, and interventions performed.
   - Prepare a brief handover summary including:
     - Mechanism of injury
     - Timeline of events
     - Vitals trends and GCS progression
     - Interventions performed (oxygen, fluids, medications)
     - Current clinical status and concerns (e.g., suspected raised ICP or airway threat)

9. *Referral and Transfer Preparation*
   - Coordinate with the referral center early once signs of moderate-to-severe TBI or facial injury are identified.
   - Ensure:
     - All paperwork and handover notes are complete
     - The child is hemodynamically stabilized before transfer (if possible)
     - Oxygen, IV access, and monitoring are maintained during transit
   - Provide caregiver with clear instructions and accompany the child if no escort is available.

10. *Recognize Indications for Specialist/Surgical Management*

    The following findings warrant urgent specialist evaluation and possible surgical intervention:
    - Penetrating injuries to the skull or face
    - Depressed skull fracture
    - Epidural/subdural hematoma (suspected with decreasing GCS, anisocoria, posturing)
    - Facial fractures with airway compromise or visual symptoms
    - Persistent vomiting, seizures, or behavioral changes

The management of pediatric maxillofacial trauma requires seamless coordination between PCPs and the trauma team. While PCPs play a crucial role in initial stabilization, early recognition of red flags, and timely referral, definitive care—including advanced imaging, airway management, and surgical interventions—is typically handled by the trauma or surgical team. Understanding this division of responsibilities ensures efficient workflow, reduces delays in care, and improves patient outcomes, especially in resource-limited or peripheral settings. Table 7.2 outlines common injury types and delineates the distinct yet complementary roles of PCPs and trauma specialists in managing each scenario.

Table 7.2 Role of PCPs and trauma team in management of maxillofacial injuries

Injury type	Primary care provider role	Trauma team role
Soft tissue injuries (e.g., *lacerations, contusions)*	Clean wounds with sterile saline or antiseptic. Apply direct pressure to control bleeding. Dress with sterile gauze. Monitor for signs of infection.	Perform surgical debridement. Suture deep or complex lacerations under sterile conditions.
Fractures (e.g., *mandibular, maxillary, zygomatic*)	Keep child NPO if surgery is likely. Administer high-flow oxygen. Elevate head to reduce swelling. Monitor for airway compromise.	Confirm diagnosis with X-ray/CT. Stabilize with maxillomandibular fixation if needed. Surgical repair for severe fractures

(continued)

Table 7.2 (continued)

Injury type	Primary care provider role	Trauma team role
Dental injuries (e.g., *avulsions, fractured teeth)*	Rinse avulsed tooth with sterile saline. Store tooth in milk or saline. Provide analgesia and reassurance. Control bleeding with gauze.	Reimplant tooth within 30 minutes if feasible. Refer to pediatric dentist for root canal or further dental care.
Orbital and nasal fractures	Apply cold compresses to reduce swelling. Advise against nose-blowing. Monitor for signs of eye trauma.	Assess for globe injuries or vision loss. Perform surgical correction for functional or cosmetic issues.
Midface fractures (e.g., *Le Fort fractures)*	Stabilize head and neck; presume C-spine injury. Watch for CSF leak from nose or ears.	Obtain CT imaging. Perform surgical repair for severe or displaced fractures.

Communicating Effectively Using the SBAR Framework

In pediatric trauma scenarios—particularly those involving potential airway compromise from facial or head injuries—clear, concise, and structured communication is critical for timely interventions. The *SBAR framework* (Situation, Background, Assessment, Recommendation) is a validated tool that enhances team coordination, improves clarity of handovers, and promotes patient safety during high-stakes situations.

SBAR stands for:

- *Situation*—What is happening right now?
- *Background*—What relevant information or history should be shared?
- *Assessment*—What do you think is going on?
- *Recommendation*—What actions do you suggest?

This tool is especially valuable for primary care providers (PCPs) working in resource-limited settings, helping them escalate concerns effectively to on-call physicians or specialists.

Example: SBAR Use in Pediatric Maxillofacial Trauma Scenario
Meera, an 8-year-old girl, was struck in the face by a cricket bat during a playground game. She presents with facial swelling, oral bleeding, and difficulty speaking.

- *Situation:*
  "Dr. Sharma, I need to discuss an urgent pediatric trauma case. Meera, aged 8, was hit on the face with a cricket bat. She has swelling, bleeding from the mouth, and is unable to speak clearly."
- *Background:*
  "She was playing when accidentally hit. There's no known history of medical issues. On arrival, we noted swelling over the left cheek, bleeding from the oral cavity, and limited mouth opening. Her vitals: RR 24 per min, SpO_2 94%, HR 112 bpm, BP 90/60 mmHg."
- *Assessment:*
  "I suspect a significant maxillofacial injury, possibly a fracture, given the impact, swelling, and difficulty in speaking. Airway compromise is a potential concern."
- *Recommendation:*
  "I recommend urgent evaluation by maxillofacial surgery. Meanwhile, we are maintaining airway precautions, initiating bleeding control, giving analgesia, and preparing for a CT scan if available."

Using SBAR in this context ensures critical details are communicated swiftly and accurately—helping the team respond with the right urgency. PCPs are encouraged to practice and adopt SBAR for referrals, handovers, and in emergencies involving pediatric trauma, especially in settings where escalation pathways must be precise and timely.

Patient and Family Education

Understanding the Injury

- *Head trauma:* Injury to brain and skull or bleeding in the brain
- *Maxillofacial trauma:* Injury to the face or jaw, such as fractures or soft tissue damage
- *Effects:* May affect consciousness, memory, limb movements, eating, speaking, or breathing

Symptoms to Watch

- Signs of worsening head injury—worsening headache, vomiting multiple episodes, seizures, altered consciousness or activity
- Difficulty speaking or eating: Change in voice, trouble moving the jaw or chewing
- Swelling and pain: Increased swelling or severe pain in the face or jaw
- Bleeding: Persistent bleeding from the mouth or nose
- Signs of infection: Fever, neck pain, redness, or pus near the injury site

Emergency Signs

Get help if:

- Child has seizures, altered consciousness, and above signs of worsening head injury.
- Breathing becomes difficult.
- Bleeding does not stop.
- Visible deformity or worsening swelling.

Activity Restrictions

- Avoid physical strain: No contact sports or activities that could risk further injury.
- Soft diet: Eat soft foods to avoid stressing the jaw.
- Rest: Allow time for healing and avoid overexertion.

Emotional Support

- Talk about concerns: Encourage your child to share how they feel.
- Seek help: Consider counseling or child support groups for coping with the injury.

Rehabilitation Services

- Provide information on accessing physical, occupational, or speech therapy as needed.
- Stress the importance of regular follow-ups with specialists to monitor recovery and address any complications.
- Provide guidance on maintaining a healthy lifestyle to support brain health.

Table 7.3 Essential caregiver education for tracheostomy, feeding tube, and catheter management

Tracheostomy care	*Cleaning and maintenance:* Teach families how to clean the tracheostomy site and change the inner cannula to prevent infections. *Suctioning:* Explain how to suction secretions safely and when it is necessary. *Humidification:* Highlight the importance of humidifying the air to prevent thick secretions. *Emergency preparedness:* Provide instructions on what to do if the tracheostomy tube becomes dislodged or blocked.
Tube feeding	*Feeding procedure:* Demonstrate how to administer feeds through the tube, including proper positioning of the child to avoid aspiration. *Cleaning the tube:* Teach how to flush the feeding tube before and after feeds to maintain patency. *Monitoring:* Advise on recognizing signs of complications, such as tube blockage or dislodgement.
Urinary catheter care	*Hygiene:* Demonstrate how to clean the catheter and surrounding area to prevent urinary tract infections. *Emptying the bag:* Teach how to empty the urine collection bag and measure output if required. *Monitoring:* Explain how to identify signs of infection, such as cloudy urine, foul odor, or fever.
General care and monitoring	*Skin care:* Emphasize the importance of preventing pressure sores by repositioning the child regularly and using cushions or pads. *Signs of infection:* Educate families on recognizing symptoms of infection at any of the sites (tracheostomy, feeding tube, or catheter). *Medication management:* Provide clear instructions on administering prescribed medications.

Patients with Tracheostomy

Educating families about caring for a pediatric head trauma patient being discharged with a tracheostomy, tube feeding, and a urinary catheter is essential for ensuring proper care and preventing complications. Table 7.3 outlines key points to cover.

Case Resolution

As the evening unfolds in the pediatric emergency area of the district hospital, 6-year-old Riyan is wheeled in—semiconscious, blood-soaked, and visibly frightened. You, a trained pediatric triage nurse, quickly initiate the ABCDE assessment, assisted by the CHO while alerting the junior resident in the trauma bay.

Airway is the first priority. Riyan is bleeding from the mouth and nose, and facial distortion is evident. The presence of gurgling sounds and facial swelling raises a red flag for impending airway compromise. Recognizing that children's airways are narrower and more collapsible, you immediately begin gentle suctioning, clearing visible blood and secretions while maintaining spinal motion restriction with manual in-line stabilization. You instruct the CHO to place rolled towels alongside the head and under the shoulders—techniques vital in infants and young children whose large occiput predisposes them to neck flexion in supine positions, potentially worsening obstruction.

Simultaneously, you ensure oxygenation with a face mask, keeping Riyan calm and in a neutral posture. These steps reflect your awareness that soft pediatric tissues, facial swelling, and oral bleeding can obstruct the airway rapidly—requiring constant reassessment and readiness for escalation.

When the junior resident arrives, the team quickly collaborates, confirming your concerns. Given the fall from height and altered mental status, there's significant concern for cervical spine injury, which is common in children due to their larger head-to-body ratio and weak neck musculature. Spinal motion restriction is continued, and preparations are made for potential intubation if Riyan's GCS drops further.

While the doctor evaluates deeper injuries, you continue monitoring Riyan's neurological status, watching for irritability, unequal pupils, or signs of raised ICP. Your documentation includes AVPU response, vitals, bleeding sites, and airway interventions—essential data that will guide referral.

Your actions also demonstrate the importance of the trauma nurse's role—ensuring equipment readiness, clear team communication, and anticipation of clinical needs. You liaise between the family, CHO, and resident, ensuring swift intervention while reassuring Riyan's parents about ongoing steps.

Before referral, you assist the junior resident in completing a thorough transfer note, which includes:

- Mechanism of injury
- Interventions done (airway support, suctioning, spinal precautions)
- Current vital signs and neurological findings
- Need for imaging and higher care

Key Messages

- *Early recognition and systematic assessment save lives*—Use PAT and ABCDE approach for rapid triage and stabilization in pediatric trauma.
- *Children are not small adults*—Their unique anatomical and physiological features demand a tailored approach to head and facial injury management.
- *Spinal motion restriction is crucial*—Always assume cervical spine injury in pediatric head trauma, especially with high-impact mechanisms or altered sensorium.
- *Airway threats can be silent but sudden*—Facial swelling, bleeding, and soft tissues in children can rapidly compromise the airway; suction, positioning, and early escalation are critical.
- *Raised intracranial pressure must be suspected, monitored, and managed*—Look for signs like altered mental status, vomiting, unequal pupils, and bradycardia.
- *Not all injuries are visible*—Maintain high suspicion for internal injury even in mild or subtle presentations, particularly in infants or when abuse is suspected.
- *Primary care providers play a pivotal role*—Timely interventions, documentation, and coordination for referral directly impact outcomes in resource-limited settings.
- *Family support and education matter*—Equip caregivers with information about red flags, home care, rehabilitation, and emotional support for the child.

Bibliography

1. ATLS Student Course Manuel; 10th Edition; 2018 by American College of Surgeons
2. Araki T, Yokota H, Morita A. Pediatric traumatic brain injury: characteristic features, diagnosis, and management. Neurologia medico-chirurgica. 2017;57(2):82–93.
3. Cintean R, Eickhoff A, Zieger J, Gebhard F, Schütze K Epidemiology, patterns, and mechanisms of pediatric trauma: A review of 12,508 patients. Eur J Trauma Emerg Surg 2023;49:451–9.
4. Dewan MC, Mummareddy N, Wellons III JC, Bonfield CM. Epidemiology of global pediatric traumatic brain injury: qualitative review. World neurosurgery. 2016 Jul 1;91:497–509.
5. Khalifa GA, El-Kilani NS, Nasr TA. Clinical outcomes of pediatric maxillofacial fractures management in three hospital series in Egypt. J Oral Maxillofac Surg Med Pathol 2017;29:511–7.
6. Kobe IO, Qureshi MM, Hassan S, Oluoch-Olunya DL. The impact of the introduction of PECARN head CT rules on the utilisation of head CT scans in a private tertiary hospital in Sub-Saharan Africa. Childs Nerv Syst. 2017 Dec 1;33(12):2147–52.
7. Kochanek PM, Tasker RC, Carney N, Totten AM, Adelson PD, Selden NR, Davis-O'Reilly C, Hart EL, Bell MJ, Bratton SL, Grant GA. Guidelines for the management of pediatric severe traumatic brain injury: update of the brain trauma foundation guidelines. Pediatric Critical Care Medicine. 2019 Mar 1;20(3S):S1–82.
8. Kuppermann N, Holmes JF, Dayan PS, Hoyle JD, Atabaki SM, Holubkov R, et al. Identification of children at very low risk of clinically-important brain injuries after head trauma: a prospective cohort study. Lancet. 2009 Oct 3;374(9696):1160–70.
9. Kumar R, Mahapatra AK. The changing "epidemiology" of pediatric head injury and its impact on the daily clinical practice. Child's nervous system. 2009 Jul;25:813–23.

10. Kundal VK, Debnath PR, Sen A Epidemiology of pediatric trauma and its pattern in Urban India: A tertiary care hospital-based experience. J Indian Assoc Pediatr Surg 2017;22:33–7.
11. Lui A, Kumar KK, Grant GA. Management of severe traumatic brain injury in pediatric patients. Frontiers in toxicology. 2022 Jun 24;4:910972.
12. Macwan CS, Deshpande AN Unfolding the hidden facts of paediatric maxillofacial trauma. J Clin Diagn Res 2014;8:E01–2.
13. Mukhopadhyay S, Galui S, Biswas R, Saha S, Sarkar S Oral and maxillofacial injuries in children: A retrospective study. J Korean Assoc Oral Maxillofac Surg 2020;46:183–90.
14. Neha Thakur, Samir Misra. Pediatric Trauma Resuscitation Module (PTRM). First edition. New Delhi: Jaypee Brothers Medical Publishers (P) Ltd; 2024. p. 23–39
15. Okoje VN, Alonge TO, Oluteye OA, Denloye OO Changing pattern of pediatric maxillofacial injuries at the accident and emergency department of the university teaching hospital, Ibadan – A four-year experience. Prehosp Disaster Med 2010;25:68–71.
16. Serpa RO, Ferguson L, Larson C, Bailard J, Cooke S, Greco T, Prins ML. Pathophysiology of pediatric traumatic brain injury. Frontiers in neurology. 2021 Jul 15;12:69651
17. Sharma M, Lahoti BK, Khandelwal G, Mathur RK, Sharma SS, Laddha A Epidemiological trends of pediatric trauma: A single-center study of 791 patients. J Indian Assoc Pediatr Surg 2011;16:88–92.
18. Sharma M, Pandey S, Kumar P, Singh K, Kumar P, Jha RP Epidemiological and clinico-radiological evaluation of head injury in pediatric population. J Pediatr Neurosci 2020;15:386–92.
19. Singaram M, G SV, Udhayakumar RK. Prevalence, pattern, etiology, and management of maxillofacial trauma in a developing country: a retrospective study. J Korean Assoc Oral Maxillofac Surg 2016;42:174–81.

Pediatric Neck Trauma

8

Rajesh Kumar
and Muhammed Elhady Muhammed Elgasim

Learning Objectives

By the end of this chapter, the reader should be able to:

- Recognize key clinical signs and red flags in pediatric neck trauma that warrant urgent surgical or airway intervention.
- Apply the ABCDE approach to assess and manage pediatric patients with blunt or penetrating neck injuries.
- Interpret imaging and diagnostic findings relevant to vascular, airway, and spinal injury in neck trauma.
- Implement safe practices for foreign body stabilization, airway protection, and hemorrhage control in resource-limited settings.
- Educate patients and families on injury prevention, early warning signs of complications, and discharge safety planning.

R. Kumar
All India Institute of Medical Sciences (AIIMS), Rishikesh, India

M. E. M. Elgasim (✉)
Medical Educator & Emergency Medicine Specialist – Cork University Hospital, Cork, Ireland

N. T. Rai (ed.), *Pediatric Trauma Resuscitation Manual (PTRM) for Primary Care Providers*, https://doi.org/10.1007/978-981-95-4979-5_8

Introduction

Pediatric neck trauma is a relatively rare but potentially life-threatening emergency due to the dense concentration of vital anatomical structures—airway, major blood vessels, esophagus, and spinal cord—within a compact region. Even seemingly minor injuries can rapidly progress to airway compromise, vascular catastrophe, or neurologic deterioration. The pediatric population presents unique challenges, as anatomical and physiological differences—including a proportionally larger head, increased ligamentous laxity, and underdeveloped musculature—make the cervical spine more vulnerable to injury even with low-impact mechanisms.

Common etiologies include motor vehicle collisions, falls, sports-related trauma, and accidental or intentional penetrating injuries. While the incidence is lower compared to adults, the consequences can be more severe in children due to their smaller anatomy and limited physiological reserves. Moreover, younger children may not be able to verbalize their symptoms, making thorough physical examination and a high index of suspicion essential for early diagnosis.

This chapter outlines a systematic, evidence-informed approach to evaluating and managing pediatric neck trauma in acute care settings. Emphasis is placed on primary survey priorities, anatomical zone-based classification, diagnostic modalities, airway and surgical considerations, and the critical role of primary care providers in initial stabilization, ongoing monitoring, and caregiver education. Early intervention can be lifesaving in these high-stakes situations.

Case Scenario

It was an ordinary morning at school when 9-year-old Aarav, an otherwise healthy and active child, tripped while hurrying back to his seat. Unnoticed by teachers, a sharpened No. 2 pencil was protruding upward from a desk corner. Aarav fell forward, and the pencil impaled the left side of his neck, just anterior to the sternocleidomastoid muscle, below the level of the ear. Panic ensued among classmates as teachers rushed to control the situation and call for emergency services.

On EMS arrival, the pencil was still embedded in situ. Aarav was conscious, tearful, and able to speak softly. There was minimal external bleeding, but his neck was visibly swollen. Paramedics carefully stabilized the pencil in place using sterile gauze and tape, avoided unnecessary manipulation, applied a cervical collar, and administered oxygen via nasal prongs.

Reflective Questions

1. What are the most common causes of penetrating neck trauma in children, and how do mechanisms differ from adult injuries?
2. In a case like Aarav's, what is the importance of leaving a penetrating object in place during transport?
3. How does one prioritize airway protection and cervical spine precautions simultaneously in such injuries?

4. Which anatomical zone has likely been injured, and what implications does this have for imaging and surgical planning?
5. What signs should raise immediate concern for vascular or aerodigestive involvement?
6. How can primary care providers prepare for such emergencies in school or rural settings?

Anatomy of the Neck

The neck is a highly complex region containing vital structures responsible for circulation, respiration, digestion, and neurological function. Due to its compact and flexible nature, injuries to this area can be life-threatening and require a systematic approach to assessment and management.

1. *Anatomical Zones of the Neck*

The neck is a compact and vulnerable anatomical region that contains numerous vital structures, including major blood vessels, the airway, the spinal cord, and critical nerves. In pediatric trauma, neck injuries—though less frequent—can be life-threatening due to the close proximity of these structures within a small space. The evaluation and management of neck trauma require a systematic approach that considers both external signs and internal anatomical relationships.

For clinical and surgical decision-making, the neck is divided into three anatomical zones. These zones help guide the urgency of intervention, imaging, and surgical accessibility when managing penetrating or blunt injuries. Table 8.1 outlines the three anatomical zones of the neck, their boundaries, key structures, and clinical implications. Recognizing the zone involved is critical for primary care providers and trauma teams to prioritize airway security, hemorrhage control, and safe referral decisions.

Table 8.1 Anatomical zones of the neck

Zone	Location	Key structures	Clinical significance
Zone I (lower neck)	From the clavicles to the cricoid cartilage	Subclavian and carotid arteries, jugular and subclavian veins, lung apices, trachea, esophagus, thyroid gland, thoracic duct	High risk of major bleeding and respiratory distress; surgical access is difficult due to the sternum and clavicles
Zone II (mid-neck)	From the cricoid cartilage to the angle of the mandible	Carotid and vertebral arteries, jugular veins, trachea, esophagus, larynx, thyroid, cranial nerves IX–XII	Most common site of penetrating trauma; surgical access is more feasible but urgent intervention may be required
Zone III (upper neck)	From the angle of the mandible to the base of the skull	Distal carotid arteries, vertebral arteries, cranial nerves, cervical sympathetic trunk	Injuries are difficult to access surgically; risk of cerebral ischemia due to vascular injury

2. *Triangular Regions of the Neck*
   The neck is also divided into two key regions for further assessment:
   - *Anterior triangle:* Houses critical structures including the trachea, larynx, carotid arteries, jugular veins, and thyroid gland. Injuries here pose significant airway and vascular threats.
   - *Posterior triangle:* Contains the spinal accessory nerve, cervical plexus, and subclavian vessels. Trauma in this region is less likely to involve life-threatening structures.

3. *Physiological Functions and Trauma Implications*
   - *Vascular system:* The carotid and vertebral arteries supply blood to the brain, while the jugular veins return blood to the heart. Injury can lead to severe hemorrhage, stroke, or shock.
   - *Respiratory system:* The trachea and larynx regulate airflow to the lungs. Trauma may cause airway obstruction, subcutaneous emphysema, or tracheal deviation.
   - *Digestive system:* The esophagus is responsible for swallowing. Injuries can lead to perforation, mediastinitis, or difficulty swallowing (dysphagia).
   - *Neurological system:* Cranial and cervical nerves control sensory and motor functions, and damage to them can potentially result in voice changes, swallowing difficulties, or loss of neck movement.

Initial Assessment and Primary Survey in Neck Trauma

The evaluation of a patient with neck trauma should begin with a systematic primary survey (ABCDE). Each life-threatening issue should be managed before proceeding to the next step. Importantly, cervical spine stabilization is integral to airway management (A) and is further assessed during the neurological examination (D) and secondary survey.

Primary Survey (ABCDE Approach)

A: Airway management with cervical spine protection—Securing the airway is critical, particularly in suspected laryngotracheal injuries. However, spinal alignment for immobilization should not be forced if it causes discomfort or pain.

B: Breathing and ventilation—Evaluate respiratory function and provide necessary support.

C: Circulation with hemorrhage control—Active bleeding should be controlled using direct pressure rather than blind clamping of vessels.

D: Disability (neurological evaluation)—Assess the patient's neurological status to detect deficits.

E: Exposure and environmental control—Fully expose the patient while preventing hypothermia.

History Taking in Pediatric Neck Trauma

A focused history should be obtained whenever possible, either from the child or a caregiver. The AMPLE mnemonic provides a structured approach:

A—Allergies
M—Medications
P—Past medical history
L—Last meal
E—Events and environmental factors related to the injury

Physical Examination in Pediatric Neck Trauma

Pediatric cervical spine injuries differ from adults due to anatomical and physiological variations, including:

- A proportionally larger head, leading to greater flexion and extension forces
- Weaker paraspinal muscles
- Increased ligamentous laxity, making the spine more flexible
- The immature vertebral column, which can elongate without rupture in infants
- Incomplete development of uncovertebral (uncinated) processes until around 10 years of age
- Since children may not reliably report symptoms, all pediatric trauma patients should be presumed to have cervical spine injuries until proven otherwise. Most children arrive at the emergency department with prehospital cervical spine immobilization, which should be maintained until a spinal injury is definitively ruled out.
- If a cervical collar is too large for a small child, sandbags and tape can be used as an alternative to immobilization.
- While stabilizing the cervical spine with the assistance of another provider, conduct a midline palpation to check for deformities or tenderness.
- Perform a comprehensive motor and sensory evaluation. Isolated sensory complaints are more common in children. Many children may be asymptomatic or uncooperative, making a detailed examination challenging. In such cases, input from family members or child life specialists can be valuable.

It is important to note that *decision rules like NEXUS and Canadian C-Spine should be used cautiously in pediatric cases* as children were underrepresented in the original study populations.

Neck trauma is generally classified into blunt and penetrating injuries, both of which can lead to life-threatening complications:

1. *Blunt trauma*—Can result in laryngeal fractures, tracheal disruption, expanding hematomas, or esophageal injuries
2. *Penetrating trauma* May cause damage to major blood vessels, the pharynx, larynx, trachea, or esophagus

Penetrating Neck Trauma

Penetrating neck injuries carry a high risk of severe damage due to the concentration of vital structures in a confined space. Any wound that breaches the platysma muscle is at significant risk of affecting deeper tissues and requires thorough evaluation.

Before assessing the specific presentations of such trauma, PCPs must recognize key physical exam indicators of severe injury (Table 8.2). Patients exhibiting hard signs should promptly be taken to the operating room for definitive surgical management.

Traditionally, penetrating neck trauma is classified into three zones to guide diagnostic and treatment strategies.

- *Zone III:* Located above the angle of the mandible. Recommended evaluation includes angiography.
- *Zone II* extends from the angle of the mandible to the cricoid cartilage. Management may involve surgical exploration, observation, Doppler ultrasound, or CT angiography (CTA).
- *Zone I* has the highest mortality rate, situated below the cricoid cartilage. Diagnosis involves angiography, esophagogastroduodenoscopy (EGD), and esophagoscopy (Fig. 8.1).

Table 8.2 Hard and soft signs of neck trauma

Type of sign	Clinical signs
Hard signs	Airway obstruction or compromise
	Rapidly expanding or pulsating hematoma
	Active, profuse bleeding
	Hemorrhagic shock
	Vomiting blood (hematemesis)
	Neurological impairment
	Extensive subcutaneous emphysema
	Air visibly or audibly escaping through the wound
Soft signs	Coughing up blood (hemoptysis)
	Presence of blood in the oropharynx
	Difficulty breathing (dyspnea)
	Trouble swallowing (dysphagia)
	Changes in voice (dysphonia)
	Stable, non-expanding hematoma
	Persistent air leak from a chest tube
	Air in subcutaneous or mediastinal tissues (crepitus, subcutaneous emphysema)
	Audible vascular sounds (bruits) or palpable thrills
	Palpable crackling sensation (subcutaneous crepitus)

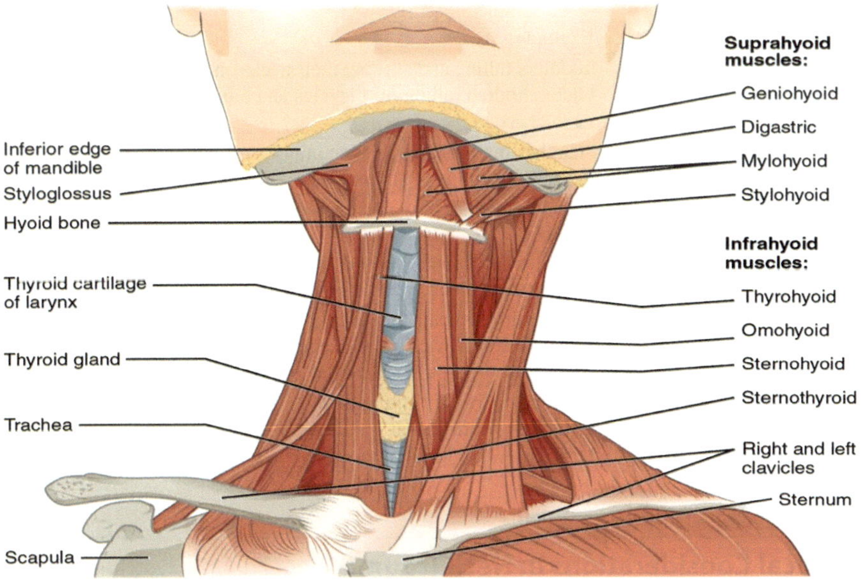

Fig. 8.1 Anatomical zones of the neck. (Image Source: OpenStax. (2016, May 18). 1110 Muscle of the Anterior Neck [Illustration]. Wikimedia Commons. https://commons.wikimedia.org/wiki/File:1110_Muscle_of_the_Anterior_Neck.jpg)

Blunt Neck Trauma

History and Mechanism of Injury

Blunt trauma to the neck can result from a direct impact or a significant force applied to the head or face (Table 8.3). Determining the exact nature of the injury and the affected regions can be challenging, especially if the event was not witnessed or if the patient has multiple traumatic injuries. These injuries may cause serious complications, including airway obstruction due to laryngeal damage, vascular injuries leading to stroke, and neurological impairment affecting the brachial plexus or spinal cord.

Table 8.3 Mechanism of blunt neck trauma

Mechanism of injury	Examples
Falls	Toddlers falling and striking their necks on the edge of a low table Older children falling off bicycles and hitting their necks on the handlebars
Motorbike injuries	"Clothesline" (garroting) type injuries from wires, ropes, or barriers encountered at speed
Motor vehicle accidents (MVAs)	Rapid deceleration of a restrained passenger with a seatbelt across the neck Unrestrained passengers striking their necks against the dashboard Hyperextension or hyperflexion injuries from sudden impact
Sports injuries	It's the direct impact on the neck from a cricket or baseball. Elbow or forearm strikes to the neck during football or basketball Blunt force trauma from martial arts strikes
Strangulation/assault	Hanging or ligature strangulation Choking or suffocation Direct blows or kicks to the neck

Clinical Considerations in Neck Trauma

Neck trauma, particularly in the pediatric population, presents a unique set of diagnostic and management challenges. The neck is a compact region rich in critical anatomical structures—including the airway, major blood vessels, spinal cord, and numerous nerves—making even minor injuries potentially life-threatening. Clinical assessment in such cases requires a high index of suspicion, especially as early symptoms may be deceptively subtle. Children may not articulate symptoms clearly, and signs such as hoarseness, mild swelling, or vague discomfort can precede catastrophic events like airway obstruction or vascular collapse.

Airway compromise in neck trauma can stem from a variety of mechanisms. Direct injury to the larynx, trachea, or pharynx may cause mechanical obstruction, while expanding hematomas, soft tissue edema, or disruption of structural integrity can progressively narrow the airway. Additionally, blunt or penetrating injuries may injure the recurrent laryngeal nerve, impairing vocal cord function and further complicating airway management. These pathologies may evolve rapidly, underscoring the need for frequent reassessment and early intervention.

Initial examination findings may be deceptively benign, particularly in zone II injuries, which are more accessible and often present with less dramatic symptoms. Therefore, careful and continuous monitoring is essential. Any change in voice, difficulty swallowing, dyspnea, stridor, or subcutaneous emphysema should prompt urgent evaluation and escalation of care.

Meticulous documentation of clinical findings—including mechanism of injury, initial vital signs, airway and neurological status, and physical examination details—is critical. This not only serves as a medicolegal record but also enables PCPs to detect clinical deterioration over time. In resource-limited settings, where imaging or specialist support may be delayed, serial examinations and vigilant clinical observation are indispensable tools in guiding safe and timely referral decisions.

Diagnostic Testing for Neck Trauma

Prompt and focused diagnostic testing is essential in pediatric neck trauma due to the close proximity of vital airway, vascular, and neurological structures. Clinical signs may be subtle or delayed, necessitating a high index of suspicion. Diagnostic tools—including imaging, endoscopy, and laboratory panels—aid in confirming injury extent and guiding interventions. The choice of tests depends on clinical presentation and suspected injury type. In cases of airway compromise or hemodynamic instability, definitive airway management and surgical intervention may take precedence over diagnostics. Table 8.4 summarizes key diagnostic approaches and their considerations in evaluating neck trauma in children.

Table 8.4 Diagnostic testing for neck trauma

Category	Diagnostic approach	Key considerations
Laboratory tests	The trauma panel includes CBC, chemistry panel, PT/INR, type and screen, and VBG/ABG.	Helpful in assessing the overall condition but not diagnostic for laryngotracheal trauma
Laryngeal injury	*Imaging:* CT (gold standard), CT angiography if vascular injury suspected	Provides detailed visualization of structures
	Laryngoscopy: Fiber-optic laryngoscopy for supraglottic and glottis evaluation	Limited in assessing the subglottic region. Best performed with the patient upright
	Airway considerations: Monitor for airway obstruction due to progressive swelling.	Patients with unstable or impending airway compromise should not undergo CT imaging.
Cervical spine injury	Imaging is required if any of the following are present: Focal neurological deficits Midline C-spine tenderness Altered mental status Intoxication Distracting injury	Ensures spinal injuries are promptly identified and managed
Esophageal injury	Endoscopy	Best diagnostic tool for detecting esophageal trauma
Vascular injury	*Angiography* indicated if: Active bleeding Pulse deficit GI bleeding Hoarseness Subcutaneous air Respiratory distress	Identifies vascular damage and guides further management
Surgical exploration	Can be both diagnostic and therapeutic for suspected laryngeal, esophageal, or vascular injuries	Consider when imaging is inconclusive or immediate intervention is needed

Acute Management of Neck Trauma

Airway Assessment and Stabilization

In pediatric neck trauma, airway assessment is the foremost priority. Evaluate for signs of obstruction—stridor, hoarseness, gurgling, or silence—indicating compromised airflow.

If the airway is stable:

Evaluate for aerodigestive tract injuries. Red flag symptoms include stridor, dyspnea, hoarseness, or dysphonia. ENT consultation with flexible fiber-optic laryngoscopy may be required.

- Consider vascular injury in high-mechanism trauma. If suspected, arrange a CT angiogram in coordination with radiology and vascular surgery.

If the airway is unstable:

- Initiate basic airway maneuvers such as jaw thrust.
- Deliver 100% oxygen via a high-flow non-rebreather mask.
- Provide gentle bag-mask ventilation if needed, avoiding excessive pressure to prevent air tracking and worsening emphysema.
- Seek immediate senior help for definitive airway management.

Airway Considerations in Altered Consciousness or Suspected Laryngeal Injury

- All intubations in neck trauma should be treated as potentially difficult airways. Early involvement of anesthesia and ENT is advised.
- In patients with suspected laryngeal injury, avoid paralytics to prevent complete airway obstruction. Prefer awake fiber-optic intubation or rigid bronchoscopy in theater.
- If emergency intubation is necessary (e.g., peri-arrest due to hypoxia):
  - Use a smaller-than-usual endotracheal tube.
  - Avoid forceful attempts that may worsen partial tracheal injuries.
  - Have a surgical airway kit ready for cricothyrotomy or tracheostomy.
  - Use video laryngoscopy if available.
  - Maintain cervical spine alignment throughout.

Fluid Resuscitation and Initial Stabilization

- Use warmed balanced crystalloids (e.g., Ringer's lactate) for initial fluid resuscitation.
- If indicated, administer blood products or clotting factors for hemorrhagic shock.
- Continuously assess neurological status, considering spinal cord or cerebral vascular injury.
- After stabilization, proceed to injury-specific imaging and determine if surgical intervention is necessary.

Surgical Management by Neck Zone

- Immediate surgical exploration is required for patients with active bleeding or hemodynamic instability.
- Zone I and zone III injuries are technically more challenging due to difficulty in vascular access:
  - Zone I: Proximal control is difficult.
  - Zone III: Distal vascular control is limited.

These factors contribute to higher mortality in vascular injuries in these zones.

For blunt neck trauma, subtle signs like voice changes, neck swelling, or pain with swallowing may mask life-threatening injuries such as laryngotracheal disruption or vascular dissection. In contrast, penetrating trauma—especially injuries violating the platysma muscle—requires careful assessment of anatomical zones, presence of "hard signs," and need for urgent surgical exploration.

The following management algorithms provide a step-by-step framework for both blunt and penetrating pediatric neck trauma (Figs. 8.2 and 8.3). They help standardize care across varied clinical settings—from primary stabilization by PCPs to advanced trauma center management—ensuring timely diagnosis, safe intervention, and improved outcomes.

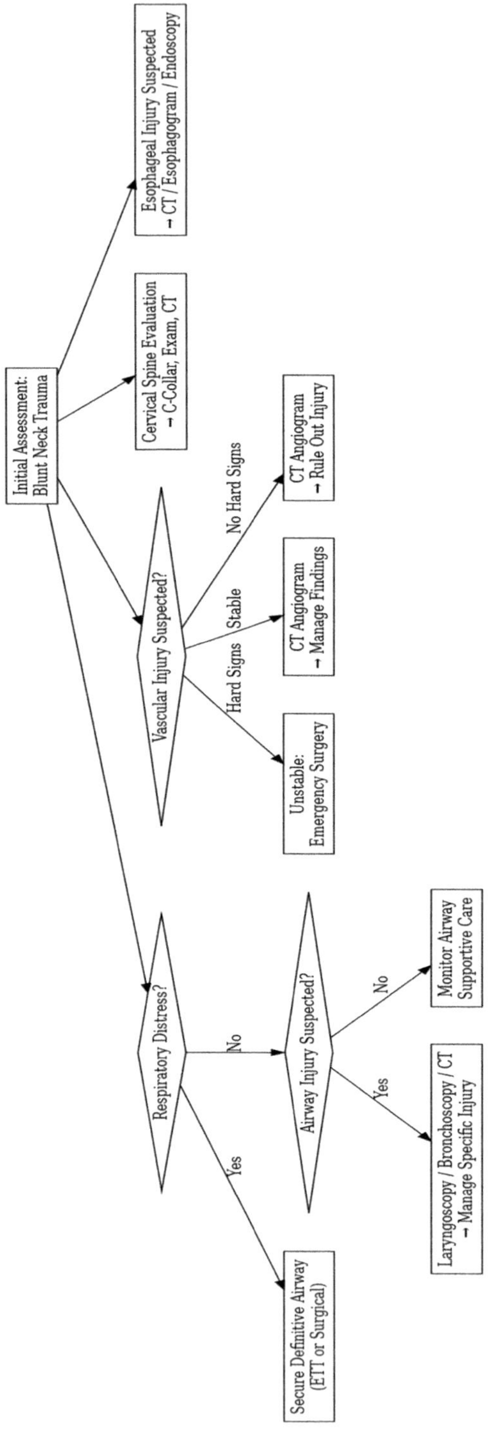

Fig. 8.2 Algorithm for management of blunt neck trauma

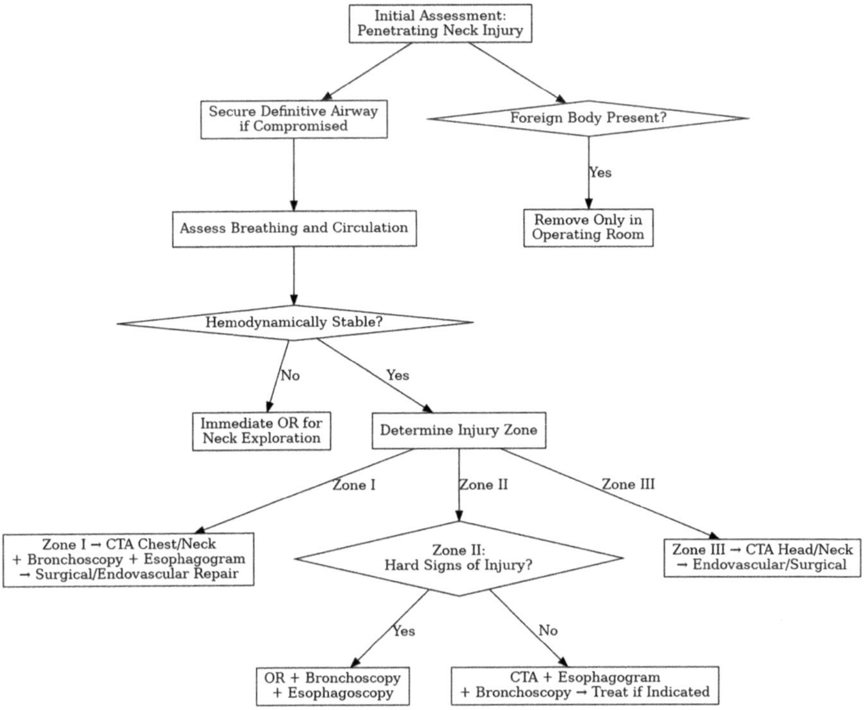

Fig. 8.3 Algorithm for management of penetrating neck trauma

PCPs Role in Pediatric Neck Trauma

PCPs are essential in the assessment, stabilization, and continuing care of pediatric trauma patients.

1. *Initial Assessment and Airway Support*
    - Use the ABCDE approach.
    - Monitor for airway compromise (stridor, hoarseness, dyspnea).
    - Maintain cervical spine precautions.
    - Assist with oxygen therapy and preparation for intubation or surgical airway.
2. *Circulatory Support*
    - Establish IV access and administer fluids or blood products as prescribed.
    - Monitor for signs of shock such as tachycardia, hypotension, or pallor.
3. *Pain Management*
    - Use age-appropriate pain scales.
    - Administer analgesics and provide comfort measures.
4. *Neurological Observation*
    - Conduct frequent assessments using GCS, pupil checks, and limb movement.
    - Monitor for signs of spinal cord injury such as numbness or weakness.

5. *Diagnostic Support*
   - Assist with imaging studies while maintaining cervical precautions.
   - Support procedures such as laryngoscopy or bronchoscopy.
   - Collect and label blood samples as ordered.
6. *Preventing Complications*
   - Monitor for hematoma expansion or airway swelling.
   - Ensure emergency airway equipment is immediately available.
   - Maintain NPO status if esophageal injury is suspected.
7. *Family Support and Communication*
   - Provide clear explanations to parents and caregivers.
   - Offer emotional support and include families in care when appropriate.
8. *Multidisciplinary Coordination*
   - Communicate effectively with ENT, trauma, anesthesia, and radiology teams.
   - Participate in handovers and ensure thorough documentation.
9. *Discharge Education*
   - Instruct families on signs of delayed complications such as breathing difficulty or neurological changes.
   - Provide wound care advice and follow-up instructions.
   - Emphasize injury prevention strategies such as supervision and safety equipment.

Case Resolution

Prehospital Interventions On EMS arrival, Aarav was conscious, oriented, and hemodynamically stable—indicating that no immediate compromise of the airway, major vessels, or neurological pathways had occurred. The pencil was visibly embedded in zone III of the neck, a region notorious for its surgical inaccessibility and proximity to major vascular structures such as the distal carotid artery and cranial nerves.

Recognizing the dangers of premature object removal, the EMS team appropriately stabilized the foreign body in situ using gauze and tape, avoiding manipulation that could precipitate hemorrhage. This step aligns with best practice: Never remove an impaled object outside the operating theater unless it's compromising the airway or CPR is needed. Oxygen was administered, and cervical spine precautions were initiated—a vital step since spinal injuries should be presumed until ruled out.

Emergency Department Assessment On arrival to the trauma bay, Aarav remained stable with GCS 15 and normal vital parameters. Physical examination confirmed no signs of airway compromise (stridor, hoarseness), voice change, or dysphagia—suggesting that major aerodigestive structures were spared. The trauma team correctly applied the ABCDE approach and maintained strict cervical spine immobilization while continuing to monitor for delayed airway compromise.

Imaging and Intervention A contrast-enhanced CT scan of the neck was performed, revealing the pencil tip abutting the external carotid artery, yet without causing a tear or thrombosis—highlighting the value of CT angiography in zone III penetrating injuries. Given the foreign body's location and proximity to critical vessels, surgical removal was indicated.

Aarav was taken to the operating theater under general anesthesia for controlled removal of the pencil. The surgical team exercised caution to avoid vessel injury during extraction. The wound was irrigated, examined, and closed. No neurovascular compromise was identified—confirming a fortunate trajectory that spared vital structures.

Postoperative Course The child recovered uneventfully in the pediatric HDU and was monitored for signs of delayed complications such as hematoma formation or infection. He was discharged after 48 hours with follow-up arranged with ENT. His caregivers were counseled on red flag symptoms (e.g., dysphagia, voice change, fever), wound care, and injury prevention strategies, including safe classroom environments and supervision.

Key Messages

- Pediatric neck trauma is rare but high risk due to the density of critical structures in a small anatomical space.
- Always suspect cervical spine injury in pediatric trauma patients until cleared, even in minor mechanisms.
- Use the ABCDE framework consistently during initial assessment; airway obstruction is the leading cause of mortality.
- Penetrating injuries that violate the platysma warrant detailed evaluation; hard signs like airway compromise or pulsatile bleeding require immediate surgery.
- Blunt neck trauma can be subtle and must not be underestimated. Watch for expanding hematomas and dysphonia.
- Avoid blind removal of penetrating objects; stabilize in situ and refer for controlled surgical removal.
- Zone-based approach (I, II, III) guides imaging and surgical strategy—zone II injuries are most common and accessible.
- PCPs play a vital role in airway protection, monitoring for decompensation, and preparing for a surgical airway if needed.
- Include caregivers in care by offering clear explanations and anticipatory guidance on discharge risks.
- Prevention is key—educate on school safety, supervision, and avoiding sharp objects in unsupervised environments.

Bibliography

1. Alao T, Waseem M. Neck Trauma. Stat Pearls [Internet]. 2025. [PMID: 29261998]
2. American College of Surgeons. **Advanced trauma life support (ATLS®): Student course manual**. 10th ed. Chicago: American College of Surgeons; 2018
3. American Heart Association. **Basic life support: Provider manual**. Dallas (TX): American Heart Association; 2020.
4. Fox SM. Pediatric Penetrating Neck Injury. Pediatric EM Morsels. 2018.
5. OpenStax. (2016, May 18). 1110 Muscle of the Anterior Neck [Illustration]. Wikimedia Commons. https://commons.wikimedia.org/wiki/File:1110_Muscle_of_the_Anterior_Neck.jpg
6. Sperry JL, et al. Western Trauma Association: Penetrating Neck Trauma. J Trauma Acute Care Surg. 2013;75(6):936–940.
7. Royal Children's Hospital Trauma Service. Blunt and penetrating neck trauma. Accessed 2024.
8. Stone ME Jr., et al. Penetrating neck trauma in children: A National Trauma Data Bank study. J Trauma Acute Care Surg. 2016;80(4):604–9.

9 Pediatric Thoracic Trauma

Poonam Joshi
and Muhammed Elhady Muhammed Elgasim

Learning Objectives

By the end of this chapter, the reader should be able to:

- Outline the priorities in the initial management of pediatric thoracic trauma, including rapid assessment using the Pediatric Assessment Triangle (PAT) and ABCDE approach; stabilization of airway, breathing, and circulation; and timely initiation of supportive care measures.
- Recognize the clinical presentation and key warning signs of life-threatening thoracic injuries in children, such as tension pneumothorax, open pneumothorax, and massive hemothorax, and understand their implications for immediate intervention.
- Describe the procedural steps and safety considerations for chest tube insertion in pediatric patients, including indications, equipment preparation, anatomical landmarks, aseptic technique, and post-insertion care.
- Communicate effectively with patients and caregivers about thoracic trauma, providing education on the nature of the injury, warning signs for deterioration, pain management strategies, activity precautions, and the importance of follow-up care and emotional support.

P. Joshi
AIIMS Kalyani, Kalyani, West Bengal, India
e-mail: poonam.nursing@aiimskalyani.edu.in

M. E. M. Elgasim (✉)
Cork University Hospital, Cork, Ireland

N. T. Rai (ed.), *Pediatric Trauma Resuscitation Manual (PTRM) for Primary Care Providers*, https://doi.org/10.1007/978-981-95-4979-5_9

Introduction

Pediatric thoracic trauma, though relatively uncommon compared to adult populations, presents a significant risk of morbidity and mortality when it does occur. Accounting for approximately 5–12% of pediatric trauma cases, these injuries are often the result of high-impact events such as motor vehicle collisions, falls from height, or bicycle-related accidents. Unlike adults, children have a more pliable chest wall due to increased rib cage elasticity. As a result, significant internal injuries such as pulmonary contusions, pneumothorax, or hemothorax may occur without obvious external signs like rib fractures, making timely recognition more challenging.

Blunt trauma is the predominant mechanism in pediatric chest injuries, constituting nearly 90–95% of cases, with road traffic accidents being the leading cause in India. Penetrating injuries, including stab or firearm wounds, are far less common in this age group but can be rapidly fatal due to smaller body size and proximity of vital structures. The presence of associated injuries—particularly to the head, abdomen, or spine—is frequent in children and complicates overall management. Nearly all children with thoracic trauma exhibit some form of multisystem involvement, emphasizing the importance of a holistic and coordinated approach to care.

Early identification and management of life-threatening injuries such as tension pneumothorax, massive hemothorax, and cardiac tamponade are crucial. The unique anatomical and physiological features of children demand careful clinical assessment, appropriate imaging, and timely interventions tailored to pediatric needs.

Primary care providers (PCPs) play a pivotal role in the acute management of pediatric thoracic trauma—especially in resource-limited or rural settings where specialized care may be delayed. Their responsibilities span from initial assessment and stabilization to assisting with lifesaving procedures and effectively communicating with the trauma team and families. This chapter equips PCPs with the practical knowledge needed to identify, manage, and refer thoracic trauma in children efficiently and safely.

Case Scenario

You are the attending PCP at a community hospital emergency unit with limited specialist support when a 14-year-old boy named Rakesh is brought in by local bystanders. A taxi driver witnessed him lying on the side of a busy road next to a fallen motor scooter, implying a possible road traffic accident.

Rakesh is conscious but visibly anxious and struggling to breathe. He is clutching his left chest, where his shirt is torn and reveals abrasions and soiling with road debris. He was initially resisting help but now lies supine, appearing increasingly pale and lethargic.

You begin your assessment:

- Airway: Patent
- Breathing: RR 48 per min, shallow with visible distress
- Circulation: HR 135 bpm, BP 110/70 mmHg, CRT 3 s, cold extremities
- SpO_2: 91% on oxygen via face mask

Given the signs of tachypnea, chest pain, and hypoxia, you suspect a significant thoracic injury like a pneumothorax or pulmonary contusion. The nearest tertiary trauma center is 90 min away.

Reflective Questions

1. What signs in this case suggest a potentially life-threatening thoracic injury?
2. How should the Pediatric Assessment Triangle (PAT) and ABCDE framework guide your initial evaluation?
3. As a PCP, what are your immediate priorities in managing Rakesh's condition while awaiting definitive care?
4. What basic investigations (e.g., chest X-ray or ultrasound) can you request, and how will the results influence next steps?
5. What is your role in assisting or preparing for chest decompression or intercostal drain insertion in a resource-limited setting?

Anatomical Considerations

- Children's ribs' increased elasticity affects chest wall compliance, which differs from that of adults. This increases chest wall flexibility before rib fractures. Thus, severe internal injuries can occur without chest wall damage.
- Due to their higher cardiopulmonary reserve, children can compensate for low blood volume and difficulty breathing.
- Decreased blood pressure in children indicates imminent death. The mediastinum's mobility reduces airway and blood vessel damage. However, the mediastinum shift may cause rapid respiratory and circulatory impairments.
- Children often experience aerophagia and reflex ileus after injury. This can cause acute gastric distension and respiratory impairment. Orogastric or nasogastric placement is advised. We advise orogastric placement when a head injury is suspected.
- Knowledge of the key structures assists in identifying injuries.

Mechanisms of Injury

Understanding the mechanisms by which thoracic trauma occurs in children is critical to anticipating internal injuries, directing focused assessments, and planning appropriate interventions. In India, the leading cause of pediatric chest trauma continues to be road traffic accidents (RTAs). These include scenarios where children are unrestrained passengers in motor vehicles, pedestrians struck by vehicles, or riders of two-wheelers without adequate protection. High-speed impact or lack of seat belts and helmets often results in a combination of blunt thoracic injuries and multisystem trauma.

Falls, whether from bicycles, stairs, rooftops, or trees, represent another common mechanism. The risk of thoracic injury increases with height and landing position. Younger children, due to their relatively larger head size and immature protective reflexes, often land headfirst or chest-first, making them vulnerable to lung contusions, rib fractures, or even flail chest in high-impact falls.

Penetrating injuries, though less common in the pediatric population, still occur in both rural and urban settings. These may result from accidental stab wounds during play with sharp objects or, in more concerning scenarios, from violent encounters involving knives or even firearms. These injuries are often severe and can involve vital structures such as the lungs, heart, or great vessels, requiring rapid identification and surgical intervention.

Lastly, healthcare providers must maintain a high index of suspicion for non-accidental trauma, particularly in younger children. Child abuse may present with inconsistent injury history, delayed presentation, or patterns of injury not aligned with the reported mechanism. Thoracic injuries in these contexts may result from blunt force to the chest or compression injuries and often coexist with injuries in other body regions.

Each of these mechanisms carries unique implications for injury patterns, and a thorough understanding helps PCPs anticipate complications and mobilize timely care.

Life-Threatening Thoracic Injuries

During the primary survey, it is essential to identify and manage the following thoracic injuries:

1. *Tension pneumothorax*:

   This immediately life-threatening injury occurs when air accumulates in the pleural space, compressing the lung on the affected side. The gradual accumulation of air causes the mediastinum to move and compress the lung on the opposite side. This condition leads to a decrease in blood flow returning to the heart and a decrease in heart function.
2. *Open pneumothorax*:

   This injury is caused by penetrating wounds in the chest. It occurs when the wound exceeds two-thirds of the trachea's diameter. When the wound reaches this size or larger, the chest's movement during inspiration creates negative pressure, causing air to enter the pleural space through the wound instead of the upper airway. A tension pneumothorax will develop if the air does not escape during expiration.

3. *Massive hemothorax*:
   This is a rare injury among pediatric patients. A rapid, large-volume accumulation of blood in the pleural space can happen because of a blunt or penetrating injury, such as a cardiac or significant vessel injury. Each hemithorax can waste 40% of blood volume.
4. *Flail chest*:
   This is the result of a blunt injury. It is less common in children than adults because the pediatric rib cage has greater elastic properties, allowing for more plastic deformation upon impact without causing broken ribs. However, the underlying lung tissue is still susceptible to contusion. When two or more adjacent ribs fracture, it disrupts the bony continuity of the thoracic wall, resulting in a flail chest.
5. *Pulmonary contusion*:
   The most common thoracic injury in children is often associated with other injuries, such as fractures and hemothorax. It may occur even without an apparent chest wall injury. Hemorrhage and edema are usually present within the affected lung segment.
6. *Cardiac tamponade*:
   Bleeding into the pericardium can occur as a result of a blunt or penetrating injury. In the case of a myocardial contusion, the blood may come from a cardiac chamber, a great vessel, or the myocardium. This condition causes the heart to fill out less, reducing stroke volume and shock.

Management of Pediatric Thoracic Trauma

Initial Assessment

The initial assessment of a child with chest injuries involves two main steps: the Pediatric Assessment Triangle (PAT) and the primary survey (ABCDE). These steps help identify and manage life-threatening conditions quickly.

Pediatric Assessment Triangle (PAT)

The PAT is a quick way to assess the severity of a child's condition. It looks at three things:

1. *Appearance*: Check if the child is alert, responsive, and interacting normally. Look for signs of distress, such as crying or lethargy.
2. *Work of breathing*: Observe how hard the child is working to breathe. Look for fast or slow breathing, use of accessory muscles, and abnormal sounds like wheezing or grunting.
3. *Circulation to skin*: Check the skin color and temperature. Look for signs of poor blood flow, such as pallor (pale skin), mottling, or cyanosis (blue skin).

Primary Survey (ABCDE)

The primary survey is a more detailed assessment focusing on identifying and managing life-threatening conditions. The ABCDE approach stands for Airway, Breathing, Circulation, Disability, and Exposure.

1. *Airway (A)*: Ensure the airway is open and transparent. Look for signs of obstruction, such as choking, stridor (high-pitched breathing sound), or gurgling.
2. *Breathing (B)*: Check the child's breathing. Look for rate, rhythm, depth, and effort. Listen for abnormal sounds and check oxygen saturation.
3. *Circulation (C)*: Assess circulation by checking the pulse, heart rate, blood pressure, capillary refill time, and skin condition. Look for signs of shock, such as rapid heart rate, weak pulse, or low blood pressure.
4. *Disability (D)*: Evaluate the child's neurological status. Check their level of consciousness using the AVPU scale (Alert, response to Voice, response to Pain, Unresponsive). Assess pupil size and reaction to light. Check the blood glucose level.
5. *Exposure (E)*: Fully expose the child to look for other injuries while preventing hypothermia. Check for signs of trauma, bleeding, and other injuries.

Clinical Features

- *Hypoxia*: Low oxygen levels
- *Severe breathing difficulty*: Struggling to breathe
- *Change in alertness*: Altered level of consciousness or awareness
- *Tracheal/mediastinal shift*: Trachea or center of the chest shifts to the opposite side.
- *Distended neck veins*: Swollen veins in the neck
- *Reduced breath sounds*: Little or no breath sounds on one side of the chest
- *Hyperresonance*: Hollow sound when tapping the chest, indicating air pockets
- *Hypotension*: Low blood pressure due to decreased blood flow to the heart
- *Rapid heartbeat and shock*: Fast heart rate, narrowing blood vessels in the extremities, and low blood pressure leading to shock

Investigations

- *Chest X-ray*: First-line investigation to assess for pneumothorax, hemothorax, rib fractures, etc.
- *Ultrasound (USG)*: This may be used to assess pleural effusion quickly in some settings.
- *CT scan*: For complex cases or suspected vascular injuries (consider radiation exposure risks)

General Management

- *High-flow oxygen*: Provide to maintain adequate oxygen levels.
- *Analgesia*: Administer pain relief as needed.

Specific Interventions

In pediatric thoracic trauma, prompt identification and collaborative intervention between the primary care provider (PCP) and the trauma team are essential. While definitive management often lies with surgical teams, PCPs play a vital role in early recognition, resuscitation, supportive care, and preparation for interventions. Table 9.1 below outlines common life-threatening thoracic injuries, the role of the PCP, and the expected actions from the trauma team.

Special Considerations

- *Resource limitations*: Be prepared to adapt care plans based on available equipment and medications.
- *Nutritional deficiencies*: Malnutrition is common in India and can impair healing. Advocate for proper nutrition.
- *Cultural sensitivities*: Communicate effectively with families, considering their language and beliefs.

Table 9.1 Life-threatening thoracic injuries with roles of PCP and trauma team

Thoracic injury	PCP role	Trauma team role
1. Tension pneumothorax	Administer high-flow oxygen. Provide analgesia. Monitor vitals and signs of deterioration.	Perform immediate finger thoracostomy in 4th/5th intercostal space. Insert intercostal catheter. Needle thoracocentesis if needed (2nd intercostal space, midclavicular line)
2. Open pneumothorax	Provide high-flow oxygen and analgesia Cover minor wounds with an occlusive dressing	Close larger wounds with sutures/staples. Insert intercostal catheter. Can use three-sided dressing as a temporizing measure but do not delay ICD insertion
3. Massive hemothorax	Administer high-flow oxygen and analgesia. Provide ventilatory support if indicated. Assist with rapid volume resuscitation.	Insert chest tube in 4th/5th intercostal space. If bleeding persists, prepare for urgent surgical thoracotomy.
4. Flail chest and pulmonary contusion	Provide aggressive pain relief. Administer high-flow oxygen. Support ventilation. Position patient on injured side.	Initiate positive pressure ventilation/ intubation if needed. Consider rib fixation and chest physiotherapy.
5. Cardiac tamponade	Administer high-flow oxygen. Provide fluid resuscitation to enhance preload. Start ECG monitoring.	Perform open surgical drainage. If surgery is unavailable, consider needle pericardiocentesis (preferably under ultrasound guidance).

Guidance for PCPs: Communicating Effectively with the Trauma Team
Primary care providers are vital members of the trauma response team. Effective communication can prevent errors, improve outcomes, and foster a culture of safety. When concerns arise, PCPs should feel empowered to speak up—*always prioritizing patient safety.*

- *Acknowledge the importance of your observations*—you are often the first to notice clinical changes.
- *Frame communication using the SBAR approach* (Situation, Background, Assessment, Recommendation) for clarity and structure.
- *Be timely*—raise concerns as soon as they arise, without delay.
- *Stay composed and professional*, even during high-stress situations.
- *Use assertive, respectful language*. For example: "I'm concerned that…" or "Could we recheck…?"
- *Engage colleagues or a supervisor* if you are uncertain and need support.
- *Be persistent if necessary*, especially if patient safety is at risk.
- *Ensure concerns are addressed*—follow up after speaking up.
- *Reflect on communication encounters* to identify areas of improvement.
- *Support a safety culture* by encouraging peers and junior staff to voice concerns when needed.

Patient and Family Education: Thoracic Injury in Children
Clear communication with families after a pediatric chest injury is essential. Understanding the injury, recognizing danger signs, and supporting recovery can improve outcomes and reduce anxiety. These simple, clear steps help families feel empowered and involved in the recovery process.

Understanding the Injury:
- A thoracic (chest) injury may involve bruising, rib fractures, lung collapse (pneumothorax), or internal bleeding.
- These injuries can affect breathing and heart function and may not always be obvious from the outside.

Symptoms to Monitor:
- Difficulty breathing or rapid, shallow breaths
- Worsening chest pain
- Blue lips or fingertips (low oxygen)
- Fever, swelling, or pus at wound sites (signs of infection)

Seek Immediate Help If:
- Your child has sudden or worsening difficulty breathing.
- Chest pain becomes severe or constant.
- There are changes in heart rate—very fast, very slow, or irregular beats.
- The child becomes drowsy, confused, or unresponsive.

Activity and Recovery:
- Limit physical exertion—avoid running, sports, or lifting until cleared by the physician.

- Allow gradual return to routine activities based on follow-up evaluations.
- Ensure proper nutrition and hydration to support healing.

Emotional Support:

- Encourage the child to express fears or discomfort.
- Reassure siblings and family members—it's normal to feel anxious after trauma.
- Consider referral to a counselor or support group if emotional distress persists.

Role of PCP in Pediatric Thoracic Trauma

In emergency settings, primary care providers (PCPs) are often the first line of support in managing pediatric thoracic injuries. Their role is integral to early recognition, resuscitation, coordination, and communication during trauma care.

1. *Rapid Initial Assessment*: Utilize the Pediatric Assessment Triangle (PAT) to assess the child's general appearance, work of breathing, and circulation to the skin. This triage tool enables quick identification of children who are critically ill or unstable.
2. *Systematic Evaluation (ABCDE)*: Conduct a focused primary survey following the ABCDE approach:
   - *Airway (A)*: Ensure the airway is patent; assess for obstructions, foreign bodies, or altered consciousness that may compromise ventilation. Use jaw thrust or suctioning as required.
   - *Breathing (B)*: Observe chest rise, auscultate for breath sounds, and assess respiratory rate and effort. Initiate high-flow oxygen via non-rebreather mask.
   - *Circulation (C)*: Palpate central and peripheral pulses, monitor blood pressure, assess capillary refill time, and observe for signs of hypoperfusion. Establish IV access for fluid administration.
   - *Disability (D)*: Assess neurological status using the AVPU scale or Glasgow Coma Scale (GCS). Evaluate for pupil symmetry and responsiveness.
   - *Exposure (E)*: Fully expose the child to identify hidden injuries while ensuring warmth to prevent hypothermia.
3. *Airway and Breathing Support*: Assist in positioning, oxygen delivery, and preparing airway adjuncts (e.g., OPA/NPA) while anticipating potential intubation in cases of severe respiratory distress or altered consciousness.
4. *Circulatory Management*: Support fluid resuscitation with isotonic crystalloids as per pediatric protocols. Monitor for signs of hemorrhagic shock and prepare for potential blood product administration if needed.
5. *Neurological Observation*: Regularly assess for any deterioration in consciousness or onset of seizure activity. Recognize subtle signs of increased intracranial pressure or spinal injury.
6. *Family Engagement and Emotional Support*: Communicate empathetically with parents or caregivers. Provide reassurance, explain procedures, and involve them in the child's care plan when appropriate.

7. *Procedural Assistance and Readiness*: Be prepared to assist the trauma team with emergency procedures such as chest tube insertion, needle decompression, or pericardiocentesis. Anticipate equipment needs and ensure sterility and safety protocols.
8. *Communication and Documentation*: Use structured tools like *SBAR (Situation, Background, Assessment, Recommendation)* to relay findings and updates to the trauma team. Meticulously document vital signs, interventions, time of assessments, and the child's response to treatment.
9. *Ongoing Monitoring*: Continuously reassess the child's airway, breathing, circulation, and neurological status. Be vigilant for clinical deterioration, and escalate care when necessary.
10. *Handoff and Coordination*: Coordinate with the trauma team, pediatric specialists, or higher centers during handover or transfer, ensuring all clinical data and management steps are accurately conveyed.

Case Resolution

Upon arrival at the district hospital's emergency department, Rakesh—a 14-year-old boy—was assessed immediately using the Pediatric Assessment Triangle (PAT) and the ABCDE approach, as indicated for any child presenting with trauma and respiratory distress.

Initial Assessment and Prehospital Management: Rakesh was found conscious but visibly dyspneic, with a respiratory rate of 48 per min, heart rate of 135 bpm, and oxygen saturation of 91% on supplemental oxygen. His capillary refill time was delayed at 3 s, and blood pressure was maintained at 110/70 mmHg. He had abrasions and embedded dirt over the left chest wall, but no active external bleeding. These clinical features—especially tachypnea, hypoxia despite oxygen, and signs of respiratory compromise—raised strong suspicion for life-threatening thoracic injuries such as pneumothorax or pulmonary contusion.

During prehospital care, oxygen was administered via a non-rebreather mask, and the child was positioned supine with continuous basic monitoring during transport. No analgesia or IV access was initiated en route due to limited resources.

Emergency Department Evaluation: At triage, a detailed ABCDE reassessment was performed. Airway was patent, but breathing was compromised—notably with reduced breath sounds on the left hemithorax and mild tracheal deviation suggesting a developing pneumothorax. IV access was established, and analgesia and high-flow oxygen were initiated promptly.

Investigations and Diagnosis: A chest X-ray confirmed the presence of a moderate left-sided pneumothorax with associated pulmonary contusion, validating the PCP's initial suspicion. An eFAST scan was performed and found negative for any intra-abdominal or pericardial fluid, ruling out other coexisting internal injuries.

Intervention and Procedure Assistance: Recognizing the need for chest decompression, the trauma team performed an intercostal chest drain (ICD) insertion in the 5th intercostal space at the midaxillary line, under sterile conditions. The PCP actively supported this procedure by preparing sterile equipment, ensuring continuous monitoring, and assisting with patient positioning.

Post-Intervention Response: Following the ICD placement, Rakesh's oxygenation and respiratory effort improved significantly, indicating the successful resolution of the pneumothorax. Pain control was optimized, and vital signs stabilized.

Hospital Course and Discharge: Rakesh was monitored in the pediatric high-dependency unit (HDU) for 48–72 h. His management included chest physiotherapy, routine vital monitoring, and family education regarding recovery and home care. He was transferred to the general ward on day 3 and discharged on day 6 with complete instructions for follow-up and activity restrictions.

Key Messages

- *Start with PAT and ABCDE*: Use the Pediatric Assessment Triangle followed by the ABCDE approach for rapid triage. Early recognition saves lives—time lost is tissue lost.
- *Don't rely on visible injuries alone*: Children's flexible chest walls can absorb blunt force without external bruising, masking serious internal trauma.
- *Look for subtle danger signs*: Be alert for indicators like tracheal deviation, asymmetric breath sounds, and distended neck veins—these may signal critical conditions such as tension pneumothorax or cardiac tamponade.
- *Prioritize early oxygenation*: Administer high-flow oxygen immediately on arrival to stabilize breathing and prevent hypoxia.
- *Position purposefully*: In cases like flail chest, lateral positioning may improve ventilation and patient comfort.
- *Manage pain aggressively*: Timely and effective analgesia is vital to prevent respiratory fatigue, especially in rib fractures or contusions.
- *Prepare for interventions*: PCPs should anticipate and assist in procedures like chest tube insertion by setting up equipment and maintaining sterility.
- *Engage with families*: Actively involve caregivers by explaining the child's condition, answering questions, and offering reassurance throughout treatment.
- *Document thoroughly and in real time*: Accurate, ongoing documentation of vitals, interventions, and response to treatment ensures continuity of care and supports clinical decisions.

Bibliography

1. American College of Surgeons. Advanced Trauma Life Support (ATLS) Student Course Manual. 10th ed. Chicago, IL: American College of Surgeons; 2018.
2. Davies DA, Pearl RH. Paediatric thoracic trauma. Semin Pediatr Surg. 2004;13(2):98–105. https://doi.org/10.1053/j.sempedsurg.2004.01.005
3. Gates RL, Welborn MB, Cotton BA. Paediatric thoracic trauma: The differences from adult patients. Curr Opin Pediatr. 2002;14(3):292–296. https://doi.org/10.1097/00008480-200206000-00014
4. Nataraja RM, Palmer CS, Arul GS. Paediatric thoracic trauma: A 10-year retrospective review. J Trauma Acute Care Surg. 2013;74(1):268–271. https://doi.org/10.1097/TA.0b013e3182788f2d
5. Stewart TC, Mckechnie PS, Tremblay LN, et al. Thoracic trauma in children: A review of 206 cases. J Pediatr Surg. 2005;40(1):128–132. https://doi.org/10.1016/j.jpedsurg.2004.09.031

Pediatric Abdominal and Pelvic Trauma

10

Rupinder Deol, Debmoy Ghatak, Prachi Sinha,
and Amit Priyadarshi

Learning Objectives

By the end of this chapter, readers should be able to:

- Apply a structured initial assessment of pediatric abdominal and pelvic trauma using the Pediatric Assessment Triangle (PAT) and ABCDE approach to identify life-threatening conditions early.
- Recognize key clinical signs and symptoms of abdominal and pelvic injuries in children, including red flag indicators for solid organ injury, hollow viscus injury, and pelvic fractures.
- Differentiate between stable and unstable pediatric trauma presentations to guide appropriate management decisions and timely referrals.
- Assist in the initiation of essential diagnostic procedures and emergency interventions, such as fluid resuscitation, oxygen therapy, pelvic binding, and preparation for imaging or surgical referral.
- Support effective communication and documentation, including structured handovers (e.g., MIST format), caregiver counseling, and medicolegal considerations in suspected child abuse.

R. Deol
College of Nursing, AIIMS Rishikesh, Rishikesh, Uttarakhand, India

D. Ghatak
Trauma & Emergency Medicine, AIIMS Kalyani, Kalyani, India

P. Sinha
Department of Neonatology, AIIMS Bhopal, Bhopal, India

A. Priyadarshi (✉)
Trauma & Emergency Medicine, AIIMS Bhopal, Bhopal, Madhya Pradesh, India

N. T. Rai (ed.), *Pediatric Trauma Resuscitation Manual (PTRM) for Primary Care Providers*, https://doi.org/10.1007/978-981-95-4979-5_10

- Educate caregivers on home care and danger signs following initial stabilization, focusing on nutrition, activity restriction, wound care (if applicable), and follow-up needs.

Introduction

Abdominal and pelvic trauma in children presents a unique diagnostic and management challenge due to the distinct anatomical and physiological characteristics of the pediatric population. Children are more vulnerable to serious internal injuries, even from seemingly minor mechanisms of trauma, owing to their compliant rib cage, proportionally larger solid organs, and underdeveloped musculature. Unlike adults, children may not reliably verbalize pain or localize symptoms, making clinical evaluation more complex. Furthermore, signs of internal injury may be subtle or delayed, increasing the risk of missed diagnoses and complications.

In India, common causes of pediatric abdominal and pelvic trauma include road traffic accidents, falls from height, bicycle handlebar injuries, and occasionally, non-accidental trauma. While many injuries can be managed nonoperatively, prompt recognition of life-threatening conditions such as solid organ laceration, hollow viscus perforation, or pelvic fractures is critical to prevent morbidity and mortality.

Primary care providers (PCPs) often serve as the first point of contact in rural or peripheral healthcare settings. Their role in triage, initial stabilization, and timely referral is vital. Using structured frameworks such as the Pediatric Assessment Triangle (PAT) and the ABCDE approach, PCPs can rapidly identify critical signs, initiate lifesaving interventions, and communicate effectively with higher-level trauma centers. Additionally, PCPs play an essential role in pain control, caregiver communication, recordkeeping, and recognizing signs of child abuse.

This chapter equips PCPs with practical guidance to assess, manage, and coordinate care for pediatric patients with abdominal and pelvic trauma. Emphasis is placed on early recognition, efficient stabilization, appropriate use of diagnostic tools, and caregiver education, enabling PCPs to optimize outcomes even in resource-limited settings.

Case Scenario

It is a busy afternoon in the emergency department of a community hospital when Khushi, an 8-year-old girl, is brought in by her parents. Two hours ago, she was riding her bicycle when she was struck by a car. There are no visible external injuries, but Khushi appears anxious and distressed. She is conscious, is crying inconsolably, and complains of abdominal pain. Her mother reports that she had one episode of vomiting at home and has been restless since. There are no signs of bleeding or limb deformities.

The triage nurse initiates oxygen therapy with a non-rebreather mask and begins a rapid assessment.

Initial clinical findings:

- Level of consciousness: Alert and verbal
- Respiratory rate (RR): 48 breaths/min
- Oxygen saturation (SpO_2): 91% on supplemental oxygen
- Heart rate (HR): 135 beats/min
- Capillary refill time (CRT): 3 s
- Blood pressure (BP): 110/70 mmHg
- Abdomen: Tender on palpation, with guarding in the left lower quadrant

The clinical picture raises suspicion of blunt abdominal trauma, possibly involving internal organ injury or pelvic fracture. There are no obvious external wounds, yet the signs of tachypnea, tachycardia, delayed CRT, and abdominal tenderness warrant urgent evaluation for internal bleeding or hollow viscus injury.

Reflective Questions

1. What are the key components of the primary assessment (ABCDE) you will initiate first in this child with suspected internal trauma?
2. Which signs and symptoms would raise your concern for intra-abdominal bleeding or pelvic fractures in pediatric patients?
3. What immediate stabilization steps should be initiated while preparing Khushi for further imaging or transfer?
4. Which bedside or radiological investigations (e.g., FAST, abdominal X-ray, CT scan) are most appropriate in this case?
5. As a PCP, how can you assist the trauma team in preparing for possible procedures such as IV access, urinary catheter insertion, or surgical consultation?

Anatomical and Physiological Considerations

Children exhibit several anatomical and physiological characteristics that make them uniquely vulnerable to abdominal and pelvic trauma. Compared to adults, they possess less subcutaneous fat, underdeveloped musculature, and more pliable bones, which reduce the natural protection against external forces. The abdominal wall is thinner, and the rib cage is more compliant, offering limited shielding to vital intra-abdominal organs such as the liver, spleen, and intestines.

Additionally, pediatric patients have a lower overall body mass, which means that traumatic forces are distributed over a smaller surface area, leading to a higher risk of internal injury even from relatively low-impact mechanisms. The abdominal cavity in children is smaller and the organs are proportionally larger, particularly in infants and toddlers. This results in a more central and superficial placement of organs, increasing their exposure during trauma.

The pediatric diaphragm also lies more horizontally compared to adults, causing the liver and spleen to extend further below the rib cage and thus making them more susceptible to blunt injuries. Moreover, the urinary bladder in younger children remains an intra-abdominal organ, unlike in adults where it becomes more pelvic with age. Another consideration is the frequent use of adult-designed safety restraints, such as seat belts, which may be ill-fitted in children. Improper usage or positioning can contribute to upper abdominal deceleration injuries during road traffic accidents.

Mechanisms of Pediatric Abdominal and Pelvic Injuries

Pediatric abdominal and pelvic trauma in India commonly results from a variety of high-risk mechanisms, reflecting both environmental and socioeconomic factors.

- *Blunt Abdominal Trauma*: This is the most frequent cause of abdominal injury in children. It typically results from falls from height, road traffic accidents, bicycle handlebar impacts, sports injuries, and physical assault. Blunt trauma can lead to injuries of solid organs (e.g., liver, spleen, kidneys, pancreas), hollow organs (e.g., intestines, urinary bladder), or a combination of both. The absence of external signs can often delay diagnosis, making vigilance essential.
- *Penetrating Abdominal Trauma*: Though less common than blunt trauma, penetrating injuries can occur from stab wounds, gunshot injuries, or impalement by sharp objects such as sticks, rods, or metal shards. These injuries often demand prompt surgical exploration due to the high risk of internal organ damage.
- *Blast or Explosion Injuries*: Particularly relevant in the context of unsafe storage or handling of fireworks, firecrackers, and household gas leaks, these injuries can cause complex trauma involving both penetration and blunt force mechanisms. They are associated with a high risk of multi-organ damage and secondary infections.

Abdominal injuries in children can present with a broad spectrum of severity and symptomatology depending on the mechanism of injury. Accurate identification requires a comprehensive approach involving detailed history-taking, focused clinical assessment, appropriate imaging modalities, and, in some cases, surgical evaluation. A high index of suspicion is crucial, particularly when external signs are minimal despite significant internal injury.

Assessment of Pediatric Abdominal and Pelvic Injuries

Initial Assessment

The initial assessment of a child with abdominal injuries and pelvic injuries involves two main steps: the Pediatric Assessment Triangle (PAT) and the primary survey (ABCDE). These steps help identify and manage life-threatening conditions quickly.

Pediatric Assessment Triangle (PAT)

The PAT is a quick way to assess the severity of a child's condition. It looks at three things (Fig. 10.1):

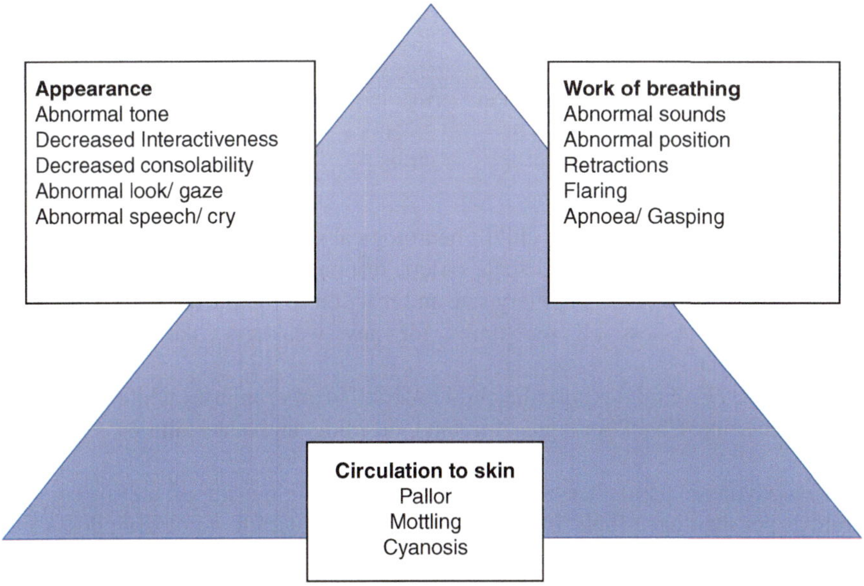

Fig. 10.1 Pediatric Assessment Triangle

1. *Appearance*: Check if the child is alert, responsive, and interacting normally. Look for signs of distress, such as crying or lethargy.
2. *Work of breathing*: Observe how hard the child is working to breathe. Look for fast or slow breathing, use of accessory muscles, and abnormal sounds like wheezing or grunting.
3. *Circulation to skin*: Check the skin color and temperature. Look for signs of poor blood flow, such as pallor (pale skin), mottling, or cyanosis (blue skin).

Primary Survey (ABCDE)

The primary survey is a more detailed evaluation that focuses on identifying and managing life-threatening conditions. The ABCDE mnemonic stands for Airway, Breathing, Circulation, Disability, and Exposure.

1. *Airway (A)*: Ensure the airway is patent and clear. Look for signs of obstruction, such as choking, stridor (high-pitched breathing sound), or gurgling.
2. *Breathing (B)*: Check the child's breathing. Look for rate, rhythm, depth, and effort. Listen for abnormal sounds and check oxygen saturation. Look for crepitus or tenderness on chest compression test (CCT).
3. *Circulation (C)*: Assess circulation by checking the pulse, heart rate, blood pressure, capillary refill time, and skin condition. Look for signs of shock, such as increased heart rate, weak thready pulse, or low blood pressure. Assess pelvic fracture with pelvic compression test (PCT).

Table 10.1 Age-wise hemodynamic parameters in children

Age	Newborn (<1 month)	Infant (<1 year)	Toddlers (1–3 years)	Children (4–12 years)	Adolescent (12–17 years)
HR (beats/min)	140–160	120–130	100–120	80–100	60–100
RR (rate/min)	40–60	26–30	26–20	20–25	12–20
SBP (mmHg)	60–70	80–90	90–95	95–105	110–120

4. *Disability (D)*: Evaluate the child's neurological status. Check their level of consciousness using the AVPU scale (Alert, response to Voice, response to Pain, Unresponsive). Assess pupillary size and reaction to light. Check the blood glucose level. Assess all the limbs for any weakness like paraplegia or quadriplegia.
5. *Exposure (E)*: Fully expose the child to look for other injuries while preventing hypothermia. Check for signs of trauma, bleeding, and other injuries.

Hemodynamic parameters vary in children age-wise; it is important to assess the child as per their age (Table 10.1). Broselow's tape is used to guide drug doses and equipment's sizes to be used in children based on the height.

Hypotension in Children

In pediatric patients, hypotension is defined using the age-adjusted formula:

$$\text{Hypotension} = \text{Systolic blood pressure}(\text{SBP}) < 70 + (\text{Age in years} \times 2)$$

This formula helps identify children at risk of circulatory shock and guides timely resuscitation.

Maintenance Intravenous Fluid Requirement

The Holliday-Segar formula is widely used to calculate daily maintenance fluid requirements in children, based on their body weight:

- *For the first 10 kg of body weight*: 100 mL/kg/day
- *For the next 10 kg (11–20 kg)*: 50 mL/kg/day
- *For weight beyond 20 kg*: 20 mL/kg/day

Example Calculation

For a child weighing 21 kg, the total fluid requirement over 24 h is calculated as follows:

- First 10 kg: 10 × 100 = 1000 mL
- Next 10 kg: 10 × 50 = 500 mL
- Remaining 1 kg: 1 × 20 = 20 mL

Total = 1000 + 500 + 20 = 1520 mL/day

This calculation aids primary care providers in planning appropriate fluid therapy for pediatric patients, especially in trauma and resuscitation scenarios.

Table 10.2 Adjuncts to primary survey

Adjuncts	Role
eFAST	Look for free fluids in peritoneal and pleural cavity and pneumothorax.
ABG	Look for acidosis and increased lactate to assess the severity of hypovolemic shock.
Pulse oximeter	Look for oxygen saturation.
Multipara monitor	Look for vitals like HR, BP, and RR.
Foley's catheter	Look for hematuria and monitor urine output.
Ryle's tube	Prevents aspiration

Adjuncts to Primary Survey These bedside investigations and instruments help in managing the life-threatening conditions (Table 10.2).

The initial management of a child with multiple traumatic injuries follows the ABCDE approach. This structured assessment ensures rapid identification and treatment of life-threatening conditions.

In children presenting with profound hypotension, nonresponsiveness to fluid resuscitation, or clinical signs of peritonitis, the recommended course of action is Damage Control Surgery (DCS)—specifically, an abbreviated exploratory laparotomy. This urgent intervention focuses on controlling hemorrhage and preventing contamination rather than performing definitive repairs. Following surgery, the child should be transferred to the intensive care unit (ICU) for further resuscitation and stabilization.

In contrast, a more detailed and cautious evaluation for abdominal injuries can be undertaken in hemodynamically stable children or those who respond positively to initial resuscitation. For such cases, further diagnostic workup is essential to rule out occult intra-abdominal injuries and to guide management decisions. This step should not be delayed, even in stable children, to avoid missed or delayed diagnoses.

Blunt Abdominal Trauma

Blunt abdominal trauma is the most frequent form of abdominal injury in children, commonly resulting from falls, road traffic accidents, or sports-related incidents. Due to the relatively unprotected nature of pediatric abdominal organs, injuries can involve both solid and hollow viscera, with the spleen, liver, kidneys, and intestines being most commonly affected.

Mechanisms of Injury

- Direct impact injuries, such as those caused by seat belt compression, bicycle handlebar impact, or a fall onto a hard surface
- Compression or deceleration injuries, often seen in motor vehicle collisions, where rapid force transmission causes shearing or crushing of internal organs

Common Blunt Abdominal Injuries

- *Spleen Injury*
  Types: Contusion, laceration, pseudoaneurysm, or rupture
  Signs: Pain in the left upper quadrant, referred shoulder pain (Kehr's sign), and signs of hypovolemic shock
  Diagnosis: Physical examination, FAST scan, or contrast-enhanced CT
- *Liver Injury*
  Types: Contusion, laceration, pseudoaneurysm, or rupture
  Signs: Right upper quadrant tenderness, palpable hepatomegaly, and signs of shock
  Diagnosis: Ultrasound for initial assessment, followed by CT scan for detailed evaluation
- *Kidney Injury*
  Types: Contusion, laceration, vascular insult, pelvic calyceal system injury, or perinephric hematoma
  Signs: Flank pain, hematuria, and costovertebral angle tenderness
  Diagnosis: Ultrasound or CT scan
- *Bowel and Mesenteric Injury*
  Types: Intestinal perforation or mesenteric tear
  Signs: Abdominal distension, vomiting, localized tenderness, presence of blood in stool, or signs of peritonitis
  Diagnosis: CT scan with contrast or diagnostic laparoscopy in case of clinical deterioration

Early recognition and prompt imaging are vital as these injuries may be subtle during initial assessment but can progress rapidly without intervention.

Identification

Timely and accurate identification of intra-abdominal injury in children is essential, particularly in the setting of blunt trauma. Clinical signs may be subtle, and a high index of suspicion is warranted.

Clinical Assessment

- *Physical Examination*: Begin by inspecting for external signs such as bruising (especially seat belt marks), tenderness, abdominal distension, or palpable masses. The presence of rebound tenderness or guarding is suggestive of peritonitis and warrants urgent escalation.
- *Focused Assessment with Sonography in Trauma (FAST)*: This bedside ultrasound tool helps rapidly detect free intraperitoneal fluid, indicating potential internal bleeding. It is especially valuable in hemodynamically unstable patients where immediate surgical decision-making is required.
- *Imaging*: A contrast-enhanced CT scan is the gold standard for evaluating internal injuries in stable patients. However, its use must be judicious in children due to the risk of radiation exposure. In minor cases, imaging may be deferred in favor of serial clinical monitoring.

Management Algorithm (Fig. 10.2)

The initial critical decision point is determining hemodynamic stability:

- If the child is unstable, an immediate FAST exam is warranted:
  - *FAST positive*: Proceed to exploratory laparotomy.
  - *FAST negative*: Maintain a high suspicion; consider continued resuscitation and repeat imaging as false negatives are possible.

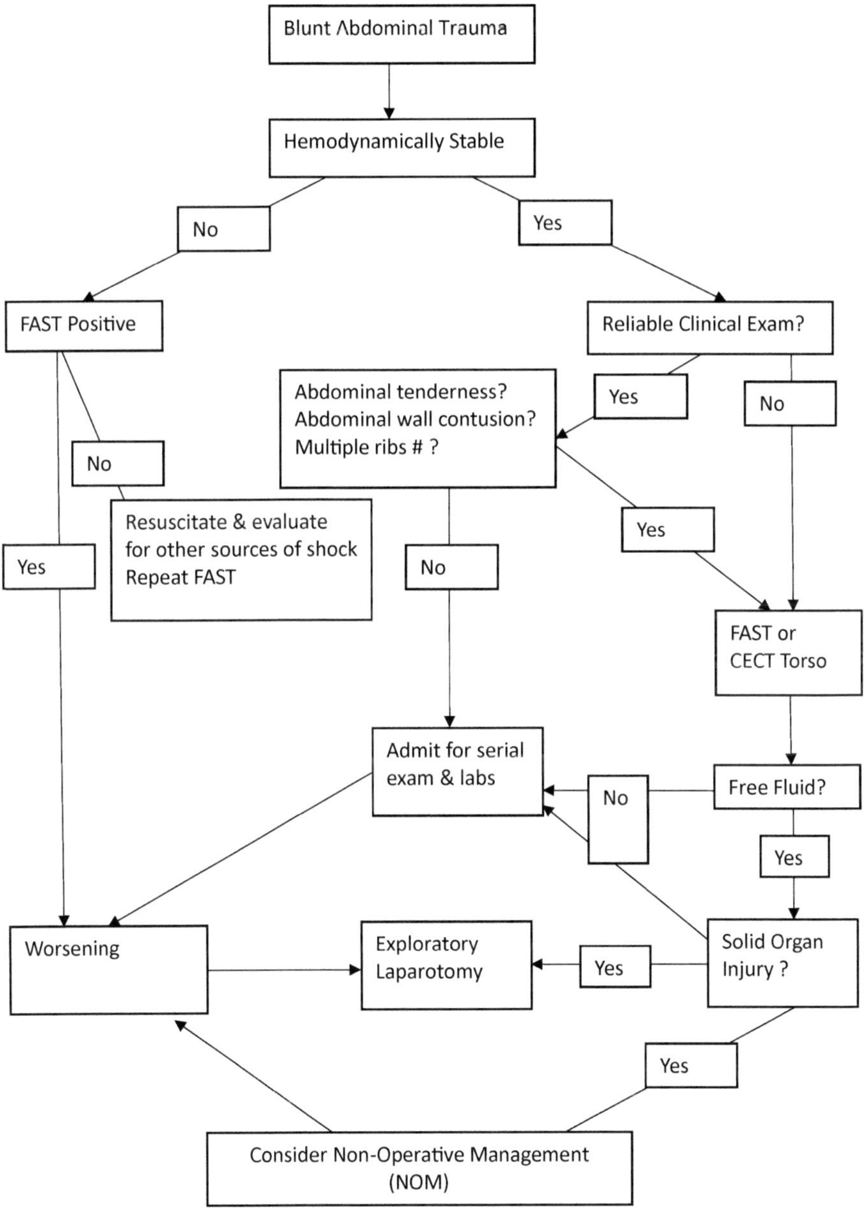

Fig. 10.2 Management algorithm for pediatric blunt abdominal trauma

- If the child is stable, evaluate the reliability of the abdominal exam:
  - If the exam is reliable and there are no high-risk features, opt for serial examinations and laboratory monitoring.
  - If high-risk features are present (e.g., lap belt sign, persistent pain, visible bruising), or the exam is unreliable, obtain a CT scan.
  - In the presence of free fluid without solid organ injury, consider laparoscopy or laparotomy to evaluate for mesenteric, bowel, or bladder injuries.

Penetrating Abdominal Trauma

Although less frequent than blunt trauma, penetrating abdominal injuries in children carry a high risk of morbidity due to the potential for multi-organ involvement. Common causes include stab wounds, gunshot injuries, and impalement by sharp or pointed objects such as rods, sticks, or glass.

Clinical Features
Key signs of penetrating abdominal trauma may include:

- Visible entry wound or multiple wounds indicating possible entry and exit tracks
- Evisceration—visible abdominal contents protruding through the wound
- Signs of hypovolemic shock—such as tachycardia, hypotension, or delayed capillary refill
- Abdominal distension, guarding, or clinical signs of peritonitis

  These findings should prompt immediate prioritization and resuscitative efforts.

Initial Evaluation and Diagnosis
- Thorough physical examination is essential to assess the trajectory and extent of injury.
- Imaging studies may include:
  - X-rays to detect retained foreign bodies or bone involvement
  - CT scan with contrast (if the child is hemodynamically stable) to evaluate organ damage and hemorrhage
  - Focused Assessment with Sonography for Trauma (FAST), particularly its pericardial view, is useful in detecting cardiac tamponade in thoracoabdominal injuries.

Management Algorithm (Fig. 10.3)
- Unstable patients with clinical signs of peritonitis or clear peritoneal violation should undergo immediate exploratory laparotomy without delay for advanced imaging.
- Stable patients with reliable clinical examination and no signs of internal injury may be observed under close monitoring, depending on:
  - Mechanism and trajectory of injury

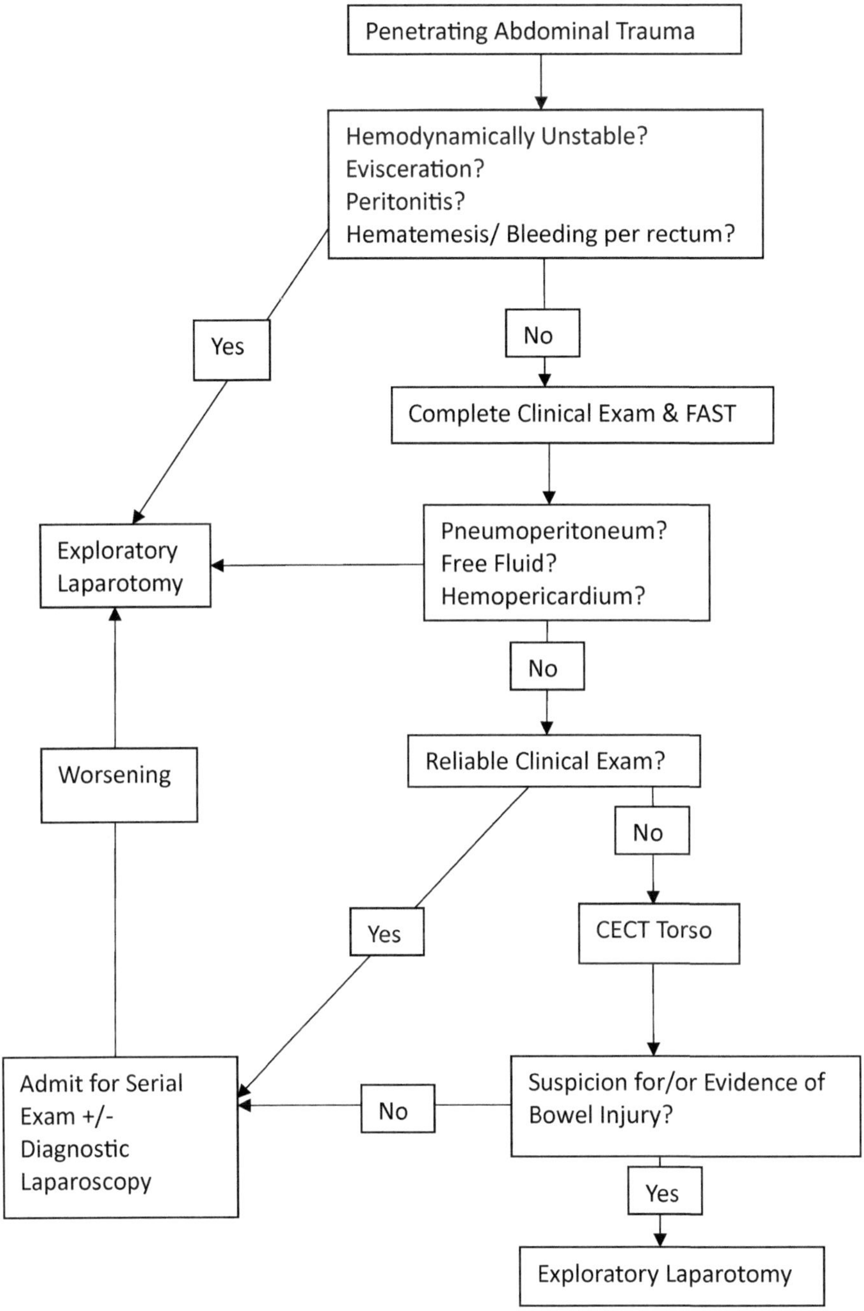

Fig. 10.3 Management algorithm for pediatric penetrating abdominal trauma

  - Institutional protocols and surgical backup
  - Surgeon's clinical judgment, including whether diagnostic laparoscopy is warranted
- Injuries within the "*cardiac box*" (bounded by the clavicle, xiphoid process, and midclavicular lines bilaterally) require particular caution as even minor-seeming wounds may involve the heart or great vessels.

Observation is appropriate in selected cases (e.g., superficial or tangential bullet trajectories) with no hemodynamic compromise or concerning imaging findings, but such decisions must be made judiciously.

Abdominal Organ Injuries

The type and severity of intra-abdominal injury in children can vary based on age, mechanism of trauma, and anatomical vulnerability. While solid organ injuries are most common following blunt trauma, hollow viscus, mesenteric, diaphragmatic, and abdominal wall injuries must not be overlooked—especially in high-impact or deceleration events. Table 10.3 provides a quick overview of key organ systems, associated clinical signs, and preferred diagnostic approaches:

Table 10.3 Common pediatric abdominopelvic injuries: mechanisms, clinical clues, and diagnostic approaches

Organ/system	Common mechanism	Key clinical signs	Preferred diagnostics
Small bowel	Shearing, compression	Abdominal pain, vomiting, signs of peritonitis (fever, tenderness)	CT scan, diagnostic laparotomy
Large bowel	Direct trauma, deceleration	Blood in stool, abdominal distension, fever	CT scan, water-soluble contrast enema
Pancreas	Blunt epigastric trauma	Abdominal/back pain, nausea, vomiting	Elevated amylase/lipase; CT scan
Diaphragm	Blunt trauma	Chest/abdominal pain, dyspnea, bowel sounds in chest	Chest X-ray, CT scan, diagnostic laparoscopy
Spleen	Blunt trauma (most common injury)	LUQ pain, Kehr's sign (shoulder pain), hypotension	FAST, CT scan
Liver	Blunt trauma	RUQ pain, hepatomegaly, hypotension, rarely jaundice	CT scan with contrast, ultrasound
Kidney	Flank impact, high-velocity trauma	Flank pain, hematuria, CVA tenderness	Ultrasound, CT scan
Mesentery	Deceleration or torsional force	Abdominal pain, blood in stool, signs of shock	CT scan (free fluid, mesenteric vessel abnormalities)
Abdominal wall	Falls, blunt trauma	Contusions, hematomas, visible bulge, fascial rupture	Physical exam, ultrasound

Clinical Evaluation and Symptoms of Pediatric Abdominal and Pelvic Injuries

Performing an accurate abdominal assessment in pediatric trauma can be challenging. Children often present with fear, pain, and distress, which may hinder cooperation. Continuous crying and agitation can lead to aerophagia, resulting in abdominal distension that further complicates clinical evaluation. Therefore, history-taking and physical examination should be conducted in the presence of caregivers, with the support of trained nurses to soothe, reassure, and administer appropriate analgesia.

History and High-Risk Mechanisms

Children with the following trauma mechanisms warrant high suspicion for abdominal injury:

- High-velocity impact or deceleration injuries (e.g., vehicular accidents)
- Direct blows to the abdomen (e.g., in assaults or physical abuse)
- Injuries above and below the abdomen, suggesting abdominal involvement
- Seat belt sign, often associated with pancreatic or duodenal injury
- Bicycle handlebar trauma, particularly in the epigastric region
- Straddle injuries involving beams or bars (perineal, urethral, or vaginal trauma)
- Penetrating injuries to the torso, especially if wounds cross the diaphragm
- Suspicion of child abuse, particularly with inconsistent history or delay in presentation

Clinical Features to Recognize

Symptoms and signs must be interpreted in the context of mechanism and timing of injury:

- Tachycardia: May reflect both pain and compensatory response to blood loss
- Hypotension: A late and ominous sign indicating cardiovascular compromise
- Abdominal distension, pain, vomiting, and localized or generalized peritonitis are hallmark findings.
- Generalized guarding or rigidity suggests peritonitis, often due to internal bleeding or hollow organ perforation.
- Tenderness over the liver, spleen, or renal angles, especially if accompanied by external bruising
- Seat belt marks, flank discoloration, or visible abrasions are critical external signs.
- Palpation: Should assess for localized tenderness, rebound, or rigidity—clues to intra-abdominal pathology
- Signs of urethral injury (e.g., blood at the meatus) and pelvic instability should be carefully examined; avoid repeated pelvic compression as it may dislodge clots and worsen bleeding.

- Neurological symptoms such as altered sensorium or hypoxia may indicate associated head or thoracic injury.
- Back and perineum inspection must be gentle, explained clearly to the child and caregivers, and performed with sensitivity.

Pediatric-Specific Shock Index (SIPA)
Primary care providers should utilize the Shock Index, Pediatric Age-adjusted (SIPA), a validated tool that better identifies children at risk for significant intra-abdominal injury, need for transfusion, or mortality compared to adult thresholds. SIPA is calculated as:

$$\text{Shock index}\,(\text{SI}) = \text{Heart rate} / \text{systolic blood pressure}$$

Age-specific SIPA cutoff values should guide urgency of intervention and escalation of care. Elevated SIPA indicates the need for prompt resuscitation and possible transfer to a higher-level trauma center.

Diagnostic Evaluation of Pediatric Abdominal and Pelvic Injuries

Early and accurate identification of intra-abdominal injuries in children is essential to guide timely interventions and avoid unnecessary procedures. Multiple diagnostic modalities—radiological, laboratory, and surgical—are used in a tiered fashion based on hemodynamic status, clinical suspicion, and resource availability.

Imaging Studies
- *Chest X-ray (CXR)* and *pelvic X-ray (PXR)*: Useful for identifying associated thoracic injuries or pelvic fractures
- *Abdominal X-ray*: Offers limited utility in blunt abdominal trauma. Diagnostic accuracy is low for intra-abdominal injuries.
- *Focused Assessment with Sonography in Trauma (FAST)*: A bedside ultrasound included in all trauma protocols. It evaluates:
  - Pericardial sac, right and left upper quadrants, and pelvis for free fluid (suggesting hemoperitoneum).
  - While FAST is quick, noninvasive, and repeatable, its sensitivity in children is limited. A negative FAST does not rule out serious injury and should be followed up with confirmatory imaging (e.g., CT scan).
  - Positive FAST, especially in unstable patients, supports surgical decision-making.

Primary care providers and nurses play a vital role in correlating FAST findings with clinical presentation, physiological status, and mechanism of injury and in supporting decisions on urgent laparotomy or further imaging.

- *Contrast-Enhanced CT (CECT)*: The gold standard for stable pediatric trauma patients after the primary survey.
  - It accurately identifies retroperitoneal injuries, grades solid organ damage, and clarifies bowel or mesenteric involvement.
  - Due to the risk of radiation-induced malignancies, especially in children, physicians should adhere to the ALARA (as low as reasonably achievable) principle.
  - Decision-support tools (e.g., PECARN abdominal rules) can help identify low-risk patients and limit unnecessary imaging.

Laboratory Investigations

During initial assessment, a trauma blood screen or Emergency Blood Leveling (EBL) should be initiated. Key tests include:

- Hemoglobin, hematocrit, base deficit, lactate—Assess hemorrhage and perfusion status.
- Coagulation profile—Evaluate bleeding risk.
- Sepsis markers (CRP, procalcitonin)—Screen for infectious complications in delayed presentations.
- Liver enzymes (ALT, AST) and amylase—Suggest hepatobiliary or pancreatic injury.
- Urine analysis—Microscopic hematuria can indicate renal or nonrenal intra-abdominal injury.

Laparoscopy in Pediatric Trauma

Laparoscopy offers a minimally invasive alternative to open surgery with lower rates of nontherapeutic laparotomy and favorable morbidity outcomes. It is particularly helpful in:

- Diagnosing diaphragmatic injuries
- Evaluating suspected bowel perforation
- Assessing penetrating injuries when imaging is inconclusive

In unstable, FAST-positive patients, diagnostic laparoscopy can rapidly transition into damage control laparotomy, making it both a diagnostic and therapeutic tool.

Indications for Exploratory Laparotomy

Immediate surgery is indicated when any of the following are present:

- Radiological evidence of hollow viscus injury (e.g., free intraperitoneal air)
- Mesenteric ischemia or gangrenous bowel
- Generalized peritonitis
- Gunshot wound to the abdomen
- Hemodynamic instability

- Evisceration of abdominal contents
- Failure to stabilize or clinical deterioration

Diagnostic Peritoneal Lavage (DPL)
DPL remains a valuable tool in resource-limited settings or when FAST and CT are unavailable. It may also be used in:

- Hemodynamically unstable patients unfit for imaging
- Polytrauma patients requiring concurrent surgery for other injuries

Angiography and Angioembolization
While its diagnostic role is limited, angiography can be used when CT imaging reveals vascular injury such as active bleeding, pseudoaneurysm, or arteriovenous fistula. In such cases, Digital Subtraction Angiography (DSA) and angiographic embolization serve as adjuncts to nonoperative management of solid organ injuries like liver or kidney trauma.

Pediatric Pelvic Fractures

Pelvic fractures account for less than 1% of all pediatric fractures but are associated with a significant risk of morbidity and mortality. Studies from Level I trauma centers report a mortality rate of up to 25% in children presenting with pelvic fractures. These injuries often result from high-energy trauma, and their evaluation must include assessment for associated abdominal, genitourinary, and vascular injuries.

Anatomical Considerations in Children
Pediatric pelvic anatomy differs significantly from adults, influencing injury patterns and management:

- Greater plasticity of pelvic bones due to ongoing ossification
- Elasticity of sacroiliac joints and a flexible pubic symphysis
- Presence of apophyses and the triradiate cartilage, where the ilium, pubis, and ischium converge, which fuses around 12–14 years of age
- Pelvic hemorrhage is less common due to robust vasoconstriction capabilities in children, unlike the friable and atherosclerotic vessels in adults.
- Pediatric fracture patterns are often more stable, despite similar mechanisms of injury to adults.

Clinical Assessment
A thorough physical examination of the pelvis and perineum is essential. Clinicians should inspect for:

- Lacerations, bruising, swelling, or abrasions
- Morel-Lavallée lesions, which present as fluctuating, soft tissue swelling due to closed degloving injuries

- Signs of associated urogenital trauma, including blood at the urethral meatus or scrotal/labial swelling

Initial Stabilization and Management
For children with unstable pelvic fractures and signs of hemorrhagic shock:

- Begin with rapid hemorrhage control and fluid resuscitation.
- Pelvic stabilization should be achieved using:
  - A pelvic binder or sheet wrap at the level of the greater trochanters
  - Internal rotation of lower limbs to reduce pelvic volume and control bleeding
  - Longitudinal skin or skeletal traction in vertical shear injuries (under orthopedic guidance)

Note: Pelvic binders are emergency interventions and must be applied correctly. Continuous monitoring is essential to prevent skin breakdown or pressure ulcers.

In resource-limited settings, these simple stabilization measures by trauma team members or PCPs can buy critical time before transfer to a trauma center.

Definitive Management
Pelvic hemorrhage may require:

- Angiographic embolization of bleeding vessels
- Preperitoneal pelvic packing or bilateral internal iliac artery ligation when angioembolization is delayed or unavailable (Fig. 10.4).

  Management often requires coordination among:

- Trauma surgeons
- Orthopedic specialists
- Vascular and interventional radiologists

Referral
Early referral to a higher-level facility is essential for:

- Hemodynamically unstable patients
- Those with associated solid organ injuries

Nonoperative vs. Operative Management
Most pediatric pelvic fractures are managed conservatively due to the child's natural capacity for bone remodeling. However, surgical fixation is indicated in:

1. Displaced or unstable fractures
2. Cases requiring improved rehabilitation or nursing care

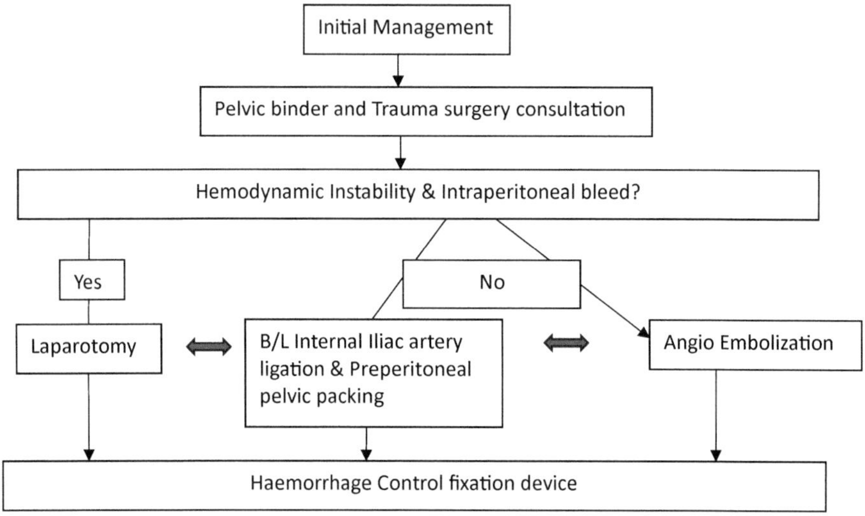

Fig. 10.4 Management algorithm of pelvic fracture

Discharge Counseling and Home Care

1. *Medications*:
   - Provide clear instructions on prescribed analgesics, including dosage and timing.
   - Advise caregivers to monitor for side effects like nausea, dizziness, or allergic reactions.
2. *Activity and Rest*:
   - Enforce rest during the initial recovery phase.
   - Gradually return to daily activities based on physician guidance and injury severity.
   - Avoid strenuous play or contact sports during recovery.
3. *Nutrition and Fluids*:
   - Promote a balanced diet to support healing.
   - Modify the diet if the child has digestive organ injuries or postsurgical limitations.
   - Maintain adequate hydration, especially after blood loss or surgery.
4. *Wound Care*:
   - Instruct parents on incision care, signs of infection, and dressing changes.
   - Prevent infection by discouraging scratching or touching the wound site.
5. *Warning Signs Requiring Urgent Attention*:
   - Increasing abdominal pain or distension
   - Bloody or tarry stools
   - Persistent vomiting
   - Breathing difficulty or chest pain
   - High fever (>38.3 °C)
   - Urinary problems or hematuria
   - Severe lethargy, fainting, or signs of shock

Case Resolution

Upon Khushi's arrival at the emergency department, the primary assessment begins with the ABCDE approach. She is alert and verbal, indicating her airway is patent (A – Airway), but her respiratory rate of 48 per min and SpO_2 of 91% despite supplemental oxygen suggests respiratory compromise (B – Breathing). The non-rebreather mask is continued, and chest rise is evaluated to rule out thoracoabdominal injury. Auscultation confirms bilateral air entry without added sounds.

Next, the focus shifts to circulation (C). Khushi's tachycardia (HR 135 bpm) and delayed capillary refill (3 s) raise concern for early compensated shock, possibly due to intra-abdominal bleeding. Blood pressure (110/70 mmHg) appears normal but is not reassuring in children—normotension may persist until late decompensation. Two large-bore IV lines are secured, and blood is drawn for initial labs including complete blood count, lactate, blood grouping, coagulation profile, and liver enzymes. Warmed isotonic fluid bolus (20 ml/kg) is initiated to maintain perfusion.

On disability (D) assessment, she remains responsive with no focal neurologic deficits. Her exposure (E) reveals no external wounds, but abdominal guarding in the left lower quadrant suggests peritoneal irritation, possibly from splenic or bowel injury.

Given these findings, Khushi's signs—tachypnea, tachycardia, abdominal pain with guarding, and delayed CRT—strongly suggest internal bleeding or hollow viscus injury. Pelvic fracture is also a differential, although no instability is felt on gentle compression.

Immediate stabilization continues with close monitoring, keeping the child warm, oxygenated, and hydrated. Analgesia is provided using IV paracetamol, carefully titrated to manage pain without masking peritonitis signs. A Foley catheter is deferred pending abdominal ultrasound due to risk of urethral injury in pelvic trauma.

Imaging decisions are guided by resource availability and hemodynamic status. A bedside Focused Assessment with Sonography in Trauma (FAST) is performed to evaluate for free fluid in the peritoneum—a surrogate for internal bleeding. Although its sensitivity is limited, it is a rapid, noninvasive screening tool ideal for this setting. Given Khushi's borderline stability, a CECT abdomen and pelvis is subsequently planned to define the injury extent, provided she remains hemodynamically responsive. An abdominal X-ray is obtained to screen for free air (suggesting hollow viscus perforation), though it is less sensitive.

Throughout this process, primary care providers play a vital supportive role: establishing IV access, communicating vital trends to the team, anticipating needs like blood crossmatch, preparing resuscitation equipment, and maintaining closed-loop communication. The PCP may assist with urinary catheterization once urethral integrity is confirmed and coordinate with surgical and radiology teams for expedited imaging and consultation.

Khushi's case highlights how early recognition, vigilant monitoring, and coordi nated teamwork led by PCPs can stabilize a pediatric trauma patient and facilitate timely referral or surgical intervention when needed.

Key Messages

- Early recognition of internal injuries in pediatric abdominal and pelvic trauma is essential as external signs may be minimal or absent.
- The ABCDE approach must be systematically applied to all pediatric trauma patients to promptly identify and manage life-threatening conditions.
- Vital signs such as tachycardia, tachypnea, and prolonged capillary refill time may be early indicators of compensated shock in children, often preceding hypotension.
- Focused Assessment with Sonography for Trauma (FAST) is a useful, rapid bedside tool to detect free fluid and guide initial decision-making, though it has limited sensitivity.
- Contrast-enhanced CT scan is the diagnostic modality of choice in hemodynamically stable children for evaluating and grading internal organ injuries.
- Most blunt abdominal injuries involving the spleen, liver, and kidneys in children can be managed nonoperatively with close monitoring and supportive care.
- Primary care providers are crucial members of the trauma team, assisting with IV access, airway support, analgesia, vitals monitoring, documentation, and communication.
- Children showing signs of peritonitis, ongoing bleeding, or hemodynamic instability should be stabilized quickly and referred to higher centers for definitive management.
- Radiation exposure must be minimized in pediatric patients using the ALARA (as low as reasonably achievable) principle, especially when selecting imaging modalities.
- Clear, empathetic communication with caregivers is an essential part of holistic trauma care, helping families understand the situation and preparing them for further treatment or transfer.

Bibliography

1. Bartscherer A, Hsiao A, Fishman J, et al. Management of pelvic fractures in children. *Pediatr Emerg Care.* 2006;22(7):448–452. https://doi.org/10.1097/01.pec.0000222482.44213.88.
2. Holmes JF, Lillis K, Monroe D, Borgialli D, Kerrey BT, Mahajan P, et al. Identifying children at very low risk of clinically important blunt abdominal injuries. Ann Emerg Med.2013; 62 (2):107–16.e2.
3. Jain S, Srivastava A, Mishra M, et al. Non-operative management of pediatric abdominal trauma. *J Indian Assoc Pediatr Surg.* 2009;14(1):6–10. https://doi.org/10.4103/0971-9261.51876.
4. Khan MA, Jawad SA, Malik AM. Blunt abdominal trauma in children: review of 3,000 cases in a pediatric trauma center. *PediatrSurg Int.* 2010;26(5):531–537. https://doi.org/10.1007/s00383-010-2664-x.
5. Lefebvre G, Hélie R, Cousineau J, et al. Pelvic fractures in children: review of 10 years' experience. *J PediatrOrthop.* 1999;19(4):457–463. https://doi.org/10.1097/01241398-199907000-00007.
6. Linnaus ME, Notrica DM, Langlias CS, St. Peter SD, Leys CM, Ostle DJ et al. Prospective validation of the shock index pediatric adjusted (SIPA) in blunt liver and spleen trauma: An ATOMAC+ STUDY. *J Pediatr Surg.*2017;52(2):340–4.

7. McDermott FT, Griffiths D, Beattie A, et al. Blunt abdominal trauma in children: a review of 131 cases. *PediatrSurg Int.* 1999;15(6):437–441. https://doi.org/10.1007/s003830050456.
8. Miller PR, Hoth JJ, Croce MA, et al. Impact of age on the outcome of pediatric abdominal trauma. *J Trauma.* 2001;51(5):930–936. https://doi.org/10.1097/00005373-200111000-00005.
9. Neha Thakur, Samir Misra. Pediatric Trauma Resuscitation Module (PTRM). First edition. New Delhi: Jaypee Brothers Medical Publishers (P) Ltd; 2024. p. 23–39
10. Rehn M, Jeppsson A, Ljungström L, et al. Pediatric blunt abdominal trauma: a population-based study. *J Pediatr Surg.* 2011;46(3):485–490. https://doi.org/10.1016/j.jpedsurg.2010.12.034.
11. Schroeder AR, Shapiro RA, Feldman KW, et al. Pediatric pelvic fractures: diagnosis, management, and outcomes. *J Trauma.* 2009;67(5):1160–1165. https://doi.org/10.1097/TA.0b013e3181b08442.
12. Sullivan T, Stewart B, Battersby T, et al. Pediatric abdominal trauma: an analysis of 4,000 injuries in children. *Ann Surg.* 2001;233(5):602–608. https://doi.org/10.1097/00000658-200105000-00005.
13. Taylor GA, Allen LM, O'Connor AR. Imaging of pediatric abdominal and pelvic trauma. *PediatrRadiol.* 2009;39(9):919–930. https://doi.org/10.1007/s00247-009-1234-x.
14. Wegner S, Colletti JE, Van Wie D. Paediatric blunt abdominal trauma. Pediatr Clin North Am.2006; 53:243–56.

Pediatric Spinal Trauma

11

A. Priscillal Devakirubai, Aravind Anand,
and Chetan Ginigeri

Learning Objectives

By the end of this chapter, the reader should be able to:

1. Identify the differences between adult and pediatric spinal columns and understand the common modes and mechanisms of injury in children.
2. Identify the sequence in primary and secondary surveys in case of pediatric spinal trauma.
3. Demonstrate the steps involved in C spine (Cervical spine) restriction and spinal immobilization while caring for a pediatric trauma patient.
4. Understand principles of management in pediatric spinal injuries.
5. Apply patient and family-centered approach to management of pediatric spinal injuries, especially regarding long-term care, rehabilitation, and psychological concerns.

A. Priscillal Devakirubai
OBG Nursing Department, St John's College of Nursing, St John's National Academy of Health Sciences, Bangalore, Karnataka, India

A. Anand
Rainbow Children's Hospital, Hebbal, Bangalore, Karnataka, India

C. Ginigeri (✉)
Pediatrics and PICU, Manipal Hospitals, Bangalore, Karnataka, India

N. T. Rai (ed.), *Pediatric Trauma Resuscitation Manual (PTRM) for Primary Care Providers*, https://doi.org/10.1007/978-981-95-4979-5_11

Introduction

Spinal injuries in the pediatric population are relatively rare but carry the potential for significant morbidity and long-term disability. Unlike adults, children have a developing musculoskeletal and nervous system, which makes their injury patterns, physiological responses, and recovery trajectories distinctly different. Their larger head-to-body ratio, ligamentous laxity, flexible spinal columns, and immature vertebrae make them more susceptible to specific types of spinal trauma—particularly upper cervical spine injuries and spinal cord injury without radiographic abnormality (SCIWORA).

The mechanism of injury plays a pivotal role in determining both the type and extent of spinal trauma. High-energy mechanisms such as motor vehicle collisions, falls from height, diving accidents, and non-accidental trauma are often responsible. These incidents may lead to isolated spinal fractures, spinal cord compression, or multisystem trauma, especially in younger children.

Understanding these differences is essential for primary care providers (PCPs), who are frequently the first point of contact in both prehospital and emergency care settings. PCPs must recognize that children with spinal injuries may present subtly—complaining of neck pain, refusing to walk, or displaying only vague neurological symptoms. Early identification, spinal immobilization, and initiation of trauma protocols are critical to prevent secondary injury.

A structured, multidisciplinary approach incorporating repeated primary and secondary surveys, strict spinal precautions, and appropriate imaging facilitates early diagnosis and intervention. PCPs also play a key role in family communication, offering support, education, and reassurance during a highly stressful period.

Ultimately, timely action by frontline providers, especially in resource-limited or rural settings, can drastically alter outcomes. This chapter outlines the anatomy, pathophysiology, mechanisms, and primary management principles of pediatric spinal trauma, equipping PCPs with the tools necessary to act swiftly, safely, and confidently when faced with these challenging cases.

Case Scenario

Aaron, a 4-year-old boy, is being brought to the emergency department by his father after having been hit by a high-speed motor vehicle at 60 km/h and thrown off by the impact, while playing near his house. The child has a laceration in the left frontal scalp and contusions over the chest and abdomen. On arrival, he responded only to painful stimuli, screamed intermittently, and did not open his eyes.

Vital Signs

Respiratory rate (RR): 40 breaths per minute
Oxygen saturation (SaO_2): 85%
Heart rate (HR): 130 beats per minute
Capillary refill: 3 s
Blood pressure (BP): 90/70 mmHg

Reflective Questions

1. What are the potential injuries in this case?
2. What is the mental status on arrival?
3. What are the implications of the vital signs recorded?
4. What diagnostic tests or imaging would be helpful in this situation?
5. How would you assist physicians in airway management and restriction of c-spine motion?

Patterns of Pediatric Spinal Injuries

Spinal injuries are uncommon in pediatric trauma, and presentation varies with age and mechanism of injury. Among pediatric spinal injuries, cervical and thoracolumbar involvement is more common. A common mode of spinal injury in infants and older children is fall from height. Other causes include motor vehicle accidents, sports injuries, and non-accidental trauma. Boys are three times more likely to be affected than girls. Children with spinal injuries have a good potential for recovery, particularly if associated neurological injuries are identified and treated in a timely and appropriate manner. Spinal injuries in children rarely happen alone and often have associated head injuries, chest injuries, or injuries to other internal organs. Among the pure forms of traumatic spinal injury, that is, spinal injury without associated bone involvement, the most common type is spinal cord injury without radiographic abnormality or SCIWORA.

Causes of Pediatric Spinal Injuries

Among the most frequent causes are falls, particularly from heights such as staircases, rooftops, playground equipment, or trees. Younger children are especially vulnerable due to their lack of coordination and underdeveloped motor skills.

Motor vehicle accidents (MVAs) represent another leading cause, especially when appropriate safety restraints like car seats or seatbelts are not used correctly. Children struck as pedestrians or those ejected during collisions are at particularly high risk for severe spinal trauma.

Sports injuries contribute to spinal trauma in older children and adolescents, particularly in contact sports such as football, wrestling, gymnastics, and diving. Hyperextension or axial loading forces during athletic activities can lead to vertebral fractures or spinal cord injury.

Finally, non-accidental trauma (NAT)—also referred to as intentional injury or child abuse—must always be considered, especially in infants and toddlers presenting with unexplained neurological signs or spinal fractures. These cases require a high index of suspicion and careful multidisciplinary evaluation, as early detection is vital for both medical and legal protection of the child.

Understanding the underlying cause of spinal injury not only aids in diagnosis but also guides preventive strategies and targeted education for caregivers and communities.

Anatomical and Physical Considerations

The gross anatomy of the spinal column in adults and children is similar; however, there are notable changes that occur from infancy to adolescence.

- Big head: Young children have relatively larger heads compared to their bodies. This makes them more prone to neck injuries.
- Flexible spine: Children's spines are more flexible than adults' because their ligaments (tissues that connect bones) are more elastic. This means the spine can stretch more, potentially damaging the spinal cord.
- Different fulcrum: In young children, the upper part of the neck (C2–C3) is the point where the spine bends the most. This area is more vulnerable to injury. In older children and adults, this point is lower down in the neck (C5–C6).
- Due to the larger head size in children, the angular momentum is greater, and the fulcrum is higher, leading to maximum injuries between the occiput and C3. Greater force is needed to affect the neck in children.
- Presence of growth plates may lead to unique injuries especially in extremity involvement.

Sciwora

SCIWORA is a condition where a child has spinal cord damage, but X-rays and CT scans do not show any broken bones or dislocations. It is more common in children under 8 years of age and in sports-related injuries. The flexibility of a child's spine while allowing a greater force to pass through the spinal column without the risk of tearing, also results in an increased risk of SCIWORA and other unusual presentations.

Neurological Problems

About half of the children with spinal injuries will have neurological problems. These can range from mild symptoms like pain and muscle spasms to severe problems like paralysis. Sometimes, the child may go into "spinal shock," where they lose muscle tone and reflexes. They may also have low blood pressure (hypotension) and a slow heart rate (bradycardia). Injuries in the neck area are more likely to cause permanent damage and can be life-threatening. A complete spinal injury means there is no movement or sensation below the level of the injury, resulting in permanent damage.

Bone Injuries

Broken bones in the spine are more common in teenagers. These fractures can occur due to excessive bending or straightening of the spine. Sometimes, the bones can also dislocate (move out of place). It's important to remember that children's X-rays can look different from adults' because their bones are still growing. Normal growth plates can sometimes be mistaken for fractures.

Mechanisms of Pediatric Spinal Injuries

Following trauma, spinal cord injury can result from compression (by surrounding vertebrae or discs), distraction (pulling the vertebrae apart), rotation (excessive twisting of the spine), hyperflexion (excessive forward bending of the spinal column), or hyperextension (excessive backward bending of the spinal column). Figure 11.1 shows these mechanisms.

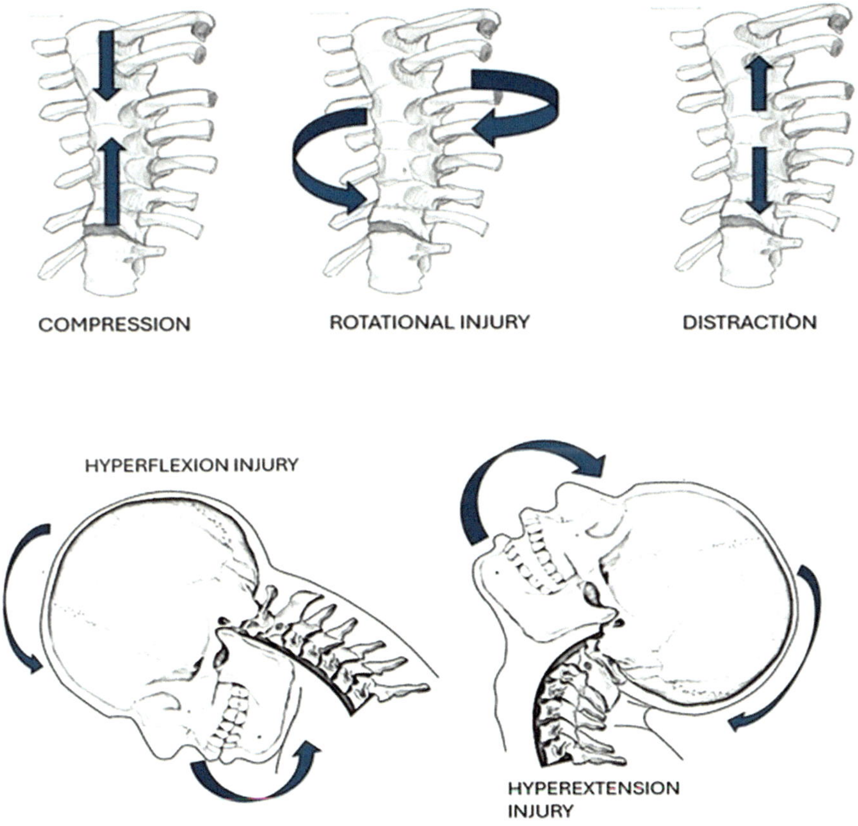

Fig. 11.1 Important mechanisms of spinal cord injury

Flexion-distraction injuries (FDI) of the spine are caused by a forward flexion of the torso with the abdomen or thorax as the fulcrum. FDI are frequently associated with seat belts which act as the anterior restraint, particularly if the shoulder strap is not properly positioned.

The affected spinal column may demonstrate contusion, compression, laceration, transection, hemorrhage/hematoma, and infarction which result in neurological injuries.

Clinical Features of Pediatric Spinal Injuries

Signs and symptoms differ widely and depend on mechanism of injury, neurological involvement, and site or organ involved.

- Pain may be generalized or may be localized in relation to skeletal injuries.
- Neck pain may be manifest in cervical spinal injuries.
- Limitation of movement of affected site or region.
- Worsening of pain on movement may indicate neurological involvement.
- Muscle weakness/spasm.
- Neurological signs are based on the level of spinal involvement and include breathing difficulty; difficulty in feeling, moving or controlling the legs and arms and bladder and bowel dysfunction. Persistent headache or loss of consciousness indicates brain involvement.
- SCIWORA is characterized by clinical signs of spinal cord injury in the absence of radiographic or CT findings of spinal fractures or instability. Symptoms may include numbness, weakness, abnormal reflexes, or loss of bladder or bowel control, along with neck or back pain.
- Spinal shock—loss of muscle tone and reflexes which may last up to 6 weeks can be seen when cervical or upper thoracic spinal cord is involved.
- Neurogenic shock—hypotension and bradycardia due to loss of vasomotor tone especially seen in cervical and thoracic vertebrae.
- Vascular injury—particularly in extremity injuries, arterial pulses should be monitored to assess for integrity of circulation and early recognition of compartment syndrome.

Management of Pediatric Spinal Injuries

The key principles of managing spinal injuries in children are as follows:

- *Systematic Approach*: Use the ABCDE approach (airway, breathing, circulation, disability, exposure) of primary survey to identify and treat life-threatening injuries quickly. Figure 11.2 highlights the flow of events during pediatric trauma resuscitation.
- *High-Risk Factors*: Be aware of the factors that make a child more likely to have a spinal injury. Recognize high-risk mechanisms of injury with increased chances of morbidity.

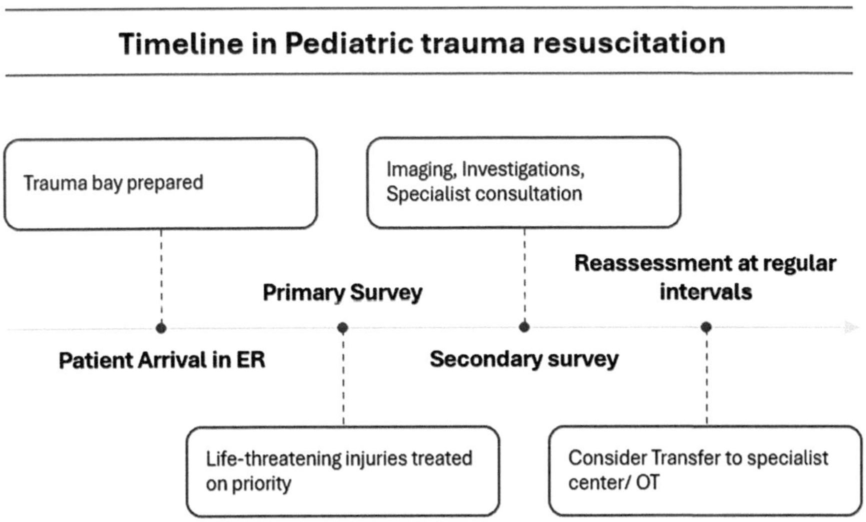

Fig. 11.2 Timeline for events in pediatric trauma resuscitation

- *Decision-Making Tools*: Use guidelines to decide when to restrict neck movement, such as the Pediatric Emergency Care Applied Research Network (PECARN) cervical spine clearance tool, and for ordering imaging tests.
- *Regular Assessments*: Monitor the child closely and document any changes in their condition.
- *Early Consultation*: Consult with a spine surgeon or neurosurgeon as soon as possible if you suspect a spinal injury.
- *Appropriate Imaging*: Get the right scans (X-rays, CT scans, MRI) to identify the type and extent of the injury after the child is stable.
- *Pain Management*: Regular assessment by validated pain scores such as FLACC scores with appropriate measures for alleviating pain should be done.
- *Nutritional Management*: Emphasis should be on early initiation of enteral feeding, and diet plans should be made in consultation with medical and dietetic teams.

Primary Survey

The initial assessment in children with spine injuries includes two steps:

1. The primary survey (ABCDE)
2. Mental status assessment using AVPU/GCS

The initial assessment of the child with suspected spinal injury should follow ABCDE protocol like any other trauma case, before assessing for the neurological deficits. Figure 11.3 shows key elements of primary survey and important priorities. Life-threatening injuries should be prioritized and treated. Neurological status assessment is to be consistent and repeated to detect early changes and initiate treatment measures. The application of ABCDE protocol is elaborated through the clinical scenario in subsequent sections.

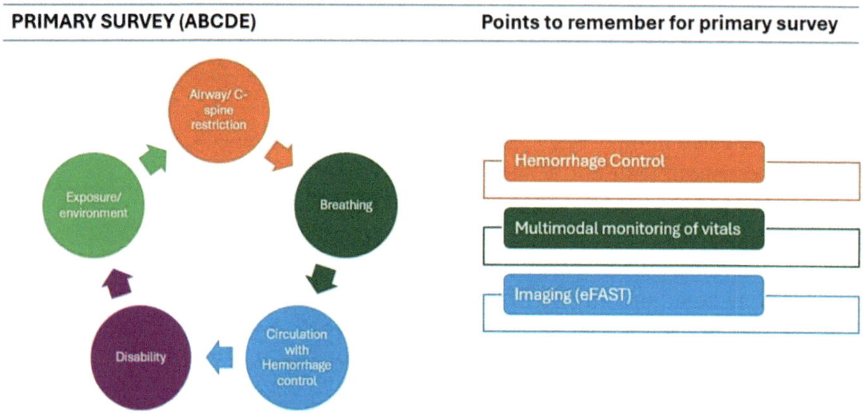

Fig. 11.3 Primary survey by ABCDE approach and key points in primary survey

AVPU Score

As in adults, a rapid initial assessment of an infant's or child's consciousness level can be made using the AVPU score. This method is particularly useful for pre-hospital and emergency room settings. Patients are assessed as alert (A), responding to voice (V), responding to pain (P), or unresponsive (U). Children assessed as P or U will have a GCS score of ≤8.

GCS, Glasgow Coma Scale or Its Modifications

Three parameters observed are the BEST eye-opening, verbal response, and motor response. Painful stimuli response can be elicited by Trapezius squeeze or supraorbital pressure; the procedure should be appropriately explained to parent/guardian and consent taken. Modified score is used in infants and children and intubated patients. In general, a score of ≤12 indicates likely traumatic brain injury, and a score ≤8 suggests the possible need for intubation as well as the need for intracranial pressure monitoring.

High-Risk Factors

Certain factors which increase the risk of mortality and morbidity are identified from history, clinical examination, or investigations and help to guide urgency of treatment and for explaining prognosis. Some of the highrisk factors associated with cervical spine injury in children are mentioned below:

- Altered mental status/associated severe traumatic brain injury
- Focal neurological deficit
- Neck pain in children above the age of 2 years

- Reduced mobility of the neck
- Respiratory distress and intubation
- Hypotension at presentation
- Other visceral involvement: chest, abdominal, or pelvic injuries
- Injury sustained during diving (sports)
- Complete cord injury at presentation

Investigations

The aims of investigations are to identify life-threatening conditions, obtain c-spine clearance, identify non-life-threatening injuries, and monitor response to treatment. These may include the following:

- Blood tests: such as CBC, blood grouping and typing, and blood gas analysis.
- Plain X-ray: as indicated by clinical examination including cervical spine, thorax and/or abdominal X-rays.
- Spine X-ray/CT scan can be used for cervical spine clearance. A diagnostic algorithm such as Pediatric Emergency Care Applied Research Network (PECARN) as shown in Table 11.1 can be used to decide on the type of imaging.
- MRI.
- USG including FAST protocol.

Important points to remember when requesting imaging tests

- Plain radiographs to be done in all patients with suspected cervical spinal injuries, awaiting c-spine clearance by other tests or by neurosurgeon.
- Bedside USG with FAST or extended FAST protocol should be done to identify visceral injuries and monitor cardiac function or need for emergency interventions.
- CT should be done in all patients with altered consciousness and if bony injuries such as atlanto-occipital dislocation or upper cervical bony injuries are suspected.
- MRI spine is a better modality for younger children and in cases of SCIWORA.
- If any new neurological injuries are noted during reassessment, appropriate repeat imaging should be done.

Table 11.1 PECARN C-spine injury risk factor-based decision for imaging

Indications for CT	Indications for X-rays
GCS 3–8 or AVPU = U	GCS 9–14, AVPU = V or P or other signs of altered mental status
Abnormal airway, breathing, or circulation	Self reported neck pain or neck tenderness on examination
Focal neurologic deficits	Substantial head or torso injury (those needing inpatient observations or surgical interventions)

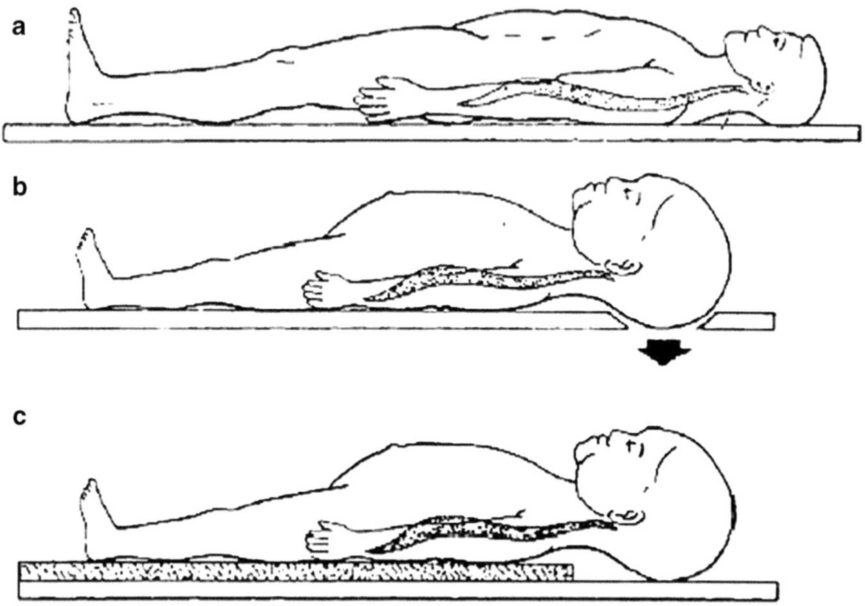

Fig. 11.4 Spine board. (**a**) Standard spine board for adults. (**b**) Backboard modifications for children with occipital recess. (**c**) Backboard with an additional padding placed from below the chest for support

Special Considerations

Modified backboard in children can be used as shown in Fig. 11.4, to accommodate for large occiput in younger children and infants; or a backboard with a double-thickness pad for the body, placed from under the shoulder may be used.

Airway maintenance with restriction of cervical spine motion:

- Airway is to be maintained using airway adjuncts or definitive airway as clinically indicated.
- Assessment: Assess the child's level of consciousness and airway grade, and check for any vomit us or blood in the mouth. Suction such content where indicated to keep the airway clear.
- Definitive Airway: A breathing tube (endotracheal tube), emergency tracheostomy, or adjuncts such as laryngeal mask airway may need to be inserted if the child is unable to protect their airway.
- C-spine must be immobilized from the point of trauma until the clearance is obtained.

Rigid spine board and logrolling: Maintain immobilization using a rigid spine board and logrolling technique to keep the spine aligned during transfers and assessments. Use padding to prevent pressure sores if the child needs to be on the spine board for a long time.

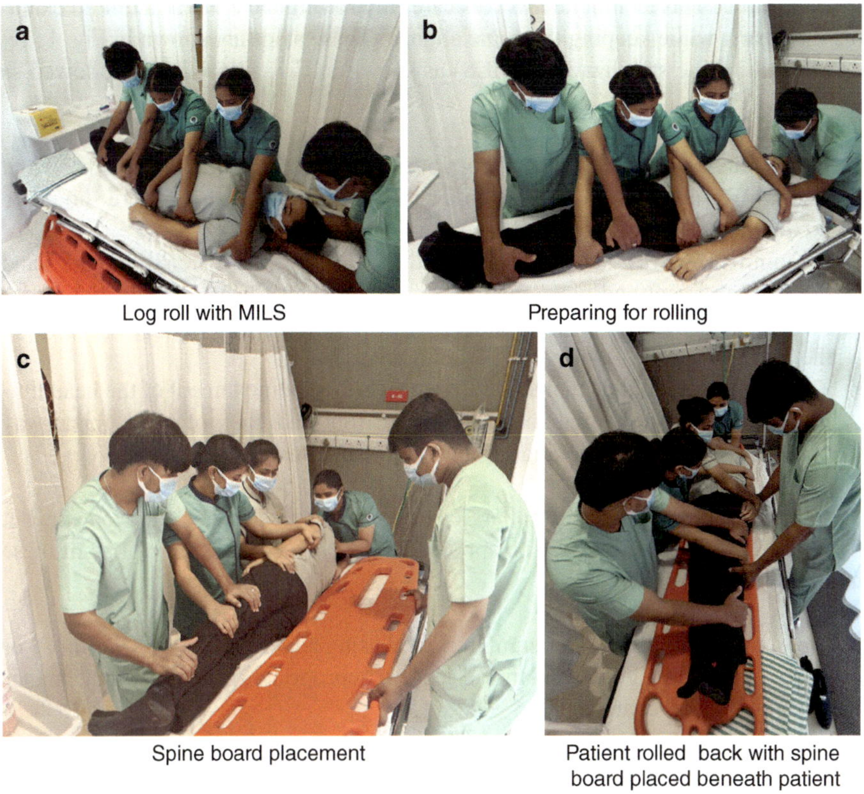

Fig. 11.5 Medical team demonstrating a log roll maneuver with MILS (Manual In-Line Stabilization)

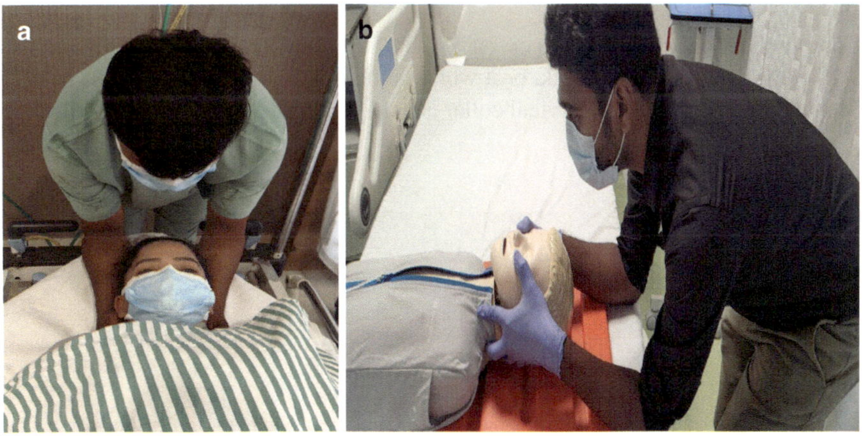

Fig. 11.6 (**a**, **b**) Manual inline stabilization technique

Logrolling: This technique involves carefully rolling the child as a unit to examine their back while keeping the spine aligned. These steps are shown in Fig. 11.5.

Manual in-line stabilization (MILS) as shown in Fig. 11.6 is to be followed as indicated.

- Healthcare professional stands behind the patient to hold the patient's head and neck firmly, ensuring the neck is in a neutral, midline position. There should be no traction to the head or neck.
- If definitive airway needs to be placed, healthcare professional should stand beside the patient and place their hands on the sides of the patient's head with their forearms resting on the patient's chest, thus not obstructing the view of the airway.
- This position should be maintained, with side-to-side movement of the head limited, to allow for examination of both the front and back of neck; for airway procedures such as suctioning; or intubation; and during logroll.

Cervical Collars: Cervical collars can prevent excessive neck movement, but they should be used carefully. The appropriate size can be assessed by one of these methods.

- Measure the child's neck circumference by using a measuring tape (Fig. 11.7) or finger lengths as a guide, and then select the appropriate size based on the manufacturer's sizing chart.
- Chin-to-shoulder length: distance from the bottom of the chin to the top of the shoulder by using finger lengths (Fig. 11.8) and then using the collar manufacturer's pediatric cervical collar sizing chart.

Once the collar is applied, the neck should not be overextended, and the patient (if fully conscious) should not be able to fully open their mouth.

Contraindications: Don't use a cervical collar if the child has a fixed neck deformity, there is swelling in the neck, or it worsens their neurological symptoms.

Manual Stabilization: If a cervical collar is not appropriate, continue to stabilize the head and neck manually.

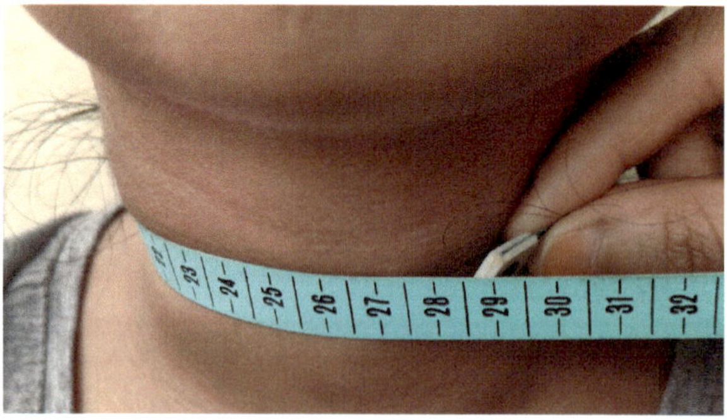

Fig. 11.7 Measurement of neck circumference using a tape measure

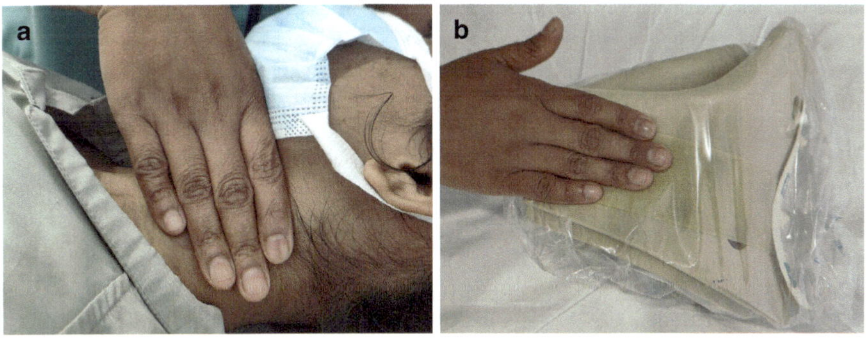

Fig. 11.8 (**a**, **b**) Measurement of chin-to-shoulder length and selection of cervical collar

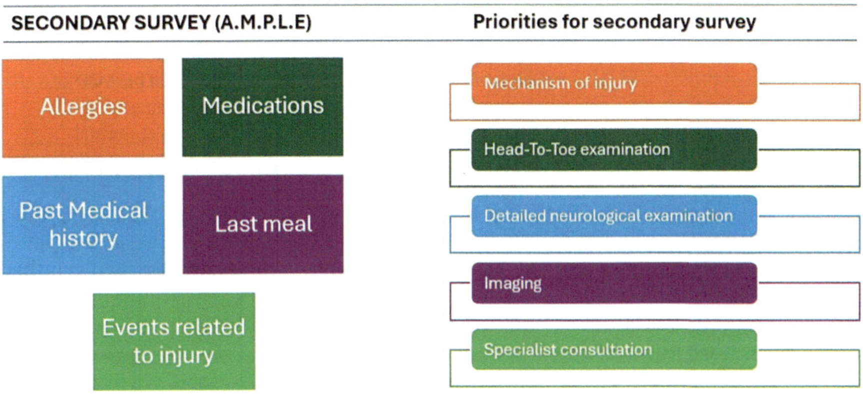

Fig. 11.9 Secondary survey

Secondary Survey

Once the immediate life-threatening problems are addressed, perform a thorough secondary survey using SAMPLE template. The aim is to identify non-life-threatening injuries, which will impact outcomes and cause morbidity. These aspects are presented in Fig. 11.9. While performing secondary survey, vital parameters and mental status need to be continuously monitored. If there is deterioration in vital parameters or mental status, immediate attention must be given to manage these new findings.

- *Secondary survey* in spinal injuries should be performed as indicated in Table 11.2, with emphasis on thorough history and examination. The PCPs' responsibilities for each step are highlighted.

Table 11.2 Secondary survey and PCPs' responsibility

Secondary survey	Assessment	Actions	PCPs' responsibility
History	*A*—Allergies *M*—Medications *P*—Past medical history *L*—Last meal *E*—Events leading to injury	Obtain focused history from a reliable source- child/parents/guardians/pre-hospital team	Collect and document the collected history using AMPLE format Communicate while transferring the child using ISBAR tool
Head examination	Size, shape, lacerations, contusions, fractures, Battle sign, Raccoon eyes, CSF leak	Inspect and palpate the head for the same Assess the signs of basilar skull fracture (Battle sign, Raccoon eyes, CSF leak)	Ensure cervical and spinal immobilization as per the pediatric age group recommendation Document the findings
Eye examination	Pupillary assessment	Assess the pupil for PERRLA—pupils equal, round, reacting to light, and accommodative	Document the assessment Perform periodic assessment Report abnormal findings immediately
Neck and cervical spine	Tenderness, deformities, tracheal deviation, jugular vein distension	Restrict cervical spine motion Check for airway compromise	Choose appropriate size of collar and apply Assess the airway and breathing
Chest examination	Use look, listen, and feel method	Assess for abrasions, bruises, cuts and cyanosis, dents, deformity, edema, fractures, equal chest wall rise, bilateral air entry by 5-point auscultation, lacerations, crepitus, rib fractures	Report abnormal findings immediately, e.g. if Chest wall rise is unequal Abnormal breath sounds heard Ensure proper oxygen support is established
Abdominal examination	Inspection and palpation, auscultation FAST as indicated	Observe for distension, bruising, tenderness, guarding Bowel sounds	Keep the child Nil per oral Periodic monitoring needed to note the changes Nasogastric tube can be inserted as a measure for gastric decompression

(continued)

Table 11.2 (continued)

Secondary survey	Assessment	Actions	PCPs' responsibility
Pelvis examination	Inspection and palpation, pelvic compression test	Observe bruising, tenderness, pelvis stable or not Note the color of the urine	Use pelvic binder Catheterize the bladder if there is no blood in the urethral meatus
Extremities examination	Inspection and palpation	Assess for abrasions, bruises, cuts and cyanosis, dents, deformity, edema, fractures	Check peripheral pulses, immobilize fractures Document findings
Back examination	Inspection and palpation	Log roll with adequate manpower Observe for abrasions, bruises, cuts and cyanosis, dents, deformity, edema, or fractures	Maintain spine alignment during log roll Document findings

- *Repeated assessment*: The primary and secondary surveys should be performed repeatedly to identify any change in the patient's status that indicates the need for additional intervention. Priority should be given to life-threatening injuries, and survey is to be completed after attending to such injuries.

Treatment Considerations

Priorities for treatment include the following:

- Identify and immediately address life-threatening injuries by systematic ABCDE approach in primary survey.
- Monitor vitals—target appropriate BP; large volume fluid resuscitation to be avoided. Include continuous ECG monitoring, pulse oximetry, and blood gases.
- Management should consist of a rapid primary survey with simultaneous resuscitation of vital functions. Use bedside tools such as USG (FAST) to guide interventions.
- Appropriate wide-bore venous access should be secured; alternatively, interosseous access should be secured for emergency treatment.
- Early identification of rapid or large volume bleeding, and initiate prompt control measures—immobilization, tourniquet application, and surgical intervention. Replace losses with appropriate blood or blood products. If necessary, early activation of massive hemorrhage protocol must be done.
- Prevent and treat: hypothermia, acidosis, and hypocalcemia.
- Initial non-operative management can be done for children with stable injuries.
- Operative management is indicated in the presence of unstable injuries. Early referrals to orthopedics, neurology, and neurosurgery must be considered. Seek early specialist opinion to clear spinal injuries and in cases of altered mental status.

- Consider the need for patient transfer to specialist center such as in burns or polytrauma; use a structured handover template (ISBAR) to convey information to the referral hospital.
- Continue post-resuscitation monitoring and re-evaluation until transfer to ICU/ OT.

Patient and Family Education

Pediatric spinal injuries place an enormous burden on the patient and their families. Patients may experience an altered perception of body image, have negative emotions besides burdening the families' economic security, and place a strain on personal relationships. Depression and anxiety are seen more often in these patients and their families. Involving the family to understand the nature and extent of injury including possible complications, by encouraging them to ask questions and clarify doubts or concerns, helps in better outcomes. Families can also be involved in the care of patients through joint decision-making for treatment and rehabilitation. A multidisciplinary team approach to management involving nurses, doctors, rehabilitative therapists, psychologists, dieticians, etc. should be emphasized and explained to the family of affected children. Information may be provided directly or through videos, leaflets, and other written content. Possibility of medical emergencies after discharge and protocol for management should be discussed. It is important to encourage the patient/family to reinforce emotional support from friends, relatives, or other support groups.

Prognosis

In general, children with spinal injuries tend to recover better than adults. The likelihood of complete recovery from neurological deficits increases with appropriate and timely management. If an MRI scan doesn't show any major damage to the spinal cord, the child is likely to have a good recovery. However, if there is damage to the blood vessels supplying the spinal cord, the child may have permanent problems. Sometimes, spinal injuries can be missed in the initial assessment, especially if there are multiple injuries in different areas of the spine. Suspicion for spinal cord injury is important in all multiple trauma cases. After initial stabilization, a detailed secondary survey with neurological examination and radiological evaluation is recommended in all cases suspected to have spinal injury. The prognosis also largely depends on associated injuries especially neurological injuries.

Case Resolution

Aaron, a 4-year-old boy, is being brought to the emergency department by his father after having been hit by a high-speed motor vehicle at 60 km/h and thrown off by the impact, while playing near his house. The child has a laceration in the left frontal scalp and contusions over the chest and abdomen. On arrival, he responded only to painful stimuli, screamed intermittently, and did not open his eyes.

Respiratory rate (RR): 40 breaths per minute
Oxygen saturation (SaO_2): 85%
Heart rate (HR): 130 beats per minute
Capillary refill: 3 s
Blood pressure (BP): 90/70 mmHg

Table 11.3 The immediate questions to be answered

Question	Findings
What are the potential injuries in this case?	Head injury, cervical spine and spinal cord injury, chest and abdominal injuries involving the internal organs, long bone fractures
What is the mental status on arrival?	*AVPU* on arrival—P (responded to painful stimuli) GCS on arrival 8 (E-1, V-3, M-4)
Are the vital signs normal for this age?	*Vital signs*: Pulse 130; BP 90/70; RR 40; CFT 3 s; saturation in room air 85% *Impression*: Tachycardia, hypotension and varying respiratory rate, low saturation
What diagnostic tests or imaging would be helpful in this situation?	Blood tests Imaging for c-spine clearance E-FAST Imaging for injuries: external and internal
How do you assist physicians in airway management and restriction of c spine motion?	Maintain MILS (manual inline stabilization), cervical collar application until c-spine clearance and airway status clear

Table 11.4 Primary survey and PCPs' responsibility

Primary survey	Assessment	Interventions	PCP's responsibility in trauma unit
Airway with c-spine restriction	AVPU—P (respond to painful stimuli), GCS—8/15 Check for patency/ secretions Need for definitive airway identified Impression: airway compromise with altered mental status	Make sure the airway is open and clear. Use techniques to open the airway while protecting the neck Suctioning Pre-oxygenation with 100% O_2 using BVM (bag valve mask) Drug-assisted intubation (DAI) done by emergency physician Gastric tube inserted to prevent gastric distention Perform neuro assessment prior to DAI—AVPU and GCS	Keep the unit ready with emergency pediatric equipment Provide manual inline stabilization (MILS), or apply cervical collar until c-spine clearance is obtained from trauma or neurosurgeon Suctioning equipment to be kept ready Keep medications for sedation, paralysis, and resuscitation loaded and ready Assist in BVM and intubation, and initiate mechanical ventilation Use length-based resuscitation tape to choose the correct size of equipment and for calculation of drugs
Breathing with ventilation	Assess rate, depth, and effort of breathing—left side of the chest hyper-extended and inflated, sluggish and unequal movement Auscultation—air entry inadequate, absent breath sounds left side of chest SPO_2—85% Impression: left pneumothorax	Needle decompression followed by chest tube insertion done in the left side of the chest Reassessment—chest wall movement is equal on both sides with adequate ventilation HR—reduced to 100/mt	Assist in needle decompression and chest tube insertion with needle size 14–18 G Site and preparation of the part—2nd intercostal space mid-clavicular line for needle decompression and 4th or 5th intercostal space along the mid- or anterior axillary line for chest tube insertion

(continued)

Table 11.4 (continued)

Primary survey	Assessment	Interventions	PCP's responsibility in trauma unit
Circulation and hemorrhage control	Assess for signs of external and internal hemorrhage—external bleeding present in the left thigh wound Use Focused Assessment Sonography for Trauma (FAST) Assess skin—color, temperature and moisture, urine output Assess for central and peripheral pulses Start 2 IV lines using large-bore cannula, and decide on the volume of fluid to be infused Impression: likely left femur fracture	Direct pressure given and compressive bandage applied Pelvis stable FAST positive for abdomen Patient skin assessment revealed pallor and cold extremities Peripheral pulses present IV cannulas inserted Fluids infused as per medical advice/unit protocol	Check for bleeding using "Floor and Four More" areas, i.e., chest, abdomen, pelvis, and extremities Utilize the hemorrhage control measures as per the requirement—direct pressure, compressive bandage, or tourniquet Select appropriate size of IV cannulas and proceed Insert interosseous access if delay in securing venous access. Keep appropriate IO needles and device ready in trauma bay Fluids including crystalloids to be kept ready for bolus/ infusion Blood bank to be alerted Activate massive hemorrhage protocol if large volume losses noted If urinary catheter placed, monitor urine output
Disability (neurologic evaluation)	Assess GCS Assess pupillary size and reactivity Any intoxicating agents Identify focal neurological deficits	Use modified GCS for intubated patient Pupils equal reacting to light	GCS or modified GCS to be used
Exposure/ environment	Perform head to toe assessment after undressing the patient; identify abrasions, bruises, cuts/cyanosis, dents, edema/ ecchymosis, fractures Assess body temperature	Multiple contusions and abrasions present in the body and extremities Dressings done Maintain normothermia, patient given warm blankets Body temperature normal	Perform head to toe examination; document all injuries Log roll the child with the help of 4 persons (refer pic on log roll) Place spine board (refer picture for the special boards for children) if not placed earlier. At this time place the pelvic binder where needed

(continued)

Table 11.4 (continued)

Primary survey	Assessment	Interventions	PCP's responsibility in trauma unit
Plan for transfer	Vitals signs stable: HR 120/mt, BP 90/50 mmHg, RR 20/mt ventilation, SPO_2 96%, child remains intubated, chest tube functioning well Venous access secure, IV fluids on flow, medications as per doctors' orders given and documented Transfer to higher referral center based on evidence of polytrauma, chest trauma, likely abdominal injury with FAST positive and for repair of likely left femur fracture For transfer, use ISBAR communication tool (identify/introduction, situation, background, assessment, and review and recommendation)		

To approach this case, life-threatening injuries should be identified immediately, followed by a detailed primary survey. Table 11.3 summarizes the immediate questions to be answered. The primary survey is detailed in Table 11.4 for the case scenario.

Key Messages

- Pediatric spinal injuries, though uncommon, can result in significant long-term disability or death. Early recognition and timely intervention by PCPs are critical to improving outcomes.
- Understanding the anatomical and physiological differences between pediatric and adult spinal columns enables PCPs to tailor assessment and management appropriately.
- A structured, stepwise approach using the ABCDE primary survey must be promptly initiated to identify and manage life-threatening injuries in children with suspected spinal trauma.
- Manual in-line cervical spine stabilization is essential during all stages of evaluation. Proper measurement and application of a pediatric-sized cervical collar and use of age-appropriate spine boards are key components of spinal motion restriction.
- The secondary survey should follow once the child is stabilized and should involve a head-to-toe assessment, focusing on identifying any hidden injuries.
- Primary and secondary assessments must be repeated regularly, especially in evolving or unstable patients, to detect any changes requiring urgent re-evaluation or intervention.
- The severity, location, and type of spinal injury, along with the presence of neurological deficits or multisystem trauma, largely determine long-term prognosis and rehabilitation needs.
- Effective communication and education for the child's caregivers by the PCP play a crucial role in psychological adjustment, adherence to follow-up care, and prevention of secondary complications.

Bibliography

1. Aitken ME, Korehbandi P, Parnell D, Parker JG, Stefans V, Tompkins E, Schulz EG. Experiences from the development of a comprehensive family support program for pediatric trauma and rehabilitation patients. Archives of physical medicine and rehabilitation. 2005 Jan 1;86(1):175–9.
2. American College of Surgeons Committee on Trauma. Advanced Trauma Life Support (ATLS) Student Course Manual, 10th ed, American College of Surgeons, Chicago, IL 2018.
3. Atesok K, Tanaka N, O'Brien A, Robinson Y, Pang D, Deinlein D, Manoharan SR, Pittman J, Theiss S. Posttraumatic Spinal Cord Injury without Radiographic Abnormality. Adv Orthop. 2018 Jan 4;2018:7060654. https://doi.org/10.1155/2018/7060654.
4. Bansal ML, Sharawat R, Mahajan R, Dawar H, Mohapatra B, Das K, Chhabra HS. Spinal Injury in Indian Children: Review of 204 Cases. Global Spine J. 2020 Dec;10(8):1034–1039. https://doi.org/10.1177/2192568219887155.
5. Basu S. Spinal injuries in children. Front Neurol. 2012 Jul 26; 3:96.
6. Brauge D, Plas B, Vinchon M, Charni S, Di Rocco F, Sacko O, Mrozek S, Sales de Gauzy J. Multicenter study of 37 pediatric patients with SCIWORA or other spinal cord injury without associated bone lesion. Orthop Traumatol Surg Res. 2020 Feb;106(1):167–171. https://doi.org/10.1016/j.otsr.2019.10.006.
7. Cunha NSC, Malvea A, Sadat S, Ibrahim GM, Fehlings MG. Pediatric Spinal Cord Injury: A Review. Children (Basel). 2023 Aug 26;10(9):1456. https://doi.org/10.3390/children10091456.
8. Elnady B, El-Morshidy E, El-Meshtawi M, Shawky A. Pediatric cervical spine injuries with neurological deficits, treatment options, and potential for recovery. SICOT J. 2017;3:53. https://doi.org/10.1051/sicotj/2017035.
9. Henry DA, Bumpass DB, McCarthy RE. Delayed diagnosis of a flexion-distraction spinal injury and occult small bowel injury in a pediatric trauma patient: Importance of recognizing the abdominal "seatbelt sign." Trauma Case Rep. 2021 Jun 16;34:100499. https://doi.org/10.1016/j.tcr.2021.100499.
10. Herzenberg JE, Hensinger RN, Dedrick DK, Phillips WA. Emergency transport and positioning of young children who have an injury of the cervical spine. The standard backboard may be hazardous. J Bone Joint Surg Am 1989; 71:15
11. Khanjari, Sedigheh; Tajik, Zahra; Haghani, Hamid. The effect of family-centered education on the quality of life of adolescents with spinal cord injuries. Journal of Family Medicine and Primary Care 8(2): p 711–716, February 2019.
12. Kim C, Vassilyadi M, Forbes JK, Moroz NW, Camacho A, Moroz PJ. Traumatic spinal injuries in children at a single level 1 pediatric trauma centre: report of a 23-year experience. Can J Surg. 2016 Jun;59(3):205–12. https://doi.org/10.1503/cjs.014515.
13. Lee LK, Farrell C. Trauma management: Approach to the unstable child. In: UpToDate, Bachur RG (Ed), Wolters Kluwer. Accessed on March 22, 2025.
14. Leonard JC, Browne LR, Ahmad FA, et al. Cervical Spine Injury Risk Factors in Children with Blunt Trauma. Paediatrics. 2019;144(1): e20183221
15. Leonard JC, Kuppermann N, Olsen C, Babcock-Cimpello L, Brown K, Mahajan P, et al. Factors associated with cervical spine injury in children after blunt trauma. Ann Emerg Med. 2011 Aug;58(2):145–55.
16. Leonard JR, Jaffe DM, Kuppermann N, Olsen CS, Leonard JC; Pediatric Emergency Care Applied Research Network (PECARN) Cervical Spine Study Group. Cervical spine injury patterns in children. Pediatrics. 2014 May;133(5):e1179–88. https://doi.org/10.1542/peds.2013-3505.
17. Mandadi AR, Koutsogiannis P, Das JM, Waseem M: Pediatric spine trauma. StatPearls. StatPearls Publishing, Treasure Island, FL; 2024.
18. Mc Auley C, Mullen S, Corley L, McDonald R, Quinn N. Secondary survey in paediatric trauma. Arch Dis Child Educ Pract Ed. 2023 Aug;108(4):253–258. https://doi.org/10.1136/archdischild-2022-324983.

19. Ryan, Denita. Handbook of Neuroscience Nursing: Care of the Adult Neurosurgical Patient. New York: Thieme, 2017. Print.
20. Skellett S, Tibby SM, Durward A, Murdoch IA. Lesson of the week: Immobilisation of the cervical spine in children. BMJ. 2002 Mar 9;324(7337):591–3. https://doi.org/10.1136/bmj.324.7337.591. PMID: 11884327; PMCID: PMC1122513.

Pediatric Extremity Injuries 12

Seema S. Chavan, Jyothiswaroop Bhaskararayuni, and Aaditya Katyal

Learning Objectives

After completing this chapter, the reader will be able to:

- Describe the unique anatomical and physiological features of the pediatric musculoskeletal system and their implications in trauma care
- Apply the principles of primary and secondary assessment using the ABCDE framework in the context of pediatric extremity trauma
- Identify common mechanisms of extremity injury in children and recognize red-flag signs of life-threatening and limb-threatening conditions such as open fractures, neurovascular compromise, and compartment syndrome
- Perform initial management of pediatric extremity trauma, including airway stabilization, bleeding control, pain assessment, wound care, splinting, and initiation of tetanus prophylaxis and antibiotics where appropriate.
- Demonstrate appropriate criteria for referral, follow-up, and documentation in extremity trauma cases, using standard clinical tools and scales.
- Communicate effectively with the trauma team and the child's caregivers using structured formats (SBAR, MIST), while providing psychological support and education to families.

S. S. Chavan
College of Nursing, AIIMS, Gorakhpur, Gorakhpur, Uttar Pradesh, India

J. Bhaskararayuni
AIIMS New Delhi, New Delhi, Delhi, India

A. Katyal (✉)
Department of Emergency Medicine, Kasturba Medical College, Manipal, Karnataka, India

Centre for Resuscitation, Acute Care and Simulation Training (CReST), Manipal Academy of Higher Education (MAHE) (An Institute of Eminence Accorded by MHRD), Karnataka, Manipal, Udupi, Karnataka, India

N. T. Rai (ed.), *Pediatric Trauma Resuscitation Manual (PTRM) for Primary Care Providers*, https://doi.org/10.1007/978-981-95-4979-5_12

- Recognize potential signs of non-accidental trauma and implement appropriate safeguarding protocols, referral pathways, and documentation procedures.
- Promote injury prevention strategies and safe return-to-activity recommendations tailored to the child's age, injury severity, and cultural context.

Introduction

Trauma is a leading cause of morbidity and mortality among children worldwide, with extremity injuries accounting for a significant proportion of these cases. In India and other low- and middle-income countries, pediatric trauma—particularly from road traffic accidents, falls, and domestic incidents—remains a pressing public health issue. These injuries not only result in immediate physical harm but can also lead to long-term disability, growth disturbances, and emotional distress for the child and their family.

Primary care providers (PCPs) are often the first point of contact in the management of pediatric injuries. Their role in early recognition, stabilization, and referral is critical to improving outcomes. Pediatric patients differ significantly from adults in terms of anatomy and physiology. Their bones are more pliable, growth plates are vulnerable to disruption, and their response to injury—including signs of shock—may be subtle and delayed. As such, a high index of suspicion and a systematic approach are essential.

This chapter provides PCPs with a practical framework to evaluate and manage pediatric extremity trauma. Using a case-based structure, it emphasizes the ABCDE approach to trauma assessment, highlights red-flag conditions such as compartment syndrome and open fractures, and outlines effective communication and documentation strategies. The chapter also addresses non-accidental trauma, a critical yet often overlooked aspect of pediatric care.

By integrating evidence-based guidelines, visual tools, and real-world scenarios, this chapter empowers PCPs to deliver timely and appropriate care—stabilizing the child, minimizing complications, and supporting the family through a potentially traumatic experience. Early intervention by informed PCPs can significantly reduce long-term disability and enhance the overall trajectory of recovery in pediatric extremity trauma cases.

Case Scenario

Anju, a 10-year-old girl, is brought to a rural primary care center following a high-speed road traffic collision. She was an unrestrained passenger who was reportedly thrown from the car. Local emergency responders have immobilized her with a cervical collar and spine board. Your center is the first point of medical contact.

On arrival, Anju is conscious but pale, confused, and in visible distress. She is actively bleeding from a deep laceration on her right thigh, where an open femur fracture is evident. Her voice is weak, and she appears tachypneic and anxious.

Vital Signs

- Respiratory rate: 42 breaths/min
- SpO_2: 90% on room air
- Heart rate: 136 bpm
- Blood pressure: 70/40 mmHg
- Capillary refill time: 2 s
- GCS: 13 (E3V4M6)

As the primary care provider on duty, you must initiate immediate stabilization before arranging for higher-level referral.

Reflective Questions

1. Based on the ABCDE framework, what should be your initial approach to assessment and stabilization at the primary care level?
2. Which clinical features in Anju suggest life-threatening hemorrhagic shock, and how can you respond with the limited resources available?
3. How will you assess and manage the open extremity injury, including bleeding control, splinting, analgesia, and infection prophylaxis?
4. What essential information must you document and communicate to the referral center using a structured handover tool like MIST?
5. How can you effectively counsel and involve Anju's caregivers in this high-stress situation while maintaining clear, compassionate communication?

Unique Features of Pediatric Extremity Injuries

Understanding the anatomical and physiological distinctions of pediatric patients is essential for accurate assessment and effective management of extremity trauma. Children are not simply "small adults"—their musculoskeletal systems are structurally and functionally different, and these differences significantly influence injury patterns, clinical presentation, and healing outcomes.

In infants and young children, the skeleton is predominantly cartilaginous, which provides flexibility but also makes it more susceptible to specific injury types. Pediatric bones are softer, more porous, and less mineralized compared to adult bones. As a result, they are more likely to bend rather than break completely, leading to unique fracture patterns such as greenstick fractures, buckle (torus) fractures, and plastic deformation. These patterns may be subtle and easily missed without a high index of suspicion and proper imaging.

A distinctive feature of pediatric bone is the presence of the physis (growth plate)—a cartilaginous zone near the ends of long bones that facilitates longitudinal bone growth. The physis is the weakest part of the growing skeleton and is highly vulnerable to trauma. Injuries involving the growth plate can disrupt normal bone development, resulting in complications such as growth arrest, angular deformities, or limb-length discrepancies, often necessitating long-term orthopedic follow-up and, in some cases, corrective surgery. Unfortunately, the epidemiology of growth plate injuries in children is still underreported compared to adult trauma data, signifying the need for more pediatric-specific research and documentation.

Beyond the skeleton, systemic physiological differences also affect trauma response. Children have a smaller body mass, less protective connective tissue, and larger organ-to-body size ratios, placing vital structures in closer proximity to potential impact. Their larger head-to-body ratio increases the risk of head injuries, especially in falls. Additionally, children possess a higher surface area-to-mass ratio, predisposing them to rapid heat loss and early onset of hypothermia—a critical concern in trauma settings.

Importantly, children may sustain significant internal injury with minimal external signs, and their compensatory mechanisms (e.g., increased heart rate) can mask early physiological deterioration. This makes it imperative for primary care providers to approach pediatric trauma with vigilance and a low threshold for escalation.

Familiarity with the key anatomical structures of the upper and lower limbs is crucial for detecting subtle signs of extremity injury. Understanding the position of major bones (femur, tibia, fibula, humerus, radius, ulna), joints, growth plates, neurovascular bundles, and common sites prone to injury is essential in pediatric trauma assessment.

Additionally, knowledge of the Salter-Harris classification system is important, as it categorizes physeal (growth plate) fractures into types I–V, based on the involvement of the physis, metaphysis, and epiphysis, helping guide appropriate diagnosis and management.

- Type I involves a transverse fracture through the growth plate.
- Type II extends through the growth plate and metaphysis (most common).
- Type III involves the physis and epiphysis, potentially affecting joint surfaces.
- Type IV traverses the metaphysis, physis, and epiphysis.
- Type V is a crush injury of the growth plate, often with the worst prognosis due to growth arrest.

Understanding this classification helps PCPs in decision-making regarding splinting, referral urgency, and long-term monitoring, as injuries involving the physis can lead to significant complications such as growth disturbances or angular deformities if not properly managed.

Common Mechanisms of Pediatric Extremity Injuries

Understanding the mechanisms that lead to extremity injuries in pediatric patients is critical for accurate diagnosis, appropriate management, and identification of red-flag situations such as non-accidental trauma. Pediatric extremity trauma often reflects the child's age, activity level, environment, and supervision. The following are the most frequently encountered causes:

1. *Road Traffic Accidents (RTAs)*: RTAs remain the leading cause of extremity trauma in children, particularly in urban and peri-urban India. Children involved in RTAs may be pedestrians, bicyclists, or unrestrained passengers. High-impact injuries from collisions or being run over can result in complex fractures, open injuries, or multi-system trauma. Primary care providers must maintain a high index of suspicion for associated internal injuries and early signs of shock in these scenarios.
2. *Falls from Height*: Falls are the second most common cause of pediatric extremity injuries, often seen in toddlers and school-age children. Injuries typically occur during unsupervised play, falls from beds, stairs, trees, rooftops, or balconies. The height of the fall, landing surface, and body position on impact influence the severity of injury. Upper limb fractures—particularly forearm and supracondylar humerus fractures—are frequent due to instinctive attempts to break the fall with outstretched hands.
3. *Sports and Recreational Injuries*: As children grow older, sports-related trauma becomes increasingly common, especially in school settings or organized sports. Contact sports, gymnastics, cycling, and playground activities can result in sprains, dislocations, or fractures. The majority of these injuries involve the upper limbs due to falls, although lower limb injuries such as ankle sprains and tibial fractures are also reported.
4. *Non-accidental Trauma (Child Abuse)*: Any unexplained or inconsistent injury history must raise suspicion for non-accidental trauma (NAT), especially in non-ambulatory infants or repeated injury presentations. Fractures inconsistent with developmental age (e.g., femur fracture in a 6-month-old) or those at unusual locations (e.g., posterior ribs, scapula) warrant detailed assessment and documentation. PCPs play a vital role in early identification, safeguarding the child, and initiating the appropriate legal and psychosocial support pathways.

Assessment of Pediatric Extremity Injuries

Initial Assessment The physical, physiological, and psychological differences between children and adults have a significant impact on the initial assessment and treatment of pediatric trauma patients. The term "golden hour" refers to an early and critical period in trauma patient care when proper management can significantly improve patients' survival rates.

Primary Survey The primary survey uses the ABCDE approach, which focuses on identifying and managing life-threatening conditions.

1. *A: Airway*

   Smaller airway poses a greater risk of airway obstruction with foreign bodies. Ensure the airway is patent and clear.

2. *B: Breathing*

   Hypoventilation is the most common cause of cardiorespiratory arrest. Diaphragmatic breathing is seen in children wherein higher oxygen demand = higher respiratory rates. Look for rate, rhythm, depth, and use of accessory muscles for breathing.
3. *C: Circulation*

   Small volumes of blood will constitute significant blood loss in small children. Hypotension is a late sign in children. Children lose 25–30% of blood volume before manifesting signs of shock. IV access in children may be challenging due to small veins. If IV access is difficult, consider the intraosseous route. Fluids can be administered as initial bolus of 20 ml/kg NS and 10 ml/kg of packed RBCs after two boluses.
4. *D: Disability*

   Children have a higher incidence of head and neck trauma. Evaluate the neurological status of the child using the AVPU scales (Table 12.1)/Glasgow Coma Scale. GCS<8 correlates with a higher rate of mortality. Additionally, check the pupillary response to light and blood glucose levels.
5. *E: Exposure*

   Children have a larger surface area-to-body mass ratio resulting in greater heat loss. This also increases the oxygen demand. Expose the child to check for any bleeding, trauma, and other injuries keeping risk of hypothermia in mind.

Secondary Survey The secondary survey comprises a head-to-toe evaluation, as well as a comprehensive history and physical examination with reassessment of all vital signs. Only after completing the initial survey and managing life-threatening injuries should a secondary survey be conducted.

AMPLE format should be used for history collection.

- A: Any allergies
- M: Medication history/taken
- P: Past medical history
- L: Last meal
- E: Events surrounding the incident

Historical points specific to extremity trauma:

- Mechanism of injury (fall, twist, direct blow)
- Pain localization (ask child to point)

Table 12.1 AVPU scale

Awake	Patient is awake
Verbal	Patient responds to a verbal stimulus
Pain	Patient responds to a pain stimulus
Unresponsive	Patient is unresponsive to stimulus

- Refusal to bear weight or use limb
- Red flags (fever, night pain, recurrent injuries)

Physical Examination

- Life-threatening injuries and its management are done in the primary survey.
- Limb-threatening injury and its management are done in a secondary survey.
- A systematic head-to-toe assessment is essential to avoid missing out on any musculoskeletal injuries.

General Examination Checking for consciousness of the patient and talking to them to check on their orientation to time, place, and person.

Extremity Assessment in Pediatric Trauma

As part of the secondary survey, a focused extremity assessment is essential to identify limb-threatening injuries that may not be immediately apparent during the primary survey. In pediatric patients, subtle findings can easily be overlooked, making a systematic approach critical. This evaluation includes four major components:

1. *Skin and Subcutaneous Tissue*: Carefully inspect the skin over the injured limb for color, perfusion, swelling, bruising, lacerations, and deformity. Special attention should be paid to identifying external bleeding or open wounds. Log-rolling the patient may help uncover hidden injuries or bleeding sites on the posterior aspect of the body, especially in high-energy trauma.
2. *Nerve Function*: Assess for sensation and motor function in the affected limb. Test for pain response and touch discrimination over distal dermatomes. Persistent numbness, tingling, or weakness may suggest nerve compression or injury, warranting urgent referral. Note that pain, tenderness, and swelling should be interpreted carefully as they may also reflect soft tissue or skeletal injury.
3. *Circulatory Status*: Evaluate peripheral perfusion by palpating distal pulses (e.g., radial, dorsalis pedis) and checking capillary refill time. Pale, cold, or cyanotic extremities, along with paresthesia or motor deficits, raise concern for arterial compromise and require immediate intervention.
4. *Musculoskeletal and Ligamentous Structures*: Look for bruises, contusions, swelling, joint deformities, and lacerations over bony prominences or joints. Gently palpate along the bone to identify areas of tenderness, especially around growth plates (e.g., distal radius, proximal tibia), which are more vulnerable in children. Ligamentous injuries may be suspected when joint line tenderness or hemarthrosis (bleeding into the joint) is present.

Checklist for Local Limb Examination

- Inspect for swelling, bruising, and visible deformities.
- Palpate for bone tenderness, especially near growth plates.
- Assess neurovascular status—pulses, capillary refill, and sensory response.

- Evaluate range of motion gently, only if the child tolerates and if fracture is not obvious.
- Always compare bilaterally with the uninjured limb for subtle asymmetries.

Clinical Features of Extremity Injury
- Pain and tenderness at the site of fracture/injury
- Swelling
- Deformity
- Limitation of a function of the extremity injured
- Laceration and bruises
- Inability to bear weight
- Bone dislocation
- Numbness
- Weakness

Diagnostic Evaluation Standard diagnostic procedures include:

- Plain X-rays.
- CT scans.
- For suspected vascular and soft tissue injuries, angiography or color Doppler scans may be performed.

Management of Pediatric Extremity Injuries

Primary care providers play a pivotal role in the initial stabilization, evaluation, and early management of pediatric extremity trauma. Early recognition and intervention can significantly reduce the risk of long-term morbidity, including deformity, infection, neurovascular compromise, and growth disturbances.

1. Fracture Management
   - *Bleeding Control*
     Actively bleeding wounds associated with fractures must be managed immediately. Apply direct pressure with sterile gauze, and if bleeding persists, consider the judicious use of a tourniquet. In situations of massive, uncontrolled hemorrhage, limb-threatening bleeding may take precedence over limb preservation. Always weigh the risk-to-benefit ratio in such cases.
   - *Pain Control (Analgesia)*
     Children in pain should receive timely and weight-based analgesia. Oral paracetamol (15 mg/kg) or ibuprofen (10 mg/kg) may be sufficient for minor injuries, while intravenous analgesics (e.g., morphine or fentanyl) may be required in severe trauma. Pain should be reassessed frequently using validated pediatric pain scales (e.g., FLACC, Wong-Baker).
   - *Neurovascular Assessment and Documentation*

Before and after any manipulation or splinting, neurovascular integrity must be assessed—including distal pulses, capillary refill, skin color, temperature, motor function, and sensation. All findings should be documented thoroughly.

- *Alignment and Splinting*
  If there is visible deformity, gentle alignment to a functional position can relieve tension and pain. Apply an appropriate padded splint to immobilize the fracture and prevent further tissue damage. Avoid forceful manipulation.

2. Management of Soft Tissue Injuries
   - *Open Fractures and Contaminated Wounds*
     These should be referred emergently for orthopedic evaluation and surgical debridement. Do not attempt wound closure at the primary level.
   - *Gross Debris Removal*
     Remove any obvious contamination (e.g., dirt, leaves, gravel) without aggressive cleaning. Avoid vigorous irrigation if transfer is planned.
   - *Wound Dressing*
     Cover the wound with saline-soaked sterile gauze, and secure gently without applying excessive pressure. The dressing should remain undisturbed until surgical review.
   - *Tetanus Prophylaxis*
     Check immunization history. If the tetanus vaccination status is unknown or incomplete, administer tetanus toxoid and tetanus immunoglobulin as per guidelines.
   - *Antibiotic Administration*
     Empirical intravenous antibiotics (e.g., ceftriaxone ± metronidazole) should be administered promptly for open fractures or contaminated wounds to reduce infection risk.
   - *Documentation*
     Note wound size, depth, bleeding, and contamination. Include time of injury and interventions performed.
3. Nerve Injuries
   - While most pediatric upper limb injuries do not cause permanent nerve damage, PCPs should still assess motor function and sensation. If nerve dysfunction is present, document findings, and refer for urgent neurological or orthopedic evaluation.
   - Management at the primary level is limited to protecting the limb, pain control, and timely referral. Definitive options—such as neurolysis, nerve repair, or grafting—are surgical decisions at specialized centers.
4. Splinting Essentials
   Before Splinting
   - Confirm and document neurovascular status.
   - Pad all bony prominences (e.g., malleoli, ulnar styloid) to prevent pressure sores.

   During Splinting
   - Choose the appropriate splint based on the injury location:
     - *Sugar-tong splint*: Forearm fractures

    - *Posterior ankle splint*: Ankle or distal tibial fractures
    - *Thumb spica splint*: Suspected scaphoid injuries
  - Ensure that joints above and below the fracture are immobilized.

   After Splinting
  - Reassess neurovascular status to rule out iatrogenic compression.
  - Elevate the injured limb, and advise intermittent ice application (15–20 min every 1–2 h).
  - Plan follow-up within 3–7 days or sooner if symptoms worsen.
5. Referral Criteria

   Emergent Referral (<24 h)
  - Open fractures with exposed bone
  - Any sign of neurovascular compromise (e.g., pulseless limb, paresthesia, paralysis)
  - Clinical suspicion of compartment syndrome (e.g., pain out of proportion, tense swelling, pallor)
  - Displaced Salter-Harris type III–V fractures

   Urgent Referral (within 24–48 h)
  - Displaced intra-articular fractures requiring reduction
  - Angulated long bone fractures not reducible at the primary level
  - Unstable or symptomatic Salter-Harris type II fractures
6. Discharge Instructions for Parents and Caregivers
   - *Limb Elevation*: Keep the injured limb raised above heart level to reduce swelling.
   - *Cold Application*: Use ice packs wrapped in cloth for 15–20 minutes every 1–2 hours (never apply directly to skin).
   - *Pain Control*: Administer prescribed analgesics—typically ibuprofen (10 mg/kg) or paracetamol (15 mg/kg)—at recommended intervals.
   - *Warning Signs—Return immediately if:*
     - Fingers or toes turn pale, cold, or bluish
     - Severe, unrelieved pain persists beyond 48 h
     - The child refuses to move the fingers or toes
     - There is increasing swelling or foul-smelling discharge from the wound
   - *Follow-up*: Re-evaluation is essential to assess healing, alignment, and potential complications, especially in growth plate injuries.

Specific Injuries of Upper and Lower Extremities

After airway, breathing, and circulation have been handled, the extremities and pelvis should be checked for orthopedic injuries. Half or more of pediatric blunt injuries are orthopedic, and blast or projectile injuries can cause open fractures and soft tissue damage.

1. *Open fractures associated with a soft tissue injury*: The evaluation begins with an investigation of distal neurovascular function.

If the neurovascular function is intact, the fracture can be splinted to reduce pain and soft tissue injury, followed by formal casting while the soft tissue edema resolves. Pediatric fractures heal more faster and with less precision than adult fractures.

If the neurovascular function is compromised, the fracture should be minimized, and the neurovascular condition re-evaluated. If they do not improve, the child will require surgery to explore the fracture site and maybe repair or graft of small artery.

2. *Distal humeral fractures*: Humerus fractures are prevalent following a fall onto an outstretched arm and can lead to brachial artery impairment. Reduction and repair of these fractures may be difficult, but if the hand is pink and warm, it may have enough blood flow to function even in the absence of radial pulses.

   Open fractures should be treated similarly, with rapid IV antibiotic treatment and complete soft tissue irrigation and debridement, with planned reoperations every 24–48 h until the wound is pronounced clean enough to seal.
3. *Compartment syndrome*: Fractures caused by a crush injury, such as those sustained after a building collapse, are associated with an increased risk of compartment syndrome and, if patient evacuation is delayed, may result in rhabdomyolysis.

   Compartment syndrome is more difficult to diagnose in children, and its presentation can be delayed by a day or more. The injuries most typically associated with compartment syndrome include tibial fractures, supracondylar humeral fractures, and femur fractures.

   Younger children may not participate with testing or communicate their symptoms, but compartment syndrome should be examined in high-risk children who exhibit the three A's: anxiety, growing agitation, and increasing analgesic demand.

Compartment Syndrome Recognition

5 P's:

- Pain out of proportion to injury
- Pallor (pale limb)
- Paresthesias (tingling/numbness)
- Paralysis (inability to move digits)
- Pulselessness (late sign)

3 A's:

- *A*nxiety
- *A*gitation
- Increased *a*nalgesic demand

Action:

- Remove all constrictive dressings/splints.
- Emergent orthopedic consultation.

The PCP's Role in Pediatric Extremity Trauma

In the management of pediatric extremity trauma, primary care providers (PCPs) are not only the first responders but often the most accessible and consistent healthcare figures in a child's journey from injury to recovery. Their role begins at the scene or point of first contact and continues through resuscitation, stabilization, and referral. This triad of responsibilities can be organized under the *"3 Rs" framework: Recognize, Resuscitate, and Refer.*

- *Recognize*: PCPs must rapidly identify life- or limb-threatening conditions by conducting a focused ABCDE assessment, followed by a neurovascular evaluation of the affected limb. They should maintain a high index of suspicion for complications like open fractures, vascular compromise, and compartment syndrome—conditions that require immediate attention and action.
- *Resuscitate*: Once critical threats are identified, PCPs must initiate stabilization. This includes airway management, bleeding control, oxygen delivery, fluid resuscitation, splinting, and pain control using age-appropriate tools. PCPs are also tasked with managing the psychological well-being of the child and family, ensuring emotional support and clear communication throughout the process.
- *Refer*: After stabilization, children must be referred to appropriate trauma or orthopedic centers. Structured communication tools such as SBAR (situation, background, assessment, recommendation) or MIST (mechanism, injuries, signs/symptoms, treatment) should be used for accurate and efficient handover. PCPs also play a key role in recognizing signs of non-accidental trauma, ensuring that child safety and safeguarding protocols are followed.

In the trauma team, PCPs must exhibit clinical vigilance, participate in closed-loop communication, and ensure that all decisions and actions are well-documented. Their ability to remain calm, communicate clearly, and execute time-sensitive interventions can be lifesaving.

Table 12.2 outlines the core roles and responsibilities of PCPs during pediatric extremity trauma resuscitation.

Managing pediatric extremity trauma requires a blend of sound clinical judgment, anatomical insight, and structured protocols—especially in settings where primary care providers are the first and often only immediate responders. To assist PCPs in making informed, high-impact decisions, the following tables provide a consolidated overview of best practices, common errors, and actionable recommendations across various domains of care.

- Table 12.3 presents clinical pearls and pitfalls across essential domains—from initial assessment and imaging to splinting, referrals, and pain management.
- Tables 12.4, 12.5, and 12.6 offer practical do's and don'ts covering key aspects of extremity trauma care, including injury management, referral timing, follow-up guidance, effective communication with caregivers, and essential documentation.

Table 12.2 Roles and responsibilities of PCPs during pediatric extremity trauma resuscitation

Domain	PCP responsibilities
Airway	Maintain airway patency; ensure cervical spine stabilization in suspected cervical injuries
Breathing	Provide supplemental oxygen; monitor and maintain oxygen saturation
Circulation	Establish IV or intraosseous (IO) access; administer fluids and monitor vital signs (pulse, BP, respiration, temperature, pain); control bleeding using pressure or tourniquets
Disability	Assess neurological status using Glasgow Coma Scale (GCS); monitor level of consciousness
Exposure	Fully expose the child to identify other injuries; prevent hypothermia by keeping the child warm
Preparation	Ensure availability and readiness of trauma equipment (tourniquets, dressings, airway tools); anticipate needs for OT transfer if indicated
Communication	Use closed-loop communication within the trauma team; update team members post-stabilization; inform and counsel family regarding prognosis
Monitoring	Continuously observe for signs of deterioration due to hypovolemia, hypothermia, or electrolyte imbalance; reassess vitals regularly
Record keeping	Document all interventions, including medications, procedures, vital signs, and clinical decisions during resuscitation
Psychological support	Provide empathetic communication and emotional reassurance to family members experiencing distress
Analgesia	Assess pain using pediatric pain scales (e.g., FLACC, Wong-Baker), and administer age-appropriate analgesics accordingly

Table 12.3 Summary of pediatric trauma extremity management

Domain	Pearls	Pitfalls
Assessment	Always palpate growth plates (e.g., distal radius, tibia) in injuries near joints. Children's physes are weaker than ligaments	Assuming "sprain" in children <10 years without imaging. Growth plate injuries mimic sprains
Imaging	Use Ottawa Ankle/Knee Rules to reduce unnecessary X-rays in children >5 years	Failing to image the contralateral limb in toddlers for comparison, missing subtle fractures
Splinting	Early splinting reduces pain and prevents displacement. Use padded splints to avoid pressure sores	Applying splints too tightly, risking compartment syndrome. Recheck neurovascular status post-application
Pain management	Ibuprofen (10 mg/kg) + acetaminophen is safe and effective for most fractures	Using NSAIDs in dehydrated patients or suspected compartment syndrome
Referrals	Emergent referral for SH III–V fractures, open fractures, or neurovascular compromise	Delaying referral for SH II fractures with >2 mm displacement, risking malunion
Follow-up	Monitor growth plate injuries annually until skeletal maturity to detect growth arrest early	Discharging without follow-up for toddler's fractures, missing delayed displacement

Table 12.3 (continued)

Domain	Pearls	Pitfalls
Non-accidental trauma	Suspect abuse in fractures in non-ambulatory infants (e.g., femur in a 3-month-old)	Overlooking inconsistent histories or recurrent injuries, missing abuse
Compartment syndrome	Recognize the 5 P's: pain out of proportion, pallor, paresthesia, paralysis, pulselessness	Misattributing pain to anxiety without reassessing the limb
Reduction techniques	Nursemaid's elbow reduction (supination-flexion) has a >90% success rate in the office	Forcing ROM testing in uncooperative children → risk of iatrogenic injury

Table 12.4 Management and treatment of pediatric extremity injuries

Do ✔	Don't ✕
Splint early to stabilize fractures and reduce pain	Apply splints too tightly (risk of compartment syndrome)
Prescribe ibuprofen + acetaminophen for pain control	Use NSAIDs in dehydrated patients or suspected compartment syndrome
Elevate the limb and apply ice (15–20 min/h)	Allow weight-bearing on unstable fractures (e.g., SH III–V)

Table 12.5 Referral and follow-up of pediatric extremity injuries

Do ✔	Don't ✕
Refer emergently for open fractures or neurovascular compromise	Delay referral for Salter-Harris III–V fractures (high risk of growth arrest)
Schedule follow-up in 1 week to reassess alignment and healing	Discharge without recheck instructions for high-risk injuries
Document red flags for non-accidental trauma (e.g., inconsistent history)	Ignore fractures in non-ambulatory infants (e.g., femur fracture in a 6-month-old)

Table 12.6 Communication and documentation

Do ✕	Don't ✕
Explain findings to parents using visual aids (e.g., X-rays)	Use medical jargon (e.g., "Salter-Harris II" without simple explanation)
Document neurovascular status pre/post-splinting	Forget to document mechanism of injury (critical for legal/abuse cases)

Case Resolution

As Anju is wheeled into the rural primary care center, the urgency is clear. She's pale, breathing rapidly, visibly in pain, and bleeding from a wound on her right thigh. You immediately initiate the ABCDE approach, knowing that timely intervention in this golden hour could make the difference between life and death.

Her airway appears patent—she is conscious and speaking weakly, though her voice is faint and her agitation concerning. You maintain cervical spine precautions with the collar in place and prepare for airway support if her mental status deteriorates. Moving to breathing, you note a respiratory rate of 42 and an SpO_2 of 90% on room air. Her breath sounds are equal bilaterally, so you begin high-flow oxygen via a non-rebreather mask to improve oxygenation.

Her circulatory status is critical: a heart rate of 136 bpm, hypotension at 70/40 mmHg, and a capillary refill of 2 s—classic signs of compensated hemorrhagic shock. You quickly recognize the gravity of her condition. In a setting where resources are limited, you establish intraosseous access, knowing that IV access might be difficult in a shocked child. You administer a 20 mL/kg bolus of isotonic saline while requesting packed red blood cells for transfusion. Bleeding from the open femur fracture is significant, so you apply direct pressure and cover the wound with a sterile saline-soaked gauze. You avoid removing debris aggressively, understanding that definitive wound cleaning must be done in a surgical setting.

Pain is addressed immediately with IV paracetamol at 15 mg/kg, and you prepare fentanyl cautiously, guided by her hemodynamics. Meanwhile, you begin empirical IV antibiotics (ceftriaxone and metronidazole) and administer tetanus toxoid, as her immunization history is unclear. These steps address not just pain and infection, but the high risk of contamination and sepsis from an open fracture.

Before splinting, you perform a focused extremity assessment, checking for distal pulses, sensation, capillary refill, and motor function. Everything is documented meticulously. You then immobilize the leg with a padded temporary splint, ensuring joints above and below the injury are stabilized. After splinting, you reassess neurovascular status—no compromise is noted.

You then turn to planning referral. Anju is too unstable for definitive care here. You draft a referral note using the MIST format:

- *Mechanism*: High-speed car crash; unrestrained passenger
- *Injuries*: Open right femur fracture, significant bleeding
- *Signs/symptoms*: HR 136, BP 70/40, RR 42, SpO_2 90%, GCS 13
- *Treatment*: Oxygen, fluids via IO, antibiotics, tetanus toxoid, wound dressing, analgesia, splinting

You follow this with a structured SBAR phone call to the trauma center, giving them a clear picture of Anju's status and your interventions. They prepare to receive her urgently.

As all this unfolds, her anxious parents arrive. They're terrified and overwhelmed. You take a moment—despite the pressure—to speak to them calmly. You explain that Anju is critically injured but stable for transfer and that she needs surgery and blood transfusion at a higher center. You avoid medical jargon, opting instead for plain language, and assure them that everything possible is being done. You encourage them to accompany her in the ambulance and provide them with written instructions and contact details for the receiving hospital.

Before the ambulance departs, you double-check your documentation—vitals, medications, interventions, and all assessments are clearly recorded. You've not only stabilized a critically injured child, but also bridged her safely to definitive care with compassion, clarity, and clinical precision.

Key Messages

- Pediatric extremity injuries are common yet often under-recognized emergencies in primary care settings. Early identification and timely management can prevent long-term disability.
- Children differ anatomically and physiologically from adults—their pliable bones, open growth plates, and distinct responses to injury demand pediatric-specific approaches to trauma assessment and care.
- The ABCDE framework remains the cornerstone of initial trauma evaluation. PCPs must rapidly assess airway, breathing, circulation, disability, and exposure, while anticipating signs of shock or neurovascular compromise.
- Open fractures, compartment syndrome, and vascular injuries are limb-threatening conditions that require urgent stabilization and referral. Delayed recognition can result in irreversible damage.
- Primary care providers (PCPs) play a pivotal role in initial stabilization—ensuring airway protection, oxygenation, fluid resuscitation, bleeding control, analgesia, and early antibiotics for open wounds.
- A focused secondary survey and extremity assessment, including skin inspection, neurovascular checks, and palpation of bones/joints, help identify injuries that may be missed during the primary survey.
- Splinting and immobilization must be performed carefully, with pre- and post-splint neurovascular assessment and appropriate padding to prevent iatrogenic harm.
- Clear documentation and structured handovers using MIST or SBAR formats ensure safe transitions to higher-level trauma centers and protect against medico-legal oversights.
- Communication with caregivers must be empathetic, clear, and culturally sensitive, especially in high-stress scenarios. Visual aids, simplified language, and reassurance are critical.
- Non-accidental trauma must always be considered in unexplained or developmentally inconsistent injuries. PCPs are key to safeguarding and initiating child protection protocols.
- Tables, checklists, and visual tools provided in this chapter serve as quick references, enabling PCPs to make informed, timely decisions—even in resource-limited environments.
- Empowering PCPs with trauma literacy, structured assessment, and referral readiness can dramatically improve outcomes for injured children across diverse care settings.

Bibliography

1. Asif S, Thaiban MA, Alghamdi A, Alqahtani M, Suliman AA, Alanazi W, et al. Management of Mangled Extremities: Upper vs Lower Limb Differences. JOHS [Internet]. 2021 [cited 2024 Nov 25];01(02):26–34. Available from: https://johs.com.sa/admin/public/uploads/187/16_pdf.pdf
2. Buckley SL, Gotschall C, Robertson W, Sturm P, Tosi L, Thomas M, et al. The relationships of skeletal injuries with trauma score, injury severity score, length of hospital stay, hospital charges, and mortality in children admitted to a regional pediatric trauma center. J Pediatr Orthop. 1994;14(4):449–53.
3. Flaherty et al., *Pediatrics* (2014); AAP (2021)
4. Ho-Fung VM, Zapala MA, Lee EY. Musculoskeletal Traumatic Injuries in Children: Characteristic Imaging Findings and Mimickers. Radiol Clin North Am. 2017 Jul;55(4):785–802.
5. Kay RM, Skaggs DL. Pediatric polytrauma management. J Pediatr Orthop. 2006;26(2):268–77.
6. Kundal VK, Debnath PR, Sen A. Epidemiology of Pediatric Trauma and its Pattern in Urban India: A Tertiary Care Hospital-Based Experience. J Indian Assoc Pediatr Surg. 2017;22(1):33–7.
7. McFadyen JG, Ramaiah R, Bhananker SM. Initial assessment and management of pediatric trauma patients. Int J Crit Illn Inj Sci. 2012 Sep;2(3):121–7.
8. Plint et al., *Pediatric EM Care* (2019); Bae et al., *Pediatrics in Review* (2020)
9. POSNA (2022); Wilkins et al., *Rockwood and Wilkins' Fractures in Children* (2020)
10. Rowland D, Baird E. Common upper limb injuries in childhood. Surgery (Oxford) [Internet]. 2014 Jan [cited 2024 Nov 22];32(1):9–16. Available from: https://linkinghub.elsevier.com/retrieve/pii/S0263931913002597
11. Verma V, Mahendra M, Rastogi D, Agarwal A, Afaque SF, M C P. Epidemiology of Pediatric Musculoskeletal Trauma Patients Admitted to a Trauma Center in Northern India: A Prospective Cohort Study. Cureus. 2023 Aug;15(8):e43327.

Pediatric Burns 13

Smita Das and N. Midhun Mohan

Learning Objectives

After completing this chapter, the reader will be able to:

- Outline the essential steps in the initial assessment and stabilization of pediatric patients with thermal burns using a structured approach
- Recognize the distinct physiological and clinical characteristics of thermal injuries in children
- Calculate fluid resuscitation requirements in pediatric burn victims based on burn size, depth, and standardized formulas
- Identify clinical indicators that warrant referral of a child with burns to a specialized burn center
- Recognize patterns and signs that raise suspicion of non-accidental burn injuries in children

Introduction

Burn injuries in children are a common and often preventable cause of both morbidity and mortality, particularly in low- and middle-income countries. Globally, the World Health Organization (WHO) identifies burns as one of the leading causes of non-fatal injuries among children, disproportionately affecting vulnerable populations. In India, pediatric burns continue to represent a significant public health challenge, frequently resulting from scalds, open flames, electrical accidents, and

S. Das
College of Nursing, AIIMS, New Delhi, New Delhi, Delhi, India

N. Midhun Mohan (✉)
Emergency Medicine, Kozhikode District Cooperative Hospital, Kozhikode, Kerala, India

N. T. Rai (ed.), *Pediatric Trauma Resuscitation Manual (PTRM) for Primary Care Providers*, https://doi.org/10.1007/978-981-95-4979-5_13

contact with hot surfaces or liquids. Following a burn incident, the initial point of medical contact for most families is often a local primary care facility or rural health center.

Primary care providers (PCPs) occupy a critical position in the early management of pediatric burn patients. Their prompt recognition of the injury, immediate stabilization measures, and timely referral to higher centers can substantially influence the patient's outcome. Initial interventions at the primary care level—such as securing the airway, providing analgesia, covering wounds, initiating fluid resuscitation, and counselling caregivers—play a pivotal role in reducing complications and improving recovery.

Pediatric burn management poses unique challenges compared to adult care due to the anatomical and physiological differences in children. These include thinner skin, a higher body surface area-to-volume ratio, and an increased vulnerability to rapid fluid shifts, hypothermia, and infections. Such factors necessitate careful monitoring and age-appropriate interventions.

This chapter provides PCPs with a structured, practical approach to pediatric burn care, emphasizing key steps including accurate assessment of burn depth and total body surface area affected, calculation of fluid requirements, anticipation of airway compromise, and identification of injuries that warrant referral to specialized burn centers. It also highlights the importance of maintaining vigilance for potential non-accidental injuries in certain burn patterns and presentations.

Beyond clinical stabilization, PCPs have a vital role in supporting families—offering education on wound care, pain management, and prevention of secondary complications, as well as initiating early psychosocial support. By adopting a systematic, child-centered approach, PCPs act as frontline guardians against the complications of burn injuries, ensuring safer transitions to higher-level care and optimizing the child's chances for functional recovery and long-term well-being.

Case Scenario

It is late evening in a semi-urban clinic when Master Ankit, a 9-year-old boy, is rushed in by his distressed parents. Moments earlier, while playing alone in a closed garage, he had accidentally ignited a box of matches. His clothing caught fire, and in a panic, he tried to extinguish the flames using his hands. Upon arrival, the child is conscious but crying in pain. A pungent smell of burnt fabric is noticeable, and large areas of skin appear reddened and blistered.

The clinic staff quickly observe circumferential burns on Ankit's right lower limb, patchy burns on the anterior surface of his left leg, and painful injuries on both palms. His clothes have already been removed by his parents, but the wounds are exposed. His weight is estimated at 35 kg and his height at 130 cm.

Initial Vital Signs

- Level of consciousness: Alert and crying
- Respiratory rate: 24 breaths/min
- Heart rate: 135 beats/min
- Blood pressure: 110/70 mmHg
- Oxygen saturation: 99%
- Capillary refill: 2 s

The treating PCP begins the initial survey and prepares to stabilize the child while considering referral.

Reflective Questions

1. What immediate actions should be taken to stop the burning process and protect the airway?
2. What are the key elements to assess during the primary survey of a child with thermal burns, and how can PCPs prioritize life-threatening issues?
3. Based on Ankit's burn distribution, how would you estimate the Total Burn Surface Area (TBSA)?
4. Should fluid resuscitation be initiated at the primary care level, and how would you calculate it?
5. What are the red flags for airway compromise or inhalation injury in this child's history?
6. When should referral to a specialized burns center be initiated, and how should you prepare the child for transfer?

Prehospital Care

In the prehospital or early primary care setting, prompt action by PCPs is critical in minimizing further tissue damage and stabilizing pediatric burn victims. The first and foremost priority is to halt the burning process while ensuring the child's airway, breathing, and circulation are stable. Any clothing that is not adherent to the skin should be gently removed to prevent continued thermal injury. Additionally, ornaments, belts, or tight accessories must be taken off immediately, as swelling may develop quickly and compromise distal circulation or cause secondary injuries.

The burned area should be irrigated with running water *(not cold or iced)* for at least 15–20 min to reduce pain and limit the depth of the burn. However, it is essential to avoid ice or ice water, as these can cause vasoconstriction and worsen tissue ischemia, increasing the depth of injury. Unscientific home remedies such as toothpaste, oil, or turmeric should be discouraged, as they can lead to infection, chemical irritation, and diagnostic delays.

Once cooling is complete, the affected area should be gently covered with a clean, dry cloth or sterile sheet to protect against contamination and minimize further heat loss. Young children are especially prone to hypothermia after burn injuries due to a higher body surface area-to-mass ratio, so care must be taken to keep the child warm during and after decontamination.

In cases where the burn occurred in an enclosed space, there is a high suspicion of smoke inhalation injury or toxic gas exposure (such as carbon monoxide or cyanide poisoning). High-flow oxygen therapy via a non-rebreather mask should be initiated immediately, even if the child appears stable, as symptoms may evolve insidiously.

For children in rural or resource-limited areas where transportation to a burn center or higher-level facility will take longer than 60 min, intravenous fluid resuscitation should be started en route. The decision to initiate fluids should be based on the estimated Total Body Surface Area (TBSA) burned and the depth of injury, using appropriate pediatric burn formulas (such as the Modified Parkland formula). Early initiation of fluids can help prevent the onset of burn shock, which can be life-threatening if left unaddressed.

Initial Assessment and Primary Survey

Thermal burns in children can be accompanied by life-threatening complications such as airway obstruction, inhalation injury, burn shock, and toxic exposures (e.g., carbon monoxide and cyanide poisoning). A systematic approach using the Pediatric Assessment Triangle (PAT) and ABCDE framework (airway, breathing, circulation, disability, exposure) is essential for early identification and stabilization of critically ill burn victims.

A—Airway with Cervical Spine Protection

Key Risks

- Edema from facial or oropharyngeal burns
- Inhalational injuries from enclosed space fires
- Systemic inflammatory response in burns >40% TBSA

Assessment

- Look for hoarseness, stridor, burns around the mouth or nares, singed nasal hairs, soot in the oral cavity, or altered mental status.
- Consider the potential for rapid airway deterioration in children due to smaller airway diameter.

Actions

- If airway involvement is suspected, early intubation is preferred before edema progresses.
- Use smaller-sized endotracheal tubes than age-predicted norms.
- Ensure manual inline cervical spine stabilization during airway management, especially in trauma cases.
- Prepare for surgical airway access (e.g., needle or surgical cricothyrotomy) in extreme scenarios.

B—Breathing and Ventilation

Common Complications

- Respiratory distress due to airway obstruction or thoracic burns
- Smoke inhalation injury, causing hypoxemia and atelectasis
- Carbon monoxide (CO) and cyanide poisoning reducing tissue oxygenation

Assessment

- Monitor respiratory rate, chest movements, accessory muscle use, and SpO_2.
- Be alert for altered consciousness or hypotension that may suggest toxic exposure.
- Recognize limitations of pulse oximetry in CO poisoning (SpO_2 may appear normal).

Actions

- Administer high-flow oxygen via non-rebreather mask immediately.
- Suspected CO poisoning should be treated with 100% oxygen, and co-oximetry should be used if available to detect carboxyhemoglobin levels.
- Obtain a chest X-ray and arterial blood gas (ABG) in children with suspected inhalation injury or respiratory compromise.

C—Circulation and Burn Shock

Hemodynamic Considerations

- Children with >15–20% TBSA burns are at risk of burn shock due to systemic capillary leak.
- Early hypotension within 1–2 h may indicate hemorrhagic shock or cyanide toxicity, not just burn shock.

Assessment

- Measure heart rate, blood pressure, capillary refill time (CRT), and urine output.
- Observe for pallor, cold extremities, or altered sensorium suggesting hypoperfusion.

Fluid Resuscitation

- Begin resuscitation if TBSA >15% or signs of hypoperfusion present.
- Use warmed isotonic crystalloid, preferably Ringer's lactate for resuscitation.
  - Add maintenance fluids with dextrose for children under 30 kg.
- Use the pediatric age-based adjusted hourly fluid rates (Table 13.1):

Practical Notes

- Prefer IV cannulation through non-burnt skin; if not possible, cannulate through burnt areas with caution.
- Avoid unnecessary fluid boluses unless hypotension is present to prevent fluid overload and worsening edema.
- Titrate fluid rate based on urine output (goal: 1 ml/kg/h) and ongoing clinical assessment.

Table 13.1 Pediatric age-based adjusted hourly fluid rates

Patient group	Fluid formula	Additional notes
Older children ≥13 years old	2 ml RL × kg × %TBSA ÷ 16	Administer continuously over 16 h
Children <13 years old	3 ml RL × kg × %TBSA ÷ 16	Administer continuously over 16 h
Infants and young children ≤30 kg	3 ml RL × kg × %TBSA ÷ 16	Administer continuously over 16 h + maintenance fluids with dextrose
Electrical injury (all ages)	4 ml RL × kg × %TBSA ÷ 16	Administer continuously over 16 h. Children <13 years old require maintenance fluids with dextrose in addition to RL calculation

D—Disability (Neurological Status)

Assessment

- Use AVPU scale: Alert, responds to Voice, responds to Pain, Unresponsive.
- Check for hypoglycemia with point-of-care glucose testing (GRBS), especially in irritable or lethargic children.

Concerns

- Altered mental status may suggest head injury, CO/cyanide toxicity, or hypoperfusion.

E—Exposure and Environment

Assessment and Actions

- Remove all clothing and constrictive items (e.g., jewelry, belts).
- Perform a full examination to identify all burn areas.
- Maintain normothermia: keep the child warm, turn off air conditioning, and cover with dry, sterile sheets.
- Assess burn depth and TBSA using the Lund and Browder chart.
- Evaluate for other injuries, particularly if there was an explosion, fall, or electrical source.

Pain Management

- Begin age-appropriate pain assessment (e.g., Wong-Baker FACES scale).
- Start analgesia promptly:
  - Mild–moderate pain: oral acetaminophen or ibuprofen
  - Severe pain: intranasal or IV opioids (e.g., fentanyl) or low-dose IV ketamine, if trained personnel available

Adjuncts to Primary Survey

Monitoring

- Continuous monitoring of:
  - Respiratory rate, SpO_2
  - Heart rate, BP
  - Level of consciousness (AVPU)
  - Temperature
  - Urine output

Investigations
- ABG with co-oximetry if inhalation injury suspected
- Chest X-ray for respiratory symptoms or closed-space exposure

Secondary Survey

The secondary survey is a comprehensive assessment performed once the child is hemodynamically stabilized and all immediate life-threatening conditions have been addressed during the primary survey. For pediatric burns, the secondary survey is essential to fully understand the extent, depth, and potential complications of the injury. It includes obtaining a focused history, performing a detailed head-to-toe physical examination, and initiating relevant diagnostic investigations to guide further treatment or referral.

1. *History Taking (SAMPLE Framework)*

   PCPs should use the SAMPLE mnemonic to guide history taking:

   S—Signs and symptoms (pain, difficulty breathing, vomiting, etc.)
   A—Allergies
   M—Medications the child is currently on
   P—Past medical history (e.g., seizures, asthma, previous burns, immunocompromised status)
   L—Last meal or oral intake
   E—Events leading to the burn (mechanism of injury)

   In addition to the above:
   - Ask about the environment of the injury: Was it in a closed or poorly ventilated space, which increases the risk of smoke inhalation or carbon monoxide poisoning?
   - Clarify how the injury occurred—if the explanation is inconsistent with the injury pattern or there's a delay in seeking care, consider non-accidental trauma (NAT).
   - Confirm immunization status, especially tetanus, as children with burns are at increased risk of wound infection.
2. *Burn Depth Assessment*

   Determine the depth of burns using clinical features such as color, moisture, blistering, capillary refill, and sensation. Burns are typically classified as follows:
   - Superficial
   - Superficial partial thickness
   - Deep partial thickness
   - Full thickness

   Table 13.2 provides a detailed classification based on these clinical features, while Fig. 13.1 demonstrates partial-thickness scald burns with intact and broken blisters.

Table 13.2 Clinical features of each class of burns

Burn description	Depth of injury	Appearance	Capillary refill	Pain/ sensation	Healing
Superficial thickness	Epidermis	Erythema e.g., sunburns	Fast	+	7–14 days. No scarring
Superficial partial thickness	Papillary dermis	Wet, pink with blisters	Fast *(blanches with pressure)*	++	2 to 4 weeks. No scarring or functional impairment
Deep partial thickness	Reticular dermis	Less wet, red +/− blisters	Sluggish or absent *(does not blanch with pressure)*	+/−	3–8 weeks with severe scarring. Needs grafting
Full thickness	Subcutaneous tissue	Dry, white, or charred and black No vesicles or blisters	Absent (do not blanch with pressure)	Absent	Severe scarring and contracture. Needs grafting

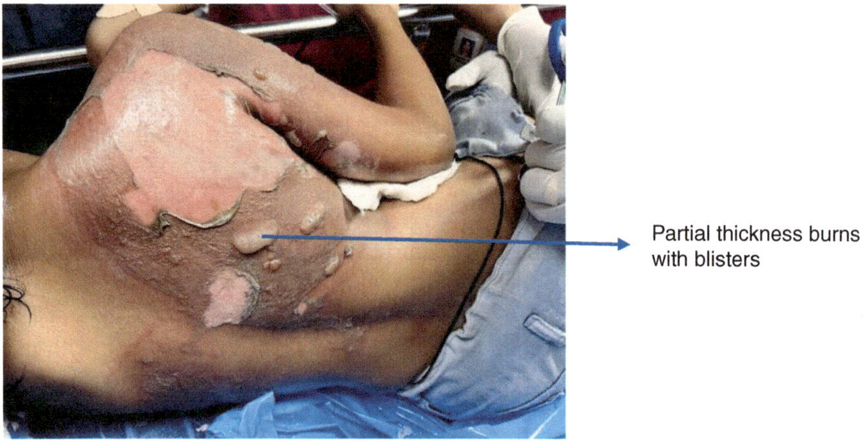

Fig. 13.1 Child having partial-thickness scald burns with broken and intact blisters

3. *Estimating Burn Extent (%TBSA)*

Accurate estimation of the Total Body Surface Area (TBSA) affected by partial- or full-thickness burns is critical to guide fluid resuscitation, monitor for systemic complications, and determine the need for specialist referral. The Lund and Browder chart (Fig. 13.2) remains the gold standard for pediatric burn estimation, as it accounts for age-related body surface area variations in children.

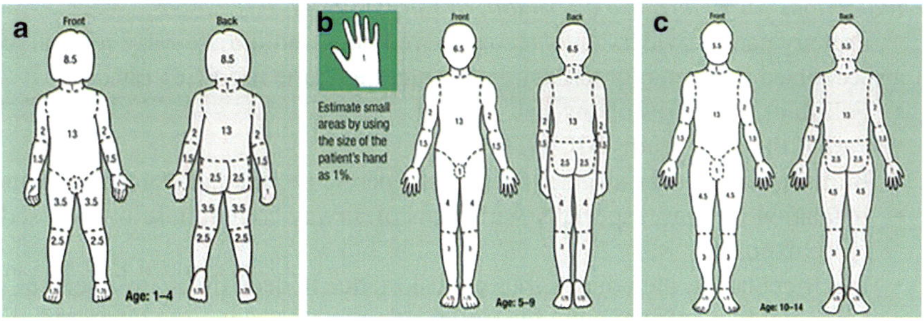

Fig. 13.2 Lund and Browder chart for calculating burns body surface area

Key Points:

- Only partial- and full-thickness burns should be included in TBSA calculation.
- Superficial (first-degree) burns should not be included in TBSA estimation for fluid calculations.

4. *Laboratory Investigations*

Routine blood tests should be initiated in the emergency department or clinic setting to assess systemic involvement, especially in children with >10% TBSA burns or deep tissue injury. Recommended baseline investigations include the following:

- *Complete blood count (CBC)* —to identify anemia, infection, or hemoconcentration
- *Serum electrolytes*—to detect electrolyte imbalance due to fluid shifts
- *Renal function tests*—for assessing baseline kidney function and detecting rhabdomyolysis
- *Liver function tests*—especially relevant in extensive burns or potential drug toxicity
- *Coagulation profile (PT, aPTT)*—to evaluate clotting status, especially in major burns
- *Blood grouping and cross-matching*—in anticipation of transfusion if indicated
- *Screening for HIV, HBsAg, HCV*—as part of hospital protocol prior to surgical intervention
- *Urine microscopy*—to assess for hematuria or myoglobinuria (suggestive of muscle damage)

Additional tests (e.g., ABG, lactate, carboxyhemoglobin levels) should be guided by clinical signs of inhalation injury, cyanide poisoning, or metabolic acidosis.

5. *Indications for Referral to a Specialized Burns Center*

   Primary care providers must recognize red flags and initiate early referral to a specialized burns unit or tertiary care center under the following conditions:

   - Full-thickness burns of any size
   - Partial-thickness burns >10% TBSA.
   - Burns involving critical areas: hands, face, perineum, genitalia, or major joints
   - Inhalation injuries, especially with signs of airway compromise or enclosed space exposure
   - Electrical burns, including lightning strikes, due to deep tissue involvement
   - Chemical burns that require decontamination or specialized management
   - Burns in children with pre-existing comorbidities (e.g., diabetes, renal failure) that may complicate healing
   - Situations where qualified personnel, equipment, or infrastructure are not available to manage pediatric burns effectively
   - Cases that demand special psychological, emotional, or rehabilitative care
   - Any suspicion of non-accidental trauma (child abuse)

Specific Considerations

I. *Wound Care in Pediatric Burns*

   Effective wound care is a cornerstone in the management of pediatric burn injuries. The goals include minimizing infection risk, promoting optimal healing, alleviating pain, and preventing long-term functional or cosmetic complications.

   Initial Wound Management

   - Immediately irrigate the burn area with cool running water for at least 20 min. This reduces the depth of injury and provides analgesic benefit by dissipating residual heat.
   - Gently remove any loose clothing or jewelry near the burned area to prevent vascular compression due to progressive edema.
   - Do not attempt to remove clothing that is adherent to the wound. Leave it in place to avoid further tissue damage.

   Dressings and Topical Care

   - After cooling, cover the burn with a clean, dry, non-adherent dressing or a clean cloth to minimize contamination and fluid loss.
   - Avoid the application of home remedies such as toothpaste, oil, ghee, or herbal pastes, as these can worsen tissue injury and promote infection.
   - Topical antibiotics (e.g., silver sulfadiazine, mupirocin) may be used based on burn depth and extent.
   - Dressings may include Vaseline-impregnated gauze or modern alternatives like hydrogel dressings, depending on availability.
   - Debridement: All large or infected blisters should be debrided. Very small, intact blisters that do not interfere with mobility or function may be left alone.
   - Emphasize aseptic technique during dressing changes to reduce the risk of infection.

Pain Management During Dressing

- Burn wound care is often painful. Prior to dressing, ensure adequate analgesia or procedural sedation is provided. Options include the following:
  - Oral analgesics (paracetamol, ibuprofen) for minor burns
  - Intranasal or intravenous opioids/ketamine for moderate to severe pain when appropriately trained personnel are available
- Distraction techniques and child-friendly communication can help reduce anxiety during dressing procedures.

Referral Considerations

- If the child is being referred to a burns center, do not apply definitive dressings. Instead, cover wounds with clean dry cloth, and focus on stabilizing the patient for transfer.

II. *Non-accidental Trauma (NAT) Considerations*

Burn injuries in children may sometimes be the result of intentional harm or neglect. PCPs must remain vigilant and consider child abuse when:

- The mechanism of injury does not correlate with the pattern or distribution of burns.
- There is delay in seeking medical care.
- Burns have clear demarcated patterns, such as immersion lines or cigarette marks.
- The history is inconsistent or changes on repeated questioning.

Any suspicion of NAT mandates thorough documentation, a detailed examination for other signs of trauma, and referral to child protection services as per institutional policy and national guidelines.

III. *Psychosocial Considerations in Pediatric Burns*

Burn injuries can have profound emotional and psychological impacts on both the child and their caregivers. Proactive engagement with the family improves compliance and contributes to a smoother recovery process for the child.

Psychological Support

- Acknowledge and address the child's pain, fear, and anxiety during evaluation and treatment.
- Use calm, reassuring language, and involve parents or guardians in the care process to provide emotional security.
- Encourage age-appropriate coping strategies, such as distraction, storytelling, or play.

Family Education

PCPs should educate the family on the following:

- Nature of thermal injuries and their potential complications
- Importance of adherence to treatment protocols including wound care, medications, and follow-up visits
- Signs of infection (increased redness, swelling, pus, foul odor, fever) that warrant immediate attention
- Pain management strategies at home
- Rehabilitation needs, including physical therapy if required for joint or functional recovery

Case Resolution

Master Ankit, a 9-year-old boy, is brought to a semi-urban clinic following an accidental thermal injury sustained while playing with matches in a closed garage. On arrival, he is alert, crying, and in significant pain. His parents report that his clothing caught fire, and he attempted to extinguish the flames with his hands. Examination reveals circumferential burns on the right lower limb, patchy burns on the anterior aspect of the left leg, and involvement of both palms. His vital signs are stable, with a heart rate of 135 bpm, respiratory rate of 24 breaths per minute, BP 110/70 mmHg, capillary refill of 2 s, and SpO_2 of 99%.

The primary care team initiates a structured approach, beginning with control of the burning process. Any remaining charred clothing is confirmed to be removed, and the affected areas are gently irrigated with cool running water to reduce further tissue damage. Hypothermia prevention is prioritized by covering non-burned areas and avoiding ice or other unscientific home remedies. The wounds are left exposed temporarily, as dressing will follow once stabilization is achieved.

Given the history of injury in an enclosed space, the team remains alert to signs of smoke inhalation or toxic exposure. Although the child is maintaining saturation and showing no immediate airway compromise, oxygen therapy is initiated as a precaution. Airway equipment is kept ready, anticipating the possibility of delayed airway edema.

A primary survey using the ABCDE framework is conducted:

- *Airway*: Patent, no soot or hoarseness noted
- *Breathing*: Symmetrical chest expansion, normal breath sounds, SpO_2 maintained
- *Circulation*: Tachycardia with maintained BP and perfusion; no active bleeding
- *Disability*: Alert and oriented; GRBS normal
- *Exposure*: Full inspection confirms partial-thickness burns on both lower limbs and palms

Using the Lund and Browder chart, the team estimates the Total Burn Surface Area (TBSA) at approximately 23%, qualifying the injury for fluid resuscitation. The Modified Parkland formula is applied: 3 mL × 35 kg × 23% = 2415 mL of Ringer's lactate, with half to be given in the first 8 h post-injury and the rest over the next 16 h. An IV cannula is placed in an unburnt area and fluids initiated. Pain is managed using intravenous fentanyl, carefully titrated to the child's response.

A clean dressing is applied using topical antibiotics and sterile gauze. Given the child's circumferential burns, palm involvement, and potential inhalation risk, referral to a burns center is indicated. The child is stabilized, documentation is prepared, and transport is arranged with IV fluids, analgesia, and monitoring en route.

This case highlights the critical role PCPs play in early stabilization, accurate assessment, and timely referral in pediatric burns. Prompt recognition of burn severity, calculation of TBSA, and fluid initiation can significantly impact outcomes while ensuring safe transition to definitive care.

Key Messages

- Pediatric burn injuries can result in life-threatening airway obstruction, respiratory failure, and shock, requiring rapid assessment and stabilization.
- A structured approach using the ABCDE principles ensures life-threatening complications are identified early.
- Enclosed space burns should raise suspicion for smoke inhalation, carbon monoxide, and cyanide poisoning, even if SpO_2 is normal.
- Prehospital care must focus on stopping the burning process with cool water irrigation and preventing hypothermia; unscientific remedies like toothpaste or ice should be avoided.
- Circumferential burns; burns involving the face, hands, genitalia, and major joints; or burns >10% TBSA in children warrant early referral to a specialized burns center.
- TBSA estimation using the Lund and Browder chart is critical for guiding fluid resuscitation; only partial- and full-thickness burns are included.
- Fluid requirements are calculated using the modified Parkland formula (3 mL × weight × %TBSA); Ringer's lactate is the preferred fluid.
- Airway compromise may be delayed; signs such as hoarseness, stridor, or altered sensorium should prompt consideration for early intubation.
- Pain management and prevention of infection are key priorities; dressings should be done under sterile precautions with appropriate analgesia.
- Systemic antibiotics are not routinely indicated unless there is evidence of infection.
- Burns in children with inconsistent history or unusual patterns should prompt suspicion of non-accidental trauma and require mandatory reporting.
- Psychosocial support and caregiver education are essential to ensure adherence to treatment, wound care, and long-term rehabilitation.
- In rural or resource-limited settings, PCPs must initiate stabilization and coordinate safe transfer while maintaining airway, breathing, and circulation.

Bibliography

1. American College of Surgeons Committee on Trauma. ATLS: Advanced Trauma Life Support. 11th ed. Chicago: American College of Surgeons; 2025.
2. de Jong AEE, Bremer M, van Komen R, Vanbrabant L, Schuurmans M, Middelkoop E, et al. Pain in young children with burns: Extent, course and influencing factors. Burns. 2014 Feb;40(1):38–47.
3. Neha Thakur, Samir Misra. Pediatric Trauma Resuscitation Module (PTRM). First edition. New Delhi: Jaypee Brothers Medical Publishers (P) Ltd; 2024.
4. Peddi M, Segu S, Ramesha K. The persistent paradigm of pediatric burns in India: An epidemiological review. Indian Journal of Burns. 2014;22(1):93.
5. Strobel AM, Fey R. Emergency Care of Pediatric Burns. Emerg Med Clin North Am. 2018 May;36(2):441–58.
6. Suman A, Owen J. Update on the management of burns in paediatrics. BJA Educ. 2020 Mar;20(3):103–10.

7. Wala SJ, Ragan MV, Mallampalli GM, Thakkar RK. Update in Pediatric Burn Care. Current Trauma Reports. 2023 Sep;9(3):101–113. https://doi.org/10.1007/s40719-023-00256-6.

Non-accidental Injuries and Child Abuse 14

A. Latha and Bharat Choudhary

Learning Objectives

By the end of this chapter, the reader should be able to:

1. Define various types of child maltreatment
2. Outline key PCP management goals for suspected child abuse, including assessment, stabilization, and ensuring safety
3. Identify clinical signs of abuse and neglect
4. Describe suitable interview techniques that establish trust and confidentiality for the child
5. Explain mandatory reporting, legal requirements, and collaboration with child protection agencies

Introduction

The World Health Organization (WHO) defines child maltreatment as "all forms of physical and emotional ill-treatment, sexual abuse, neglect, and exploitation that result in actual or potential harm to the child's health, development, or dignity." Child abuse is broadly categorized into four main types: neglect, physical abuse, psychological abuse, and sexual abuse.

A. Latha
College of Nursing, All India Institute of Medical Sciences,
Jodhpur, Rajasthan, India

B. Choudhary (✉)
Trauma & Emergency (Pediatrics), All India Institute of Medical Sciences,
Jodhpur, Rajasthan, India

N. T. Rai (ed.), *Pediatric Trauma Resuscitation Manual (PTRM) for Primary Care Providers*, https://doi.org/10.1007/978-981-95-4979-5_14

Abuse is considered "an act of commission," whereas neglect is defined as "an act of omission" in care that leads to potential or actual harm. Neglect may manifest as inadequate healthcare, insufficient education, poor supervision, failure to protect from environmental hazards, or unmet basic needs such as food, clothing, and shelter. Globally, neglect is recognized as the most prevalent form of child maltreatment.

Physical abuse refers to any act that causes bodily harm to a child, including hitting, punching, kicking, biting, burning, shaking, or other forms of intentional injury inflicted by a caregiver. Clinical manifestations can include bruises, bite marks, fractures, head injuries (including shaken baby syndrome), burns, and female genital mutilation. Accurate medical history is critical for identifying and confirming cases of physical abuse.

Psychological abuse encompasses verbal abuse, humiliation, intimidation, or terrorizing behavior, which can have long-term consequences on a child's mental health and development.

Sexual abuse involves the participation of a dependent, developmentally immature child or adolescent in sexual activities that they cannot fully comprehend, consent to, or which violate familial and social norms. Not all cases require direct physical penetration; sexual abuse may also include exposure to sexually explicit material, oral-genital contact, genital-to-genital contact, genital-to-anal contact, or genital fondling.

Abusive head trauma occurs primarily in infants under 1 year of age and is caused by violent shaking. It often results in intracranial injuries, most commonly subdural hemorrhage, which may lead to cerebral edema, permanent neurological damage, or death.

Problem Statement

Child abuse is a serious global concern affecting millions of children and is often referred to as a "silent epidemic." Worldwide, the prevalence of child abuse is estimated at 12–13%, affecting approximately 18% of girls and 8% of boys. According to the CDC (2024), 1 in 4 girls and 1 in 13 boys experience abuse, and nearly 1 billion children have faced some form of sexual violence.

In India, the National Crime Records Bureau (NCRB) reported in 2016 that a child is sexually abused every 15 min, with 53% of cases involving perpetrators who are parents, relatives, or school teachers. Between 2016 and 2022, reported cases of child sexual abuse rose by 96%, with an 8.7% increase from 2021 alone. These figures likely underestimate the true burden due to underreporting driven by social stigma, fear of retaliation, and lack of awareness, particularly in rural communities.

Different types of abuse have been documented, including physical abuse (69%), sexual abuse (53%), emotional abuse (49%), overall neglect (up to 71%), emotional neglect (up to 60%), and physical neglect (up to 58%). Alarmingly, in 90% of child abuse cases, the perpetrator is someone known to the child.

Socioeconomic factors such as poverty, limited education, and stressful living conditions further heighten the risk of violence against children. Children from low-income families are particularly vulnerable to neglect compared to their wealthier peers. Globally, 17.2 million children are engaged in domestic work, 11.5 million in child labor, with 3.7 million working in hazardous conditions (21.4%). An additional 5.7 million adolescents require protection and access to safe work opportunities. Many children are trapped in forced labor and trafficking; in 2012, the International Labour Organization (ILO) estimated that 5.5 million children were among 20.9 million victims of forced labor. Girls represent the majority of child domestic workers (67.1%), with 65.1% under 14 years of age, including 7.4 million aged 5–11 and 3.8 million aged 12–14.

Case Scenario

An 11-year-old boy, Muthu, was brought to the emergency department by his father. He informed that the child sustained injury due to fall from a 6-feet ladder. On examination, Muthu had multiple bruises of varying ages on his back, thighs, and arms. His left arm was swollen, and he flinched in pain when touched. He was malnourished, poorly groomed, and visibly fearful. His vitals are as follows:

- Pulse: 160 bpm
- Respiration: 48/min, SpO_2 88%
- BP: 60/40 mmHg, peripheries cold CRT>3, GCS was E3 V3 M4 = 10/15

Can Muthu be a victim of abuse?

On examination, he appears hemodynamically unstable, with a deep laceration over the forehead, visible bruises on his limbs and back, and a suspected left arm fracture. He is in compensated shock with signs of respiratory distress and altered sensorium. The management follows the structured trauma approach using the ABCDE framework, ensuring life-threatening conditions are identified and addressed without delay.

Initial Triage and Assessment

Based on Muthu's presentation, tachycardia, hypotension, and altered consciousness, he is triaged as needing immediate resuscitation. The first responder must alert the team leader and initiate emergency support while ensuring safety and preparation for transfer or escalation of care.

A—Airway with Cervical Spine Precaution

Assessment: Inspect for airway patency, noting any obstruction from facial trauma or bleeding. Watch for signs such as noisy breathing, inability to vocalize, or secretions.

Intervention: Position the airway appropriately, and clear any obstruction using suction. Administer high-flow oxygen via non-rebreather mask (10–15 L/min). Given the mechanism of injury, apply a cervical collar to stabilize the spine. Be prepared for advanced airway management if mental status worsens or airway compromise develops.

B—Breathing

Assessment: Evaluate respiratory rate, work of breathing, and oxygen saturation. Look for nasal flaring, intercostal retractions, or cyanosis.

Intervention: Administer oxygen to maintain $SpO_2 \geq 94\%$. If signs of deterioration are present (e.g., reduced breath sounds or chest asymmetry), consider the possibility of rib fracture, pneumothorax, or other thoracic trauma and manage accordingly.

C—Circulation with Hemorrhage Control

Assessment: Monitor heart rate, capillary refill, blood pressure, and peripheral perfusion. Look for pallor, cold extremities, or weak pulses.

Intervention: Initiate two large-bore IV lines (18G or 20G). Send blood samples for crossmatching, hemoglobin, and other investigations. Begin warm isotonic fluid resuscitation (Normal Saline or Ringer's Lactate) at 20 ml/kg over 15–20 min, repeating up to 60 ml/kg if signs of shock persist. Aim for urine output ≥1 ml/kg/h. Control external bleeding from the forehead using sterile pressure dressing. Immobilize the fractured left arm with a splint, and administer appropriate analgesia. Maintain warmth using blankets or warming devices.

D—Disability (Neurological Status)

Assessment: Use the AVPU or pediatric GCS to assess consciousness. Check for pupil reactivity, symmetry, and limb movements. Look for subtle signs of head trauma or intracranial injury.

Intervention: Rule out hypoglycemia by checking blood glucose levels and correct if necessary. Continue neurological monitoring during stabilization.

E—Exposure and Environmental Control

Assessment: Fully expose the child to evaluate for hidden injuries, ensuring privacy and maintaining temperature. Notable findings include bruises of different ages, swelling in the left arm, and superficial injuries to the thighs.

Intervention: Document all injuries carefully. Cover Muthu with warm blankets after evaluation to prevent hypothermia.

SAMPLE History for Muthu

His father informed that he was well till morning; while climbing on the ladder, his foot slipped, and he fell down. His face also hit the ladder. There is no past significant history.

He is poor in studies so he doesn't go to the school. He had breakfast in the morning. No drug allergy report.

Head-to-Toe Assessment

- *Bruising*: Multiple bruises of different colors and stages of healing noted on the back, arms, and thighs—some red/purple (recent), others yellow/brown (older), indicating repetitive injury over time.
- *Swelling and Fracture Signs*: Marked swelling in the left arm with restricted and painful movement, suggestive of an unaddressed fracture.
- *Pallor*: Generalized pale skin indicating possible anemia or chronic neglect.
- *Hair and Skin*: Thin, discolored (flag sign) hair, often associated with protein deficiency.
- *Dental Hygiene*: Presence of dental caries and poor oral hygiene, reinforcing evidence of chronic neglect.

Can This Presentation Be Because of Child Abuse?

Muthu's clinical presentation raises significant concern for non-accidental trauma (NAT). Several features collectively point toward possible child abuse and neglect. The presence of multiple bruises of varying ages, evidence of malnutrition, poor hygiene, and an anxious, withdrawn demeanor are hallmark indicators. The history of being socially withdrawn for a month, followed by a traumatic event resulting in head injury, further compounds the suspicion.

When to Suspect Child Abuse in Any Child?

As PCPs, recognizing child abuse early is crucial for protecting vulnerable children. Abuse should be suspected when injuries, behaviors, or caregiver responses are inconsistent, unexplained, or concerning. Table 14.1 explains the different signs of suspected maltreatment.

In hemodynamically stable children, The examination should be conducted in a calm and non-threatening manner to ensure their comfort and cooperation. Anthropometric measurements and vital signs should be recorded, followed by a thorough head-to-toe assessment. In adolescents, sexual maturity rating should also be documented. A comprehensive systemic examination is essential to identify serious internal injuries and ensure appropriate medical care.

Table 14.1 Signs of suspect for child abuse

Category	Signs and indicators
Physical signs	Injuries inconsistent with history (e.g., a non-mobile infant with fractures) Bruises in unusual locations (face, back, buttocks, ears, neck, abdomen) Multiple bruises of different ages (suggesting repeated trauma) Burns (cigarette burns, glove/sock-like burns from forced immersion) Fractures (spinal fractures, rib fractures in infants, skull fractures) Head injuries (intracranial bleeding, retinal hemorrhages in shaken baby syndrome) Bite marks, cuts, or strap marks
Behavioral signs in the child	Fearfulness, withdrawn behavior, flinching at touch Overly clingy or fearful of parents/caregivers Avoiding physical examination or refusing to explain injuries Regression (bedwetting, thumb-sucking) Aggressive or self-harming behaviors
Inconsistent or suspicious history	Delay in seeking medical care for serious injuries Vague, changing, or conflicting explanations from caregivers Caregiver minimizes injury severity or reacts inappropriately Previous history of similar unexplained injuries
Neglect and malnourishment	Failure to thrive (severe underweight, stunted growth) Poor hygiene, untreated medical issues (e.g., infections, lice, dental, decay) Lack of supervision, wandering alone, or frequent school absences
Sexual abuse indicators	Genital pain, bleeding, sexually transmitted infections Inappropriate sexual knowledge or behavior for age Difficulty walking or sitting Sudden fear of a particular person or place
Parental or caregiver red flags	History of domestic violence, substance abuse, or mental illness Extreme discipline or unrealistic expectations for the child's age Lack of concern for the child's well-being History of abuse in siblings or past child welfare involvement

Documentation Photographic documentation should be performed whenever possible after consent, as it holds significant medico-legal importance, particularly in case of suspected child abuse. Clear photographs should be taken of all injuries observed during the physical examination, both as a whole and individually. Images should be captured to ensure they are identifiable and understandable, even by individuals who have not directly examined the case.

Are All Unexplained Injuries Abused?

PCPs must recognize that not all unexplained injuries are due to abuse. Some may result from accidents, medical conditions, or cultural practices. However, PCPs must remain vigilant and assess each case carefully. Injuries with inconsistent explanations, multiple bruises of varying ages, or marks in unusual locations should

Table 14.2 Few conditions mimicking as abuse

Condition	Findings on examination	PCP considerations
Bleeding disorders (e.g., hemophilia, von Willebrand disease)	Easy bruising, spontaneous bleeding, prolonged bleeding from minor injuries	Assess bleeding history, monitor for excessive bruising, coordinate hematology referral
Osteogenesis imperfecta (brittle bone disease)	Frequent fractures, blue sclera, joint laxity, short stature	Handle with care, educate caregivers on fracture prevention, refer to genetics
Mongolian spots	Bluish-grey birthmarks, often on the lower back or buttocks, present at birth	Differentiate from bruises, document location and characteristics, reassure caregivers
Ehlers-Danlos syndrome	Hypermobile joints, fragile skin, easy bruising, delayed wound healing	Encourage protective measures, document skin findings, collaborate with specialists
Cupping/coining (cultural practices)	Circular or linear red marks on the skin, non-tender, no swelling	Assess cultural background, educate families on safer practices, document findings
Phytophotodermatitis (skin reaction to citrus + sun exposure)	Linear or irregularly shaped skin discolorations, may resemble burns	Take detailed history, provide skin care education, reassure caregivers
Scurvy (Vitamin C deficiency)	Perifollicular hemorrhages, swollen bleeding gums, joint pain	Assess nutrition intake educate on diet improvement, refer for supplementation
Impetigo or skin infections	Crusted, weeping skin lesions, may resemble burns	Ensure hygiene education, wound care, and infection control

raise concerns. Our role is to document findings accurately, provide compassionate care, and report any suspicions to the appropriate child protection authorities to ensure the child's safety and well-being. As PCPs, we need to differentiate the other pathological problem examples given in Table 14.2.

How to Investigate Suspected Abuse?

Any child younger than 2 years old with suspected physical abuse should undergo a skeletal survey after discussion with a physician. Additionally, any sibling under the age of two of an abused child also receives a skeletal survey. This imaging study includes 21 dedicated views, as recommended by the American College of Radiology, to thoroughly assess for occult fractures or other signs of injury. It is important to consider that the most common differential diagnosis for non-accidental injury is accidental trauma, requiring careful clinical evaluation to distinguish between the two. Investigations needed to perform on child abuse are given in Table 14.3.

Table 14.3 Investigations in children with suspected abuse

Assessment	Details	PCP considerations
Skeletal survey	Performed in all children <2 years with suspected abuse and siblings <2years of abused children	Ensure child comfort during imaging, provide emotional support to caregivers, explain procedure to family
Number of views	21 dedicated views as per American College of Radiology	Verify proper positioning, assist radiology team, document procedure
Included views	AP and lateral skull, lateral spine, AP and oblique chest, AP pelvis, AP femurs, AP legs, AP humeri, AP forearm, PA hands, AP (dorsoventral) feet	Ensure all required views are taken for accurate assessment
Follow-up imaging	If findings are abnormal or unclear, repeat in 2 weeks to assess healing patterns	Educate caregivers about the need for follow-up; monitor for pain or distress
Laboratory investigations	Done to rule out medical conditions that mimic abuse	Ensure proper sample collection, educate family on the need for tests
Bone panel	Calcium, Magnesium, Phosphate, Alkaline Phosphatase	Monitor for bone disorders; ensure supplementation if needed
Hematology panel	Complete Blood Count (CBC)	Check for anemia or infection
Coagulation panel	PT, PTT, INR	Rule out bleeding disorders
Metabolic panel	Glucose, BUN, creatinine, albumin, protein	Assess overall health and nutritional status
Liver function tests	AST, ALT	Detect liver injury due to trauma
Pancreatic enzymes	Amylase, lipase	Identify pancreatic injury from blunt trauma
Bleeding disorders panel	von Willebrand antigen and activity, Factor VIII, Factor IX, platelet function assays	Differentiate abuse from bleeding disorders
Differential diagnosis	Most common alternative diagnosis to non-accidental injury is accidental trauma	Conduct thorough history-taking, assess injury patterns, collaborate with medical team

AP anterior and posterior, *PT* prothrombin time, *PTT* partial thromboplastin time, *INT* International Normalized Ratio, *AST* aspartate aminotransferase, *ALT* alanine aminotransferase

Anatomical and Physical Considerations

Fractures in children can result from both accidents and abuse, making detection challenging.

Abuse-related fractures are most common in infants, particularly those under 12 months. The child's age, fracture type, history, and context are key indicators. PCPs play a crucial role in recognizing abuse and taking action to protect children, as failure to intervene can lead to recurrence and increased mortality. Studies show that many fatal child abuse cases could have been prevented with early detection.

Abuse-related fractures, often caused by violent acts or neglect, frequently include rib, skull, humeral, and femur fractures. Berthold et al. reported that among 551 children under 36 months with fractures, 5.6% were confirmed as abuse-related. After soft tissue injuries, fractures are the second most common sign of physical abuse. Awareness is essential for timely diagnosis and intervention.

Children's bones are more flexible and have a higher cartilage content, making them less prone to fractures from minor trauma. A humerus fracture in children often suggests significant force and raises concerns for non-accidental injury. The periosteum (bone covering) is thicker in children, which helps fractures heal faster but can also mask signs of previous injuries on X-rays. Transverse fractures typically result from direct impact or bending forces, which are common in abuse cases. Spiral fractures are caused by twisting forces, often suspicious in non-ambulatory children. Metaphyseal fractures (bucket handles or corner fractures) are highly suggestive of abuse caused by violent shaking or pulling.

A humerus fracture in a young should always prompt a careful evaluation, as early recognition or abuse can prevent further harm and potentially save a life. Table 14.4 explains the types of abuse and its assessment findings of suspected abuse

Common symptoms include severe pain, swelling, bruising, and possible limb deformity. Immediate evaluation and appropriate treatment are important. Common risk factors for child abuse is given in Table 14.5.

Table 14.4 Assessment findings of suspected abuse

Type of abuse	Assessment findings	PCP considerations
Neglect	Poor weight gain or growth Inadequate hygiene Persistent hunger Irregular school attendance Constant fatigue Reports of lack of supervision Delinquent behavior	Monitor growth parameters Assess hygiene and nutritional status Observe for emotional distress or developmental delays Document findings accurately Report concerns to child protection services
Physical abuse	Unexplained bruises, burns, or fractures Bald patches on scalp Apprehensive or fearful child Extreme aggressiveness or withdrawal Fear of parents Older infants/toddlers not crying when approached by strangers	Perform a thorough head-to-toe assessment Observe caregiver-child interactions Document injury patterns carefully Ensure pain management and emotional support Report suspected abuse to appropriate authorities
Emotional abuse	Speech or communication difficulties Habit disorders (sucking, biting, rocking) Psychoneurotic reactions Learning difficulties Suicide attempts	Observe for behavioral and emotional distress Provide a supportive, safe environment Encourage psychosocial support and therapy Document finding and collaborate with mental health professionals

(continued)

Table 14.4 (continued)

Type of abuse	Assessment findings	PCP considerations
Sexual abuse	Difficulty walking or sitting Torn, stained, or bloody underclothing Genital pain, swelling, or itching Bruises, bleeding, or lacerations in genital/anal areas Reluctance to change clothes or participate in physical activities Poor peer relationships	Conduct a sensitive, non-judgmental assessment Ensure privacy and emotional support Assist with forensic evidence collection if required Collaborate with social workers and children protection teams
Abusive head trauma	May show no external trauma Retinal hemorrhages on ophthalmoscopic exam Full, bulging fontanels Head circumference larger than expected	Monitor for neurological deterioration (seizures, lethargy, vomiting) Support with oxygen and seizure precautions Assist with imaging (CT/MRI) and ophthalmology assessment Report findings to child protection authorities

Table 14.5 Common risk factors for child abuse

Category	Risk factors	PCP considerations
Child-related factors	*Age*: Children under 4 years or adolescents *Parent expectations*: Unwanted children or those failing to meet parent expectations *Special needs*: Persistent crying, abnormal physical, or medical conditions *Disabilities*: Intellectual disabilities or neurological disorders *Sexual orientation*: Lesbian, gay, bisexual, transgender, and queer (LGBTQ) children may face increased maltreatment	Identify vulnerable children thoroughly, and do early screening and observation Provide targeted support for children with special needs or disabilities Educate caregivers about healthy child development and positive parenting strategies
Parent or caregiver factors	*Bonding issue*: Difficulty bonding with the child *History of abuse*: Caregivers who were abused as children are at higher risk of abusive behavior *Unrealistic expectations*: Lack of understanding of child development *Substance abuse*: Alcohol or drug misuse, including during pregnancy *Mental health issues*: Poor impulse control and mental disorders *Financial strain*: Economic hardships can contribute to stress and situations	Assess parent-child interactions for signs of bonding issue or neglect Offer mental health support and counselling caregivers Provide education on child development and stress management Refer families to social service for financial or substance abuse support

Table 14.5 (continued)

Category	Risk factors	PCP considerations
Relationship factors	*Family violence*: Domestic violence or relationship breakdowns *Isolation*: Lack of community support or social networks	Promote safe family environments through counselling and intervention Collaborate, with domestic violence programs and social services
Community and societal factors	*Inequality*: Gender and social inequality contribute to maltreatment *Lack of resources*: Insufficient housing and family support services *Poverty and unemployment*: Economic instability *Substance availability*: Easy access to drug and alcohol *Cultural norms*: Societal attitudes that normalize violence, rigid gender roles, or corporal punishment	Advocate for policy changes to support vulnerable families Refer families to community-based resources for financial aid and housing Educate communities on positive parenting practices and the dangers of corporal punishment Work with public health programs to reduce substance abuse and increase child welfare awareness

Health Consequences of Child Abuse

- *Immediate physical injuries* may include head trauma, fractures, burns, or severe disabilities.
- *Long-term psychological effects* can manifest as post-traumatic stress disorder (PTSD), anxiety, depression, and other mental health conditions.
- *Adolescent girls* are at risk of gynecological problems and unintended pregnancies.
- *Cognitive and academic impact*: maltreatment can impair learning, memory, and overall school performance.
- *Increased risk of substance use*: affected children are more likely to engage in smoking, alcohol, or drug use, which in turn predisposes them to noncommunicable diseases (NCDs) such as cardiovascular disease and cancer.
- *Neurodevelopmental effects*: chronic stress from abuse disrupts early brain development, affecting nervous system maturation and immune function.
- *Cycle of violence*: children who experience maltreatment are more likely to become either victims or perpetrators of violence in the future.
- *Behavioral and health risks*: increased likelihood of depression, obesity, high-risk sexual behaviors, unintended pregnancies, and substance misuse.
- *Educational consequences*: children exposed to violence are approximately 13% more likely to drop out of school.
- *Economic burden*: child abuse contributes to substantial costs, including hospitalizations, mental health care, child welfare services, and long-term health expenditures.

How to Use the SBAR Technique to Talk to Children with Abuse?

The SBAR (situation, background, assessment, recommendation) technique is to communicate with children who may be experiencing abuse. PCPs need to remember the points.

- PCPs need to be patient so the child sets the pace.
- Use simple, gentle, and age-appropriate language.
- Do not make promises like "I will not tell anyone," but we can say that I only share with people who can help to keep you safe.
- Strictly follow the reporting laws.

S: Situation
- Make sure the child is in a private, safe, and comfortable setting.
- Build trust, be calm, and use a warm tone.
- Example: I want you to know that you are safe right now, and I am here to listen and help you.

B: Background
- Open-ended, non-leading questions.
- Do not put pressure; give them their own pace.
- Do not make assumption.
- Example: I noticed that you seem to be a little quiet today; can you tell me how you are feeling?

A: Assessment
- Explore gently what the child is experiencing.
- Validate their feelings without judgment.
- Watch for non-verbal cues.
- Example: Children are scared of others, but I want you to know that it's okay to share anything with me.

R: Recommendation
- Reassure the child.
- We are with them for any issues.
- Explain each movement in a simple and non-threatening way.
- Example: Thank you for sharing with me. I am glad you told me; my job is to help to keep you safe.

Preventing and Reporting to Child Maltreatment

Role of the Primary Care Provider (PCP)

Whenever child abuse or neglect is suspected, PCPs have a critical responsibility to act promptly. They should immediately inform the supervising physician and assist in reporting the case to the appropriate local child protection authorities or helplines, such as Childline 1098. Early reporting not only ensures the child's safety and well-being, but also helps prevent recurrence and facilitates access to necessary care and protection.

Importance of Early Interventions

Early interventions can lead to significant long-term benefits, both for the child and for society at large.

- *Benefits for the child*:
  - Improved cognitive development
  - Better behavioral and emotional regulation
  - Enhanced social competence
  - Increased educational attainment
- *Benefits for society*:
  - Reduction in juvenile delinquency
  - Lower crime rates
  - Improved community well-being

Core Interventions to Prevent Child Maltreatment

1. *Parent and Caregiver Support*
   - Home visits and group sessions aimed at building parenting skills
   - Promoting non-violent discipline strategies and emotional bonding
2. *Education and Life Skills Approaches*
   - Ensuring access to quality education to build resilience in children
   - School-based programs that teach body autonomy, consent, and help-seeking behaviors
   - Promoting positive school environments and strong student-teacher relationships
3. *Norms and Values Transformation*
   - Challenging harmful gender norms and societal attitudes that normalize violence
   - Promoting nurturing fatherhood and shared caregiving responsibilities
4. *Laws and Policy Enforcement*
   - Advocating for and upholding legislation that prohibits corporal punishment and protects children from abuse, neglect, and exploitation
5. *Response and Support Services*
   - Strengthening systems for early recognition, timely intervention, and ongoing psychosocial support
   - Providing trauma-informed care and reducing recurrence through multidisciplinary involvement

The *INSPIRE framework* provides seven evidence-based strategies to prevent and respond to violence against children. These are outlined in Table 14.6, serving as a practical guide for health providers and policymakers. This comprehensive, multisectoral approach helps ensure that interventions are sustainable, child-centered, and community-empowering.

Table 14.6 INSPIRE framework for preventing and responding to violence against children

Strategy	Approach	Sectors	Cross-cutting activities
Implementation and enforcement of laws	Enforce laws prohibiting violent punishment by parents, teachers, or caregivers Criminalize sexual abuse and exploitation of children Regulate alcohol misuse Restrict youth access to firearms and other weapons	Justice	
Norms and values	Promote changes in harmful gender and social norms Community mobilization programs Bystander intervention initiatives	Health, education, social welfare	*Multisectoral action and coordination*
Safe environments	Reduce violence by addressing "hotspots" Interrupt cycles of violence Improve the built environment in schools and at-risk areas	School and at risk areas needs to plan well and child safe	
Parent and caregiver support	Home visits Group programs in community settings Comprehensive caregiver support programs	Social welfare, health	
Income and economic strengthening	Cash transfer programs Group savings and loans combined with gender equity training Microfinance linked with gender norm interventions	Finance, labor	
Response and support services	Counseling and therapeutic interventions Screening combined with follow-up interventions Treatment programs for juvenile offenders Foster care programs coordinated with social welfare services	Health, justice, social welfare	*Monitoring and evaluation*

(continued)

Table 14.6 (continued)

Strategy	Approach	Sectors	Cross-cutting activities
Education and life skills	Increase enrolment in preschool, primary, and secondary schools Ensure safe and enabling school environments Educate children on sexual abuse prevention Life and social skills training Adolescent intimate partner violence prevention programs	Education	

Patient and Family Education in Pediatric Injury and Abuse: A Primary Care Provider's Guide

When educating patients and families about injuries and abuse, PCPs play a crucial role in ensuring understanding, promoting safety, and fostering recovery. The key teaching points are as follows:

For Injuries

- Explain the type of injury and its severity. Use simple, non-medical terms to ensure understanding.
- Provide detailed instructions on wound care, medication schedules, and follow-up appointments.
- Emphasize the importance of adhering to prescribed treatments to prevent complications.
- Teach patients and families to monitor for signs of infection (e.g., redness, swelling, fever) or worsening symptoms.
- Encourage immediate medical attention if complications arise.
- Discuss ways to avoid similar injuries in the future, such as safe practices at home or during physical activities.
- Highlight the importance of using protective gear when necessary

For Abuse

- Educate families on the physical (e.g., bruises, burns), emotional (e.g., withdrawal, fearfulness), and behavioral signs (e.g., aggression or regression) of abuse.

- Stress the fact that abuse can take many forms: physical, emotional, sexual, or neglect.
- Teach families how to create a safety plan for a victim of abuse, including identifying safe spaces and emergency contacts.
- Provide information about local shelters or hotlines for immediate assistance.
- Explain the legal and ethical responsibility to report suspected abuse.
- Reassure families that reporting is confidential and aimed at protecting victims.
- Encourage open communication within the family about feelings and experiences.
- Recommend counselling services for both victim and family members to address trauma.
- Provide resources on positive parenting techniques that avoid physical punishment or verbal harm.
- Discuss stress management strategies for caregivers to prevent abusive behaviors.
- Teach families about the safe environment in their homes (e.g., locking away medications and cleaning products).
- Emphasize the importance of supervision to prevent accidents.
- Share information about support groups, social services, and community programs that can assist with parenting challenges or financial stress.
- Educate families on how past trauma may affect behavior and relationships.
- Promote a supportive environment that fosters healing and trust.
- Encourage families to keep records of injuries or incidents for medical and legal purposes if needed.

PCPs should approach these teaching points with empathy and cultural sensitivity while ensuring that patients and families feel supported throughout their journey toward recovery and safety.

1. Provide emotional and physical support to the child throughout the comprehensive physical examination.
2. Conduct a systematic assessment to identify and document all visible and suspected injuries.
3. In cases where abusive head trauma is suspected, closely monitor for signs of neurological deterioration, such as reduced consciousness, which may indicate raised intracranial pressure (ICP).
4. Promptly report any suspicion of abuse to the supervising physician, and assist in notifying the appropriate local authority, child protection service, or child helpline (1098), in accordance with institutional protocols.
5. Ensure the child is placed in a secure and safe environment to prevent further harm.

6. Maintain objective, factual, and detailed documentation regarding all findings and statements related to the suspected abuse.
7. Evaluate the caregivers' coping strategies, emotional stability, and availability of supportive relationships or systems.
8. Identify existing family stressors, resource gaps, and potential avenues of psychosocial or community support.
9. Refer the child and family to relevant support services, such as mental health counseling, parenting programs, or social work interventions.
10. Understand and fulfill the legal obligation to report all suspected cases of child abuse to designated local or state law enforcement or protection agencies.

Management of Suspected Child Abuse in the Emergency Department

In the context of pediatric emergency care, timely recognition and appropriate response to suspected child abuse are critical to ensuring both the immediate safety and long-term well-being of the child. Primary care providers (PCPs), especially those at the frontline in emergency and outpatient settings, must be equipped with a clear, structured approach to evaluate, manage, and escalate cases where abuse is suspected. Given the diverse presentations of non-accidental injuries—ranging from subtle bruises to severe neglect and trauma—a standardized algorithm serves as an essential guide for clinical decision-making. The following algorithm (Fig. 14.1) outlines a stepwise pathway for PCPs to follow when encountering a child with suspected abuse. It incorporates initial assessment, stabilization, documentation, safeguarding procedures, mandatory reporting responsibilities, and referral to child protection services. Adhering to such a protocol not only ensures clinical accountability but also strengthens the child protection framework within the healthcare system.

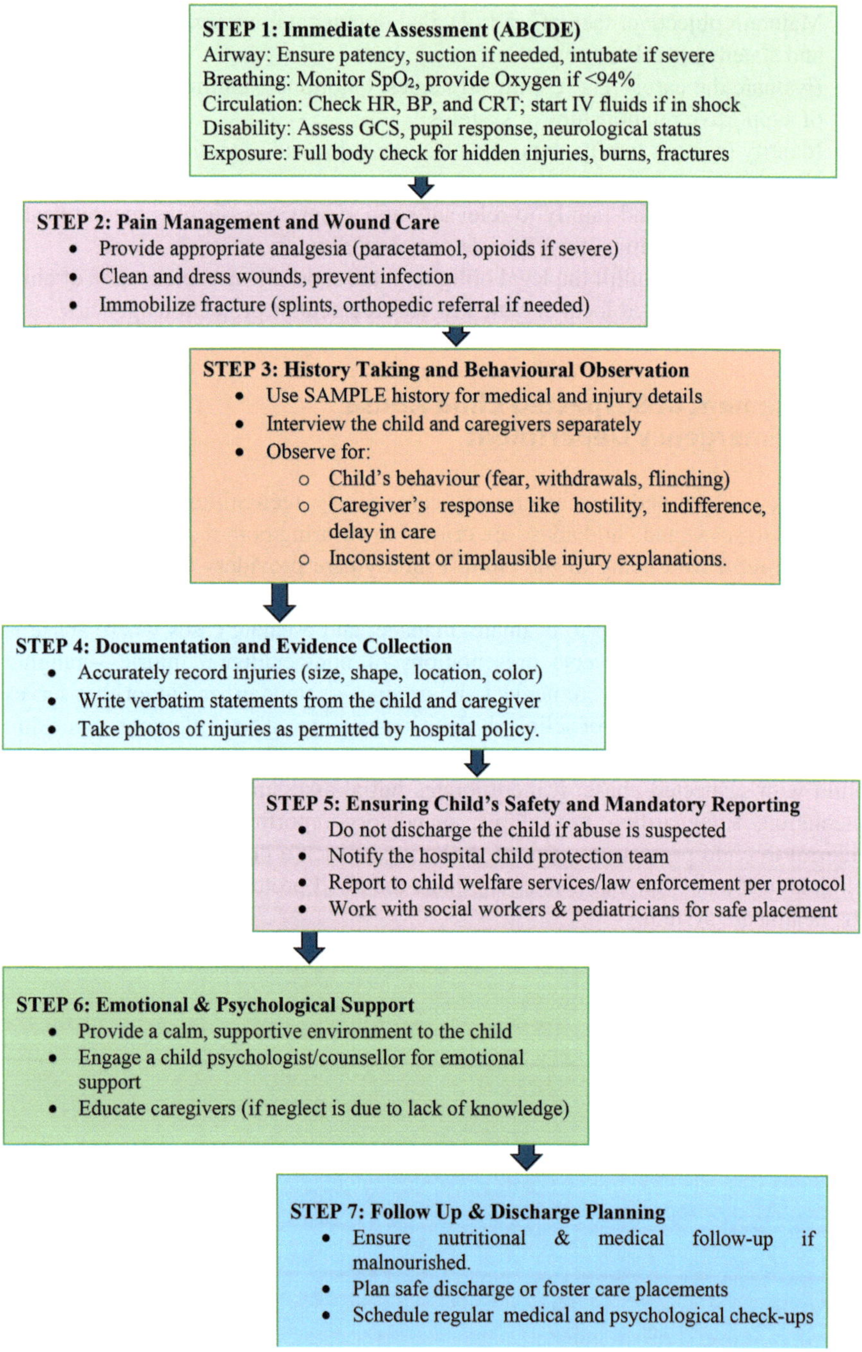

Fig. 14.1 Algorithm for managing suspected child abuse in the emergency department

Case Resolution

Muthu's arrival at the primary care center presented not only a medical emergency but also a potential safeguarding concern that required keen observation and timely action. As a PCP, the first priority was to stabilize the child using a structured trauma assessment protocol while simultaneously remaining alert to red flags for non-accidental trauma.

On examination, Muthu was pale, visibly in pain, and in compensated shock. There was active bleeding from a scalp wound and swelling of the left arm, which appeared to be fractured. Vital signs revealed tachycardia, borderline hypotension, and delayed capillary refill—all indicators of impaired perfusion. The ABCDE approach was initiated promptly. His airway was intact but monitored closely for any signs of compromise, especially considering the potential for traumatic brain injury. High-flow oxygen was administered, and a cervical collar was applied to protect the spine.

Breathing was supported while observing for any respiratory effort or trauma-related compromise. For circulation, two peripheral IV lines were established, and warm isotonic fluid boluses were given at 20 ml/kg. Bleeding from the scalp was managed with direct pressure and sterile dressing. Analgesia was provided in accordance with pediatric dosing protocols, and a padded splint was applied to immobilize the injured arm.

Upon full exposure, what became more concerning were the numerous bruises in varying stages of healing—on the back, thighs, and upper arms—along with signs of chronic neglect such as malnutrition (weight-for-age Z score of –2), thin and discolored hair, poor dental hygiene, and visibly dirty clothes. Muthu was notably withdrawn, avoiding eye contact, hesitant to speak, and showing signs of fearfulness—behavioral patterns that often point toward an abusive environment.

As a frontline clinician, the PCP recognized these indicators of possible child maltreatment and took immediate action. The clinical findings and behavioral cues were documented objectively. The case was escalated appropriately by notifying the physician in charge and initiating a referral to the local child protection helpline (1098), as per legal obligation. A fundoscopy was performed to assess for retinal hemorrhages, which were absent, and imaging studies confirmed a compound humerus fracture and scalp injury.

Beyond acute management, the PCP coordinated with a social worker and ensured that the child received holistic support. Nutritional rehabilitation was initiated, and hygiene concerns were addressed with caregiver education. A referral for psychological support was made to address the likely emotional trauma Muthu had endured.

Throughout the episode, continuous monitoring of vital signs, neurological status, and perfusion was maintained. The child's safety was prioritized while facilitating a safe referral for definitive care and psychosocial protection. Importantly, the PCP's role did not end with stabilization but extended into advocacy and safeguarding—ensuring the child entered a safe pathway of recovery and protection.

This case highlights the essential role of PCPs not only in initial trauma management but also in recognizing and acting upon signs of child abuse. Timely identification, compassionate communication, meticulous documentation, and intersectoral coordination form the backbone of care for children like Muthu.

Key Messages

- Child abuse is often hidden but not rare; primary care providers must stay alert for both obvious and subtle signs.
- Child maltreatment includes physical, emotional, and sexual abuse, as well as neglect—each with distinct clinical and behavioral indicators.
- The ABCDE trauma approach remains crucial for stabilizing the child while simultaneously assessing for signs of non-accidental trauma.
- A detailed and consistent medical history is essential, especially when caregiver explanations are vague, inconsistent, or delayed.
- Some clinical conditions such as Mongolian spots, osteogenesis imperfecta, and bleeding disorders can mimic signs of abuse and must be carefully differentiated.
- Objective and detailed documentation of all findings, including injury patterns and caregiver-child interactions, is critical for legal and clinical follow-up.
- Children under 2 years with suspected abuse should undergo a skeletal survey, and appropriate laboratory workups should be done to rule out mimicking conditions.
- Use trauma-informed communication techniques like SBAR when speaking with the child, ensuring a supportive and non-threatening approach.
- Reporting suspected child abuse to the appropriate child protection authorities is both a legal and ethical responsibility for PCPs.
- Management does not end with stabilization—ensure referrals to psychosocial, mental health, and social support systems for holistic care.
- PCPs also play a role in prevention through parental education, community awareness, and advocacy for policies that support child protection.

Bibliography

1. Addressing the silent epidemic of child maltreatment in India. Available from:URL:https://www.bristol.ac.uk/policybristol/policy-briefings/child-maltreatment-india. Accessed March 16, 2025.
2. Austin AE, Lesak AM, Shanahan ME. Risk and protective factors for child maltreatment: A review. Curr Epidemiol Rep. 2020 Oct 7;7(4):334–342. https://doi.org/10.1007/s40471-020-00252-3. PMID: 34141519; PMCID: PMC8205446.
3. Bandyopadhyay S, Das S, Mondal S. Assessment of Undernutrition Among the Under-5 Children in a Slum of Kolkata: A Comparison Between z Scores and the Conventional System. Childhood Obesity and Nutrition. 2013;6(1):52–57. https://doi.org/10.1177/1941406413513154

4. Berthold O, Frericks B, John T, Clemens V, Fegert JM, Moers AV. Abuse as a Cause of Childhood Fractures. Dtsch Arztebl Int. 2018 Nov 16;115(46):769–775. https://doi.org/10.3238/arztebl.2018.0769. PMID: 30602409; PMCID: PMC6329369.
5. Child Abuse and Neglect Available from: URL:https://www.utmb.edu/pedi_ed/CoreV2/Abuse/page_08.htm. Accessed March 20, 2025.
6. Child abuse on the rise in India | Fair Planet. Available from:URL:https://www.fairplanet.org/editors-pick/child-abuse-on-the-rise-in-India/. Accessed March 25, 2025.
7. Child labour and domestic work: Available from:URL:https://www.ilo.org/international-programme-elimination-child-labour-ipec/sectors-and-topics/child-labour-and-domestic-work. Accessed March 21, 2025.
8. Child maltreatment. Available from:URL:https://www.who.int/news-room/fact-sheets/detail/child-maltreatment. Accessed March 20, 2025.
9. Child Protection. Available from:URL:https://www.unicef.org/india/what-we-do/child-protection. Accessed March 21, 2025.
10. Csorba R, Atas Elfrink Z, Tsikouras P. Diagnosis of Child Sexual Abuse. J Clin Med. 2024 Nov 30;13(23):7297. https://doi.org/10.3390/jcm13237297. PMID: 39685755; PMCID: PMC11642304
11. Fernandes G, Fernandes M, Vaidya N, et al. Prevalence of child maltreatment in India and its association with gender, urbanisation and policy: a rapid review and meta-analysis protocol. BMJ Open. 2021 Aug 9;11(8):e044983. https://doi.org/10.1136/bmjopen-2020-044983. PMID: 34373291; PMCID: PMC8354262.
12. Focardi M, Gori V, Romanelli M, et al. "Mimics" of Injuries from Child Abuse: Case Series and Review of the Literature. Children (Basel). 2024 Sep 9;11(9):1103. https://doi.org/10.3390/children11091103. PMID: 39334635; PMCID: PMC11430524.
13. Fractures and trauma. Available from: URL: https://melbvetortho.com.au/fractures-trauma/ Accessed March 21, 2025.
14. Global Perspectives Child Abuse and Neglect in India: Prevalence. Available from: URL: https://istss.org/global-perspectives-child-abuse-and-neglect-in-India-prevalence-and-policy-recommendations-ruby-charak-phd.Accessed March 16, 2025.
15. Gonzalez D, Bethencourt Mirabal A, McCall JD, et al. Child Abuse and Neglect (Nursing) [Updated 2023 Jul 4]. In: StatPearls [Internet]. Treasure Island (FL): StatPearls Publishing; 2025 Jan-. Available from: https://www.ncbi.nlm.nih.gov/books/NBK568689/
16. Haq I, Shah MS, Bachh AA, Ansari MA. Validity of Weech's formulae in detecting undernutrition in children. Nepal Med Coll J. 2010 Dec;12(4):229–33.
17. INSPIRE: Seven strategies for Ending Violence Against Children. Available from:URL:https://www.who.int/publications/i/item/inspire-seven-strategies-for-ending-violence-against-children. Accessed March 20, 2025.
18. Jacobi G, Dettmeyer R, Banaschak S, Brosig B, Herrmann B. Child abuse and neglect: diagnosis and management. Dtsch Arztebl Int. 2010 Apr;107(13):231–39; quiz 240. https://doi.org/10.3238/arztebl.2010.0231. Epub 2010 Apr 2. PMID: 20396522; PMCID: PMC2855177.
19. Jarraya M, Hayashi D, Roemer FW, Crema MD, Diaz L, Conlin J, Marra MD, Jomaah N, Guermazi A. Radiographically occult and subtle fractures: a pictorial review. Radiol Res Pract. 2013;2013:370169. https://doi.org/10.1155/2013/370169. Epub 2013 Mar 17. PMID: 23577253; PMCID: PMC3613077.
20. National Children's Alliance Available from:URL:https://www.nationalchildrensalliance.org/media-room/national-statistics-on-child-abuse/. Accessed March 16, 2025.
21. Pandya NK, Baldwin K, Kamath AF, Wenger DR, Hosalkar HS. Unexplained fractures: child abuse or bone disease? A systematic review. Clin Orthop Relat Res. 2011 Mar;469(3):805–12. https://doi.org/10.1007/s11999-010-1578-z. PMID: 20878560; PMCID: PMC3032841.
22. Seay KD, Kohl P. Caregiver Substance Abuse and Children's Exposure to Violence in a Nationally Representative Child Welfare Sample. J Soc Work Pract Addict. 2013 Jan 1;13(1):70–90. https://doi.org/10.1080/1533256X.2013.756335. Epub 2013 Feb 19. PMID: 23440502; PMCID: PMC3579640.

23. The Effects of Parents' History of Childhood Maltreatment on Child Maltreatment Behaviours and Relationship Quality. Available from:URL:https://scholarworks.waldenu.edu/cgi/viewcontent.cgi?article=16594&context=dissertations. Accessed March 20, 2025.
24. Toghian Chaharsoughi N, Ahrari S, Alikhah S. Comparison the Effect of Teaching of SBAR Technique with Role Play and Lecturing on Communication Skill of Nurses. J Caring Sci. 2014 Jun 1;3(2):141–7. https://doi.org/10.5681/jcs.2014.015. PMID: 25276757; PMCID: PMC4134175.
25. Violence against children – World Health Organization (WHO) Available from:URL:https://www.who.int/news-room/fact-sheets/detail/violence-against-children. Accessed March 16, 2025.
26. Violence against Children in India – Social Welfare – Vikaspedia. Available from:URL:https://socialwelfare.vikaspedia.in/viewcontent/social-welfare/women-and-child-development/child-development-1/violence-against-children-in-India?lgn=en. Accessed March 16, 2025.

Pediatric Sedation and Analgesia

15

Mahesh G. Devasthale, Sachin Dwivedi, and Jayaraj Mymbilly Balakrishnan

Learning Objectives

- Understand the indications and importance of sedation and analgesia in the management of pediatric trauma.
- Gain foundational knowledge of the pharmacological agents commonly used for pediatric sedation and analgesia, including their indications, dosages, and side effects.
- Equip primary care providers (PCPs) with the skills to support clinicians in pre-sedation assessment, preparation, administration techniques, and post-sedation care.
- Emphasize the importance of continuous monitoring and safety protocols to minimize sedation-related complications.
- Explore various pharmacologic and non-pharmacologic strategies for effective pain management in pediatric trauma cases.
- Enable PCPs to effectively educate patients and families about the sedation process, its benefits, potential risks, and post-sedation care.

M. G. Devasthale
Trauma Centre, AIIMS, Rishikesh, India

S. Dwivedi
Center for Excellence in Nursing Education and Research, All India Institute of Medical Sciences, Rishikesh, Uttarakhand, India

J. M. Balakrishnan (✉)
Department of Emergency Medicine, Kasturba Medical College and Hospital, Manipal Academy of Higher Education (Institution of Eminence and Deemed to be University), Manipal Government of Karnataka Bioincubator, Manipal, Karnataka, India
e-mail: jayaraj.mb@manipal.edu

N. T. Rai (ed.), *Pediatric Trauma Resuscitation Manual (PTRM) for Primary Care Providers*, https://doi.org/10.1007/978-981-95-4979-5_15

Introduction

Pain and anxiety are universal responses to trauma, and in pediatric patients, they are often amplified due to developmental, cognitive, and emotional factors. Effective sedation and analgesia are essential components of pediatric trauma care—not only to manage distress and facilitate procedures but also to minimize the psychological sequelae that may persist if pain is under-treated. While procedural sedation is typically initiated and overseen by trained emergency physicians or anesthesiologists, primary care providers (PCPs) play a pivotal supportive role throughout the care continuum.

PCPs often serve as the first point of contact in acute or semi-acute trauma scenarios, especially in resource-limited or decentralized settings. Their involvement in pre-sedation assessment, preparation, monitoring, and post-procedural care can significantly influence the safety and success of the sedation process. This requires a clear understanding of the child's developmental stage, weight-based drug dosing, common sedative and analgesic agents, and the principles of safe procedural sedation.

This chapter is designed to equip PCPs with essential knowledge and skills to collaborate effectively in pediatric trauma care involving sedation and analgesia. It covers the pharmacology of commonly used agents, assessment protocols like SOAPME, monitoring standards including capnography and pulse oximetry, and the importance of documentation and ethical considerations such as informed consent. It also highlights the nuances of pain assessment in children, ranging from behavioral tools like FLACC to self-reported scales for older children.

By bridging knowledge gaps and enhancing coordination with the clinical team, PCPs can contribute meaningfully to reducing procedural trauma, optimizing pain relief, and ensuring child safety. Ultimately, the chapter aims to foster a shared understanding among healthcare providers to promote compassionate, competent, and coordinated care in pediatric trauma settings.

Case Scenario

A 10-year-old boy, Rohan, is brought to the emergency department after falling off his bicycle onto a gravel road. He has sustained an open scalp laceration measuring approximately 6 cm and has multiple superficial abrasions on his limbs. Rohan is visibly distressed—crying loudly, clutching his mother's hand, and recoiling from medical staff attempting to examine the wound. He is alert and oriented but refuses to cooperate with any assessment or wound cleaning. His vitals are stable, with a heart rate of 130 bpm, respiratory rate of 28/min, SpO_2 at 98%, and BP of 100/60 mmHg. The emergency physician determines that procedural sedation is required for wound cleaning and suturing.

As a PCP assisting in the pediatric trauma bay, you are asked to help prepare for and monitor the child during the sedation process. You are also expected to help counsel the mother, assist with medication readiness, and ensure appropriate documentation of the procedure and monitoring events.

Reflective Questions

1. What elements of Rohan's behavior and vitals suggest that sedation is warranted rather than simple distraction or restraint?
2. What pre-sedation assessments should you assist with as a PCP, and why are they important in this case?
3. Which sedation options are likely to be preferred in this scenario, and what are your responsibilities during their administration?
4. What equipment should you verify is present and functional before initiating sedation?
5. How will you communicate with Rohan's mother to provide reassurance and explain the steps ahead?
6. What signs of respiratory or cardiovascular compromise will you monitor for during the sedation process?
7. How will you contribute to the documentation and post-sedation handover?

Understanding Need for Sedation and Analgesia in Pediatric Trauma

Pediatric trauma accounts for a substantial burden of illness globally and remains one of the leading causes of death and disability in children. Unlike adults, children often experience and express pain differently due to developmental, cognitive, and emotional variations. As such, managing pain and anxiety in pediatric trauma is not only about reducing discomfort but also about preventing long-term psychological sequelae such as procedural anxiety, post-traumatic stress, and behavioral disturbances.

In an emergency or trauma setting, the child's experience is often overwhelming. The unfamiliar environment, separation from parents, distressing injuries, and presence of strangers in medical attire all contribute to heightened fear and resistance. Painful procedures—such as wound debridement, fracture reductions, or catheter insertions—become difficult to execute safely without adequate sedation or analgesia.

Sedation and analgesia serve multiple important functions in pediatric trauma care. First, they ensure humane, ethical care by alleviating pain and anxiety. Second, they enable necessary diagnostic and therapeutic procedures to be conducted efficiently and with minimal movement, thereby improving procedural success rates and reducing complications. Third, appropriate sedation protocols reduce the need for physical restraint, thus minimizing additional psychological trauma.

For primary care providers, understanding the indications, safety considerations, and monitoring protocols surrounding sedation is crucial. PCPs often act as the first point of contact or play a supportive role in emergency care teams. Their ability to identify candidates for sedation, prepare equipment, explain procedures to families, assist in monitoring, and recognize adverse effects makes them vital to the child's overall care and safety. A team-based, well-informed approach helps optimize outcomes and fosters trust between the care team, the child, and their caregivers.

Unique Challenges and Indications for Sedation and Analgesia in Pediatric Trauma

- Children respond to pain and sedative medications in highly variable ways, influenced by their age, stage of neurological development, temperament, and cultural background. These factors make standardized approaches less reliable and demand individualized care.
- Drug dosing in children is not a scaled-down version of adult protocols. Differences in body composition, organ maturity, and metabolic pathways result in unique pharmacokinetics and pharmacodynamics. Doses must always be calculated precisely based on the child's weight and age. The principle that "children are not miniature adults" is especially critical in the context of sedation safety and efficacy.
- Fear and anxiety are almost universal in pediatric trauma. The emergency setting, separation from caregivers, and presence of unfamiliar faces and equipment contribute to heightened distress. In some cases, parents themselves may be injured or unavailable, leaving children without emotional support and compounding the stress.
- Young children and those with developmental delays often cannot express pain verbally. Conventional pain scales may be inadequate, requiring the use of age-appropriate observational tools like the FLACC scale or behavioral cues to assess discomfort accurately.
- Both over-sedation and under-sedation carry risks. *Inadequate sedation* may result in procedural failure, heightened anxiety, and long-term trauma. *Excessive sedation*, on the other hand, may lead to respiratory depression, airway compromise, or cardiovascular instability, especially in trauma patients with coexisting injuries.

Indications for Sedation and Analgesia in Pediatric Trauma

1. *Pain Management:* Essential to reduce suffering, prevent chronic pain sensitization, and facilitate healing. Indicated for acute injuries such as lacerations, fractures, and burns.
2. *Anxiety Reduction:* Helps manage the emotional distress associated with trauma and invasive procedures, improving cooperation and patient experience.

3. *Diagnostic Facilitation:* Necessary for imaging studies (e.g., CT, MRI), wound evaluation, and minor interventions where patient stillness is critical.
4. *Therapeutic Procedures:* Required during painful treatments such as fracture reductions, wound closure, or burn care, where procedural success depends on patient immobility and comfort.
5. *Optimizing Clinical Outcomes:* Properly administered sedation and analgesia reduce procedural complications, enhance provider efficiency, and improve satisfaction for both the child and caregivers.

Pharmacology of Sedation and Analgesia in Pediatrics Trauma

Effective management of pain and sedation in pediatric trauma patients requires a thorough understanding of the pharmacological agents used. The selection of medication depends on the child's specific need, injury type, and the procedure being performed (Table 15.1).

Table 15.1 Sedative and analgesic medications in pediatric trauma care

Name of drug and dose	Clinical use	Adverse effect	PCPs responsibilities
Midazolam 0.5 to 0.75 mg per kg oral 0.025 to 0.05 mg/kg intravenous 0.2 mg per kg intranasal	Anxiolysis, sedation, amnesia	Respiratory depression leading to hypoxia or apnea, hypotension and paradoxical agitation (rare)	Monitor for any adverse reactions. Ensure continuous cardiorespiratory monitoring Keep a close watch on blood pressure and pulse oximetry
Ketamine 3 to 4 mg per kg intramuscular 1 to 2 mg per kg intravenous	Sedation, analgesia, amnesia	Excessive salivation and laryngospasm, tachycardia, hypertension, and raised intracranial pressure	Evaluate the patient's breathing, and promptly inform the physician should there be any disruption in the respiratory rate (apnea) or indications of respiratory depression
Propofol 1 mg per kg intravenous followed by 0.5 mg; repeat if needed	Deep sedation, general anesthesia	Respiratory depression, apnea, Hypotension, and pain on injection	Regular and frequent monitoring is necessary for blood pressure, heart Rate, oxygen saturation, and ventilation
Etomidate 0.3 to 0.5 mg per kg intravenous 0.1 mg per kg; repeat if needed	Sedative Hypnotic with little hemodynamic change	Respiratory Depression, myoclonus, nausea, and vomiting	Throughout etomidate therapy, keep a close eye on blood pressure, pulse, and respiratory status. May result in transient apnea

(continued)

Table 15.1 (continued)

Name of drug and dose	Clinical use	Adverse effect	PCPs responsibilities
Morphine 0.05 to 0.2 mg per kg per dose Maximum dose 2 to 4 mg intravenous, PO 0.2–0.5 mg per kg per dose	Moderate to severe pain	Anxiety reduction, sleepiness, mental fogging, orthostatic hypotension, and depression of the respiratory system	Before administering, keep an eye on the patient's breathing rate For up to 24 hours following morphine administration, regularly check for respiratory depression and Hypotension
Fentanyl 1 μg/kg intravenous Repeat every 30 minutes	Severe pain, adjunct to sedation	Respiratory depression, hypotension, and bradycardia	After 15 minutes, repeat regular observations with the sedation score and respiratory rate every 5 minutes. Pulse oximetry for infants younger than 6 Months, if indicated
Acetaminophen (paracetamol) 10 to 15 mg per kg per dose (maximum dose ≤2 years, 60 mg per kg per day; ≥ 2 years, 75 mg per kg per day maximum 4 grams per day)	Mild to moderate pain, antipyretic	Skin rash, hypersensitivity reactions, nephrotoxicity	Seek medical advice before giving the medication to a child younger than 2 years old. Remember that acetaminophen treatment is only administered temporarily

Assessment and Preparation for Sedation and Analgesia in Pediatric Trauma

The administration of effective and safe sedation to pediatric trauma patients necessitates meticulous evaluation and preparation. This procedure encompasses a thorough pre-sedation assessment, risk stratification, and the establishment of clear communication and consent with the child's parents or guardians. A frequently employed acronym that aids in the planning and preparation of a procedure is *SOAPME*, which stands for the following:

- *S—Suction:* Suction catheters of appropriate sizes (e.g., Yankauer tip) with a fully functional suction apparatus.
- *O—Oxygen:* Adequate oxygen supply with properly working flow meters or alternative oxygen delivery devices.
- *A—Airway Equipment:* Includes Ambu bag, suction catheters, oropharyngeal and nasopharyngeal airways, laryngeal mask airways, laryngoscope with blades, endotracheal tubes, stylets, and face masks.

- *P—Pharmacy:* A stocked inventory of essential emergency medications, including antagonists when indicated, to manage and sustain life.
- *M—Monitoring Devices:* Devices such as pulse oximeters, end-tidal CO_2 monitors, and other relevant monitoring tools (e.g., non-invasive blood pressure monitors, ECG machines, stethoscopes).
- *E—Emergency Equipment:* Additional equipment or medications for complex scenarios, such as a defibrillator.

Conducting a Thorough Pre-sedation Assessment

Trauma-Specific History

Before administering sedation or assisting the emergency team, PCPs play a critical role in gathering a focused and trauma-relevant history. This not only aids in clinical decision-making but also ensures patient safety.

1. *Mechanism and Context of Injury:* Elicit a detailed account of the trauma—how it occurred, the time elapsed since injury, and initial symptoms. This helps anticipate potential internal injuries or complications.
2. *Medical History:* Review past illnesses, surgical interventions, hospitalizations, and especially any known cardiac, respiratory, neurological, or bleeding disorders that may increase sedation-related risks.
3. *Allergies and Medications:* Identify all current medications (including over-the-counter and herbal remedies) and any allergies, particularly to medications, latex, egg, or soy products—important due to their relevance in certain sedative agents.
4. *Previous Sedation or Anesthesia Exposure:* Ask about prior procedures involving sedation, including any history of airway difficulty, adverse reactions, or delayed recovery.
5. *Fasting Status (NPO):* Document the time of last food and fluid intake. Follow standard fasting guidelines: *6 hours for solids, 4 hours for breast milk, and 2 hours for clear liquids* to reduce aspiration risk.

Physical Examination

A targeted yet comprehensive physical exam is crucial before sedation. PCPs should assess the following:

1. *General Appearance and Cooperation:* Note the child's distress, consciousness level, and ability to follow commands. Uncooperative behavior may require adjustments in sedation strategy.
2. *Vital Signs:* Record heart rate, respiratory rate, blood pressure, and oxygen saturation. Do not attribute tachycardia or agitation solely to anxiety—explore possible pain, shock, or hypoxia.

3. *Airway Assessment:* Examine for features that could complicate airway management—micrognathia, macroglossia, limited neck mobility, or midface anomalies. Also, check for loose deciduous teeth, especially in children aged 5–12.
4. *Respiratory System:* Listen for wheezing, stridor, or signs of respiratory distress. Be alert to upper respiratory infections or reactive airway disease, which heighten the risk for laryngospasm.
5. *Cardiovascular System:* Evaluate perfusion through heart sounds, peripheral pulses, capillary refill, and signs of circulatory compromise.
6. *Neurological Status:* Assess consciousness (e.g., using AVPU or GCS), pupil responses, limb strength, and mental development. Subtle deficits may indicate evolving head injury.
7. *Injury-Specific Examination:* Examine wounds, deformities, or swelling in detail. Document the site, depth, and severity, especially if the procedure involves these areas.

Risk Stratification

1. *ASA Classification:* Use the ASA Physical Status Classification to identify patients at higher procedural risk. Children rated ASA III or above may need anesthesiologist involvement or more intensive monitoring.
2. *Sedation-Related Risk Factors:* Be vigilant for features such as difficult airway anatomy, known obstructive sleep apnea, gastroesophageal reflux, or significant systemic illness.
3. *Procedure Complexity:* Consider the nature and expected duration of the procedure. Invasive or prolonged interventions (e.g., orthopedic reductions, extensive debridement) warrant deeper sedation (Table 15.2) and increased preparedness for complications.

Table 15.2 Sedation levels in pediatric trauma care

Sedation/ anesthesia level	Description	Typical uses
Minimal sedation (anxiolysis)	A drug-induced state in which the patient remains awake, alert, and able to respond normally to verbal commands	Suitable for minor procedures or diagnostic studies
Moderate sedation (conscious sedation)	A drug-induced depression of consciousness where the patient responds purposefully to verbal commands or light tactile stimulation	Used for procedures such as fracture reductions, laceration repairs, or moderately complex imaging studies
Deep sedation	A drug-induced state of depressed consciousness in which the patient is not easily aroused but responds purposefully to repeated or painful stimulation	Applied for more painful or invasive procedures, such as complex fracture reductions or foreign body removal
General anesthesia	A drug-induced coma-like state in which the patient cannot be aroused, even with intense stimulation	Reserved for major surgeries or procedures requiring complete immobility and comprehensive pain control

Routes Administering Sedation and Analgesia

Understanding the various routes of sedation delivery is essential for selecting the most appropriate method based on the child's age, clinical condition, and the procedure involved:

- *Oral Sedation:* Used primarily for mild to moderate sedation in cooperative children. Commonly administered agents include midazolam, triclofos, and chloral hydrate. Onset is slower, and titration is less precise, but it is non-invasive and well tolerated.
- *Intranasal Sedation:* Suitable for rapid onset without IV access. Agents like midazolam and fentanyl are delivered via spray or drops into the nostrils. PCPs must verify the drug concentration and dose delivered per actuation to ensure accurate administration.
- *Intravenous (IV) Sedation:* Preferred for precise titration and rapid onset, especially during painful or prolonged procedures. Common agents include midazolam, ketamine, propofol, and fentanyl. Continuous monitoring is mandatory due to higher risk of adverse events.
- *Intramuscular (IM) Sedation:* Useful when IV access is difficult or not immediately available. Frequently used agents are ketamine and midazolam. Anticholinergic premedication (e.g., atropine) is often added to reduce salivation when ketamine is administered.
- *Inhalational Sedation:* Involves agents like nitrous oxide, administered via a face mask. Provides rapid onset and offset and is particularly effective for minor procedures or short-duration analgesia.
- *Combination Techniques:* In certain scenarios, combinations are employed for better sedation and pain control—for example, IV ketamine for deep sedation alongside local anesthetic infiltration at the wound site.

Monitoring and Safety in Sedation and Analgesia in Pediatric Trauma

In pediatric trauma settings, effective monitoring is essential to ensure the safety of sedation practices. Children undergoing sedation may face heightened risks due to their unique physiology and the nature of their injuries. A structured and vigilant approach helps detect early signs of deterioration and ensures timely intervention.

1. *Continuous Monitoring of Vital Signs.*
    - *Heart Rate:* Track continuously to identify tachycardia (which may indicate pain, anxiety, or hypoxia) or bradycardia (a possible sign of over-sedation or hypoxia).
    - *Blood Pressure:* Monitor at regular intervals. Hypotension could suggest sedative overdose, shock, or bleeding, while hypertension may result from pain or distress.

- *Respiratory Rate:* Continuous observation is crucial. A decline may indicate respiratory depression—a known complication of sedative medications.

2. *Oxygen Saturation (SpO_2).*
   - Use pulse oximetry to monitor oxygenation levels in real time. A falling SpO_2 reading may precede or accompany airway obstruction or hypoventilation and requires immediate action.
3. *End-Tidal CO_2 Monitoring ($EtCO_2$).*
   - Capnography is valuable for early detection of hypoventilation or apnea—often before a drop in oxygen saturation is observed. It is particularly important in deeper levels of sedation or high-risk patients.
4. *Trauma-Specific Clinical Parameters.*
   - *Neurological Status:* Regularly assess using tools such as the Glasgow Coma Scale (GCS), especially in cases of suspected head injury. Monitor for any deterioration in consciousness.
   - *Pain Assessment:* Utilize age-appropriate pain scales (e.g., FLACC, Wong-Baker FACES) to ensure adequate analgesia, and adjust doses accordingly.
   - *Site-Specific Observation:* Monitor wound sites or fractured limbs for signs of bleeding, swelling, or compartment syndrome. Timely recognition can prevent serious complications.

Strategies for Ensuring Patient Safety and Managing Potential Complications

Pre-sedation Preparation

- Conduct a thorough pre-sedation assessment, including a focused medical history, physical examination, and risk stratification using tools like the ASA classification.
- Ensure informed consent is obtained from the parent or guardian, clearly outlining the procedure, benefits, risks, and available alternatives.
- Confirm that all essential equipment is available and functional—this includes oxygen supply, suction, airway devices, resuscitation tools, and emergency medications.
- Facilitate clear, closed-loop communication among all team members, especially between the clinician administering sedation and those performing the procedure.

Emergency Preparedness

- Keep resuscitative equipment easily accessible: bag valve mask, airway adjuncts, intubation supplies, and defibrillator.
- Ensure availability of reversal agents such as naloxone (for opioids), flumazenil (for benzodiazepines), and epinephrine (for anaphylaxis).
- Confirm that all involved personnel are trained in Pediatric Advanced Life Support (PALS) and familiar with institutional emergency protocols.

Airway Management

- Maintain airway patency using positioning techniques such as head tilt-chin lift or lateral positioning in high-risk cases.
- Use adjuncts like oropharyngeal or nasopharyngeal airways when necessary.
- Be prepared for advanced airway interventions, including intubation, if there are signs of respiratory compromise.

Continuous Monitoring

- Assign a designated provider (e.g., trained nurse or PCP) to continuously monitor the child throughout sedation.
- Track vital parameters including heart rate, respiratory rate, blood pressure, SpO_2, and end-tidal CO_2.
- Reassess sedation depth and pain levels frequently to adjust medication and maintain appropriate comfort and safety.

Pain Management in Pediatric Trauma Patients

Effective pain control is a cornerstone of pediatric trauma care. Beyond alleviating immediate discomfort, timely and appropriate analgesia promotes healing, minimizes psychological stress, and enhances cooperation with procedures. However, assessing and managing pain in children—especially in high-stress trauma settings—poses unique challenges. Children may under-report or be unable to articulate their pain, necessitating the use of age-appropriate assessment tools and vigilant clinical observation. For PCPs, understanding these diverse strategies enhances their ability to support the emergency care team, advocate for the child's comfort, and participate meaningfully in trauma-informed pediatric care.

Pain Assessment Tools

- *Infants and Non-verbal Children:* The FLACC (Face, Legs, Activity, Cry, Consolability) scale offers a reliable, behavior-based method to evaluate pain in preverbal or developmentally delayed children.
- *Toddlers and Young Children:* Tools such as the Wong-Baker FACES Pain Rating Scale help children point to the face that best expresses their level of discomfort.
- *Older Children and Adolescents:* Numeric Rating Scales (0–10) and Visual Analog Scales (VAS) are effective for self-reporting in children mature enough to understand abstract scoring systems.

Multimodal Analgesia Strategies

Adopting a multimodal approach—combining different classes of medications and supportive techniques—can optimize pain relief while minimizing drug-related side effects.

Pharmacologic Options

- For mild to moderate pain, medications like acetaminophen and ibuprofen are first-line choices due to their safety and efficacy profiles.
- For moderate to severe pain, agents such as morphine or fentanyl may be necessary, but must be used with careful monitoring for respiratory depression.
- Ketamine can serve as a valuable adjunct for procedural pain or in situations where opioids are contraindicated. Local anesthetics or regional nerve blocks may be particularly useful for limb injuries.

Non-pharmacologic Techniques

- Distraction tools (e.g., toys, music, cartoons), guided imagery, and breathing exercises can significantly reduce pain perception and anxiety.
- Physical methods such as ice packs, limb elevation, and splinting help in managing soft tissue injuries and fractures.
- The presence of a calm, reassuring caregiver can have a powerful analgesic effect—leveraging the comfort of touch and familiar voices.

Post-sedation Care for Pediatric Trauma Patients

Ensuring safe and effective recovery after sedation is a vital component of pediatric trauma care. PCPs must remain vigilant in monitoring recovery parameters, managing side effects, and detecting potential complications. Post-sedation care begins immediately after the procedure and continues until the child returns to their pre-sedation baseline. Primary care providers play a pivotal role in early recognition of recovery readiness, monitoring for side effects, educating caregivers about home care, and ensuring safe transition from procedural areas to wards or discharge. Clear discharge instructions—including warning signs and follow-up recommendations—must be shared with families to support continued recovery at home.

Criteria for Recovery and Safe Discharge

1. *Stable Vital Signs:* Heart rate, respiratory rate, blood pressure, and oxygen saturation should be within normal age-appropriate limits and stable over time.
2. *Return of Protective Reflexes:* The child should regain airway reflexes, including the ability to cough and swallow effectively, indicating a reduced risk of aspiration.
3. *Level of Consciousness:* The child should be alert, responsive to verbal commands or tactile stimulation, and oriented appropriately for their age.
4. *Effective Pain Control:* Pain should be well managed using appropriate pain scales, with the child appearing calm and comfortable.
5. *Motor Coordination:* The child should demonstrate purposeful movement of all extremities. If appropriate based on injury, assess the ability to sit up or maintain balance.

6. *Oral Intake Tolerance:* The child should be able to tolerate small sips of clear fluids without vomiting. Solid food can be offered gradually if the child is not expected to remain NPO for medical reasons.

Managing Common Post-sedation Issues

- *Nausea and Vomiting:* Use antiemetics like ondansetron as needed. Offer small, frequent sips of clear fluids to prevent dehydration.
- *Respiratory Depression:* Maintain continuous monitoring of respiratory rate and oxygen saturation. Provide supplemental oxygen as required. Be prepared to initiate assisted ventilation with a bag valve mask if needed.
- *Hypotension:* Monitor blood pressure regularly. Administer isotonic IV fluids if hypotension is observed. In persistent cases, vasopressors may be considered under physician guidance.
- *Agitation or Emergence Delirium:* Calm the environment and reduce sensory stimulation. Reassure the child. For severe cases, low-dose sedatives (e.g., midazolam) may be used cautiously under appropriate supervision.

Ethical and Legal Aspects of Providing Sedation and Analgesia in Pediatric Trauma

Primary care providers must approach sedation and analgesia in pediatric trauma with a strong understanding of ethical responsibilities and legal obligations. These considerations ensure the safety, dignity, and rights of the child while also protecting the provider and institution. By incorporating ethical sensitivity and legal vigilance into sedation practices, PCPs can uphold high standards of pediatric trauma care and build trust with families.

- Always obtain informed consent from a parent or legal guardian before administering sedation or analgesia. Clearly explain the procedure, its intended benefits, potential risks, and available alternatives in understandable terms.
- When developmentally appropriate, seek assent from the child, using age-appropriate language to describe the procedure, and involve them in decision-making.
- In life-threatening emergencies, where delay could harm the child and consent cannot be obtained in time, implied consent may be applied. Document the medical necessity and the circumstances justifying the immediate intervention without formal consent.
- Documentation is critical—record all communication regarding consent, the sedation plan, drugs administered, and any deviations from standard protocols with clear rationale.
- Treat every pediatric patient with compassion, dignity, and respect. Ensure emotional support is offered throughout the sedation process to minimize fear and distress.

- Maintain strict confidentiality regarding the child's health information. Share details only with authorized personnel directly involved in care.
- Cultural and religious values may influence decisions about sedation and pain management. Engage in respectful conversations with families, acknowledging their beliefs while prioritizing the child's medical needs and safety.
- Exercise extra caution when sedating children with special healthcare needs or comorbidities, carefully balancing risks and benefits.
- Adhere to institutional protocols and national regulations when handling controlled substances (e.g., fentanyl), ensuring proper storage, documentation, and staff training to prevent misuse or legal breaches.
- Engage in open communication with the family, seeking to understand and accommodate their cultural or religious preferences while ensuring the child's safety and well-being.
- Weigh the potential benefits of sedation against the risks, especially in children with complex medical conditions or special healthcare needs.
- Stick to narcotic drug usage policies and safety precautions when handling drugs like fentanyl to maintain legal and ethical compliance and workplace safety.

Communication and Documentation

In pediatric trauma care, clear communication and thorough documentation are essential for safe sedation practices. Effective communication ensures shared understanding among the care team, supports informed parental consent, and promotes the child's comfort. Accurate, timely documentation safeguards clinical decisions, ensures continuity of care, and provides legal protection. Figures 15.1 and 15.2 illustrate the key principles of communication within the healthcare team and with patients and families, respectively.

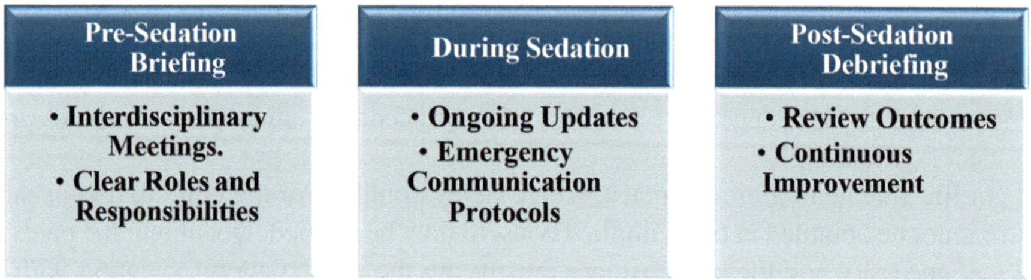

Fig. 15.1 Communication with the healthcare team

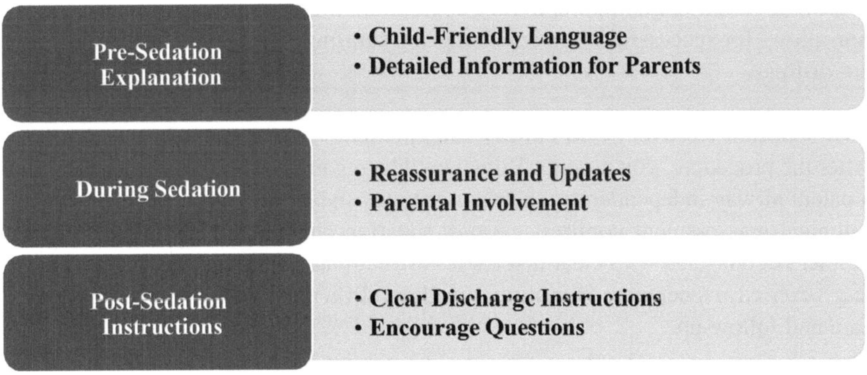

Fig. 15.2 Communication with patients and parents

Case Resolution

Rohan, a 10-year-old boy with a 6 cm open scalp laceration and multiple abrasions, presents to the emergency department visibly anxious and uncooperative. His vital signs—heart rate of 130 bpm and respiratory rate of 28/min—indicate physiological stress. Despite being alert and oriented, his heightened anxiety and resistance to examination suggest that distraction techniques or physical restraint would be inadequate and potentially traumatic. Thus, procedural sedation is deemed necessary to ensure both the child's comfort and procedural success.

Pre-sedation Assessment and Preparation

As a PCP, your role begins with supporting the emergency team in conducting a comprehensive pre-sedation assessment, including a focused neurological exam to rule out signs of raised intracranial pressure (ICP). Rohan's stable neurological status and lack of history suggest sedation can proceed safely, although close monitoring remains essential.

A detailed medical history is reviewed to rule out prior sedation complications, allergies, or underlying conditions. You ensure that informed consent is obtained from Rohan's mother, explaining the purpose of sedation, the safety measures in place, and what to expect during recovery.

Given the superficial nature of injuries and the child's anxiety, nitrous oxide is selected for conscious sedation, alongside local anesthetic infiltration at the wound site. Equipment for oxygen delivery, suction, airway management, and emergency medications (e.g., naloxone, flumazenil) is checked and readied.

Sedation Execution and Monitoring

Nitrous oxide is administered via mask while maintaining effective communication with Rohan to alleviate his fears. You assist in monitoring vital signs continuously, including heart rate, respiratory rate, SpO_2, and consciousness level, while observing for any signs of respiratory depression or airway obstruction. The sedation allows for successful wound cleaning and suturing under local anesthesia without distress.

Post-sedation Recovery and Family Engagement

After the procedure, you monitor Rohan until he regains full alertness, can maintain a patent airway independently, and demonstrates stable vital signs. A focused neurological reassessment confirms no post-sedation changes or complications. His mother is counseled with clear discharge instructions, including signs to watch for (e.g., excessive sleepiness, vomiting, breathing difficulty) and guidance for wound care and follow-up.

Unexpected Events and Response

If Rohan were to become unusually drowsy post-sedation, your immediate response would include airway repositioning, administering supplemental oxygen, and reassessing his neurological status. Team communication is prioritized, and you document all observations, interventions, and decisions in the patient's chart meticulously.

Key Messages

- Children's responses to pain and sedation are highly individualized and depend on their age, developmental stage, and emotional maturity.
- Anxiety and fear are common in pediatric trauma patients, often exacerbated by the unfamiliar and stressful environment of emergency care.
- Pediatric sedation and analgesia should always be decided and administered by a qualified physician with appropriate training in pediatric procedural sedation.
- A thorough pre-sedation assessment—including detailed medical history, physical examination, and risk stratification—is essential for ensuring safety.
- Primary care providers (PCPs) must inquire about the child's last oral intake to evaluate aspiration risk and adhere to fasting guidelines.
- Neurological evaluation should include an assessment of consciousness level, pupillary responses, and motor and sensory functions to detect any underlying abnormalities.
- Intranasal routes are effective for pediatric sedation; medications such as midazolam and fentanyl can be safely administered via nasal spray, with attention to dosing and delivery technique.
- Capnography (end-tidal CO_2 monitoring) provides early detection of hypoventilation or airway compromise and should be continuously used during moderate to deep sedation.
- Pain should be regularly assessed using age-appropriate tools—such as FLACC, Wong-Baker FACES, or numerical scales—to guide analgesic titration.
- Opioids like morphine or fentanyl may be necessary for managing severe pain but require close monitoring for potential side effects, particularly respiratory depression.

- Parental presence, when feasible, and verbal reassurance significantly reduce a child's anxiety and improve their cooperation during procedures.
- Every pediatric patient must be treated with empathy, respect, and sensitivity to ensure not only physical stabilization but also emotional well-being throughout the sedation process.

Bibliography

1. Bingham, R., Thomas, A.L., & Sury, M (2008). Hatch & Sumner's Textbook of Paediatric Anaesthesia Third edition (3rd ed.). CRC Press. https://doi.org/10.1201/b13331
2. Charles J. Coté, Stephen Wilson, American Academy of Pediatrics, American Academy of Pediatric Dentistry; Guidelines for Monitoring and Management of Pediatric Patients Before, During, and After Sedation for Diagnostic and Therapeutic Procedures: Update 2016. *Pediatrics* July 2016; 138 (1): e20161212. https://doi.org/10.1542/peds.2016-1212
3. Gooden, Cheryl K., and others, 'Nursing Perspective', in Cheryl K. Gooden, Lia Lowrie, and Benjamin F. Jackson (eds), *The Pediatric Procedural Sedation Handbook* (New York, 2018; online edn, Oxford Academic, 1 Nov. 2018),https://doi.org/10.1093/med/9780190659110.003.0054, accessed 12 Sept. 2024.
4. Pershad, Jay; Kost, Susanne. Clinical Pediatric Emergency Medicine; Maryland Heights Vol. 8, Iss. 4, (2007): 253–261. https://doi.org/10.1016/j.cpem.2007.08.005
5. tern J, Pozun A. Pediatric Procedural Sedation. [Updated 2023 May 22]. In: StatPearls [Internet]. Treasure Island (FL): StatPearls Publishing; 2024 Jan-. Available from: https://www.ncbi.nlm.nih.gov/books/NBK572100/
6. Thakur Neha, Misra Samir, 2024, Pediatric Trauma Resuscitation Manual PTRM, 1st Edition, Jaypee Brother Medical Publishers, New Delhi. ISBN 9789356963979.
7. Trivedy, C., Hall, M., & Parfitt, A. (2010). Mastering Emergency Medicine: A Practical Guide (1st ed.). CRC Press. https://doi.org/10.1201/b13209.

Skills Stations and Training

16

Jabeen Fayyaz
and Muhammed Elhady Muhammed Elgasim

Learning Objectives
By the end of this chapter, the reader will be able to:

- Demonstrate understanding and skills in pediatric airway management techniques, including the insertion of oropharyngeal (OPA) and nasopharyngeal (NPA) airways and effective bag-valve-mask (BVM) ventilation.
- Assist in emergency thoracic procedures, including needle thoracostomy, finger thoracostomy, and chest tube insertion, while ensuring aseptic technique and continuous patient monitoring.
- Support safe neuro-orthopedic interventions by applying cervical spine immobilization, pelvic binders, and limb splints and tourniquets for haemeorrhage control with attention to anatomical and developmental considerations.
- Monitor for and assist in the managment of post-procedural complications, including airway compromise, bleeding, infection, and pain, using structured observation and reassessment protocols.
- Communicate effectively with patients and families, providing reassurance, procedural explanations, and discharge education in a trauma-informed and culturally sensitive manner.
- Document procedural events accurately and comprehensively, including procedure time, steps of procedure, medications used during the procedures, complications, and caregiver communication.

J. Fayyaz (✉)
Division of Emergency Medicine, Department of Paediatrics; SimKIDS Simulation Program, Learning Institute , The Hospital for Sick Children (Sickkids), Toronto, ON, Canada
e-mail: jabeen.fayyaz@sickkids.ca

M. E. M. Elgasim
Medical Educator and Emergency Medicine Specialist—Cork University Hospital, Cork, Ireland

N. T. Rai (ed.), *Pediatric Trauma Resuscitation Manual (PTRM) for Primary Care Providers*, https://doi.org/10.1007/978-981-95-4979-5_16

- Apply principles of Crisis Resource Management (CRM) such as SBAR and closed-loop communication, to enhance teamwork, safety, and efficiency in high-stress pediatric trauma scenarios.

Introduction

In pediatric trauma care, the margin between life and death is often measured in seconds and skill. Primary care providers (PCPs), nurses, and emergency personnel must be equipped with not only clinical knowledge but also the procedural competence to act swiftly and confidently. Simulation-based training has emerged as a cornerstone of pediatric trauma education, offering a controlled, reflective, and hands-on environment to develop and refine these essential skills.

This chapter presents a structured, skills-based curriculum organized around the ABCDE (**A**irway, **B**reathing, **C**irculation, **D**isability, **E**xposure/**E**nvironment) approach to pediatric trauma resuscitation. Each skill station is grounded in evidence-based practice and includes detailed guidance on procedural preparation, anatomical considerations unique to children, monitoring parameters, post-procedure care, and documentation. Whether assisting in airway management, intraosseous access, or supporting a chest tube insertion, the role of the PCP is clearly delineated through checklists and role-based responsibilities.

Importantly, this chapter goes beyond procedural steps. It emphasizes the "how" of teamwork; introducing Crisis Resource Management (CRM) principles such as closed-loop communication, task prioritization, and the use of structured tools like SBAR (situation, background, assessment, recommendation). It also recognizes the emotional and psychological needs of pediatric patients and their families, integrating communication strategies that promote empathy and trust during stressful clinical encounters.

By integrating clinical acumen with communication, documentation, and simulation-enhanced practice, this chapter equips primary care providers with the critical tools needed to deliver timely, safe, and effective trauma care. The ultimate goal is not just procedural mastery but improving outcomes and preserving the lives and dignity of children in crisis.

BASIC Airway Skills

Oropharyngeal Airway (OPA) Insertion

General and Anatomical Considerations:An oropharyngeal airway (OPA) helps keep the upper airway open in an unconscious patient by preventing the tongue from blocking airflow. In emergencies, especially when a child has reduced consciousness or ineffective breathing, an OPA allows primary care providers to maintain ventilation, support oxygenation, and buy time until definitive airway management is available. It is quick to insert, easy to use, and essential for basic airway stabilization.

- Large tongue and floppy epiglottis in babies and children increase the obstruction risk.
- A shorter airway length requires accurate sizing.

Preparation:

- *Indications:* Unconscious child with no gag reflex.
- *Contraindications:* Gag reflex present, suspected skull base fracture, or oral trauma.
- *Equipment:* OPA (various sizes), tongue depressor, PPE.
- *Child and Family Preparation:* Explain to the family that the child is unconscious and requires airway protection.
- *Positioning and Monitoring:* Supine, neutral neck. Monitor O2 saturations, ETCO2 monitoring and heart rate.

Procedure Steps:

- Select the correct size (corner of mouth to jaw angle).
- Use a tongue depressor to displace the tongue.
- Insert OPA with curve-facing tongue.
- Monitor for obstruction; ensure airway patency.

Monitoring:

- *Pre-procedure:* Baseline SpO_2, ETCO2 and heart rate.
- *During Procedure:* Continuous monitoring of SpO_2, heart rate, ETCO2 and airway patency.
- *Post-procedure:*
  - Reassess airway patency and oxygenation.
  - Monitor for gagging, vomiting, or obstruction.
  - Regular checks every 5 min initially, then every 15 min once stable.

Post-procedure Care:

- *Ensure the airway remains patent and secure.*
- *Monitor for return of gag reflex or signs of vomiting.*
- *Reposition or remove OPA if airway compromise occurs.*
- *Maintain suction readiness for secretions or vomit.*
- *Educate caregivers on potential complications and signs of obstruction.*

Documentation:

- *Procedure Details:* Indication, OPA size, and technique used.
- *Response:* Airway patency achieved, SpO_2, and heart rate post-insertion.
- *Adverse Events:* Gagging, vomiting, obstruction, or distress, with interventions documented.
- *Family Communication:* Explanation about airway management and potential risks was provided.

Nasopharyngeal Airway Insertion

General and Anatomical Considerations:A nasopharyngeal airway (NPA) helps maintain an open airway in patients who are semi-conscious or have a gag reflex, where an oropharyngeal airway may not be tolerated. It prevents soft tissue collapse, supports airflow, and allows effective ventilation in emergencies.

For primary care providers, knowing when and how to insert an NPA can stabilize breathing quickly while preparing for further airway management or transport.

1. The nasal passages in children are narrow, therefore be extra careful.
2. Prominent adenoids and turbinates increase resistance, therefore dont forefully push to avoid any trauma.
3. Avoid use in suspected basal skull fracture, facial and nasal trauma.

Preparation:

1. *Indications:* Partial airway obstruction with preserved gag reflex, that is in semiconsious babies and children.
2. *Contraindications:* Facial trauma, suspected skull base fracture.
3. *Equipment:* NPA (various sizes), water-based lubricant, PPE.
4. *Child and Family Preparation:* Explain to the caregiver that an airway adjunct is being used to help breathing.
5. *Positioning and Monitoring:* Supine, neutral neck position. Monitor O2 saturation and respiratory effort.

Procedure Steps:

1. Select appropriate NPA size (nostril to tragus).
2. Lubricate the tip well.
3. Gently insert into the nostril along the floor of the nose.
4. Confirm airway patency by observing chest rise and breath sounds.

Monitoring:

- *Pre-procedure:* Baseline SpO_2, ETCO2 and respiratory effort.
- *During Procedure:* Continuous monitoring of SpO_2, ETCO2, respiratory effort, and airway patency.
- *Post-procedure:* Reassess airway patency, respiratory rate, ETCO2, and SpO_2. Monitor for bleeding, obstruction, dislodgment, or discomfort. Regular checks every 5 min initially, then every 15 min once stable.

Post-procedure Care:

- Reassess airway patency and respiratory status.
- Monitor for bleeding or displacement.
- Check for signs of discomfort or distress.
- Educate family/caregivers about monitoring and signs of airway compromise.

Documentation:

- *Procedure Details:* Indication, side (left/right), size of NPA, technique used.
- *Response:* Airway patency achieved, SpO_2, and respiratory rate post-insertion.
- *Adverse Events:* Bleeding, dislodgment, obstruction, or discomfort with corrective actions documented.
- *Family Communication:* Explanation given regarding the procedure and ongoing monitoring.

Advanced Airway Skills

Bag Valve Mask (BVM) Ventilation

Anatomical Considerations:Bag-valve-mask (BVM) ventilation is a critical skill that allows providers to deliver lifesaving breaths to patients who are not breathing adequately or at all. For infants and children, effective BVM use supports oxygenation, maintains ventilation, and buys crucial time until advanced airway support is available. Mastery of proper mask seal, head positioning, and gentle ventilation is essential for preventing hypoxia and improving survival in emergency situations.

- A small face and short nose require appropriate mask sizing that is a mask size that cover the bridge of the nose to the chin area.

Preparation:

- *Indications: Respiratory arrest, ineffective spontaneous breathing, apnea .*
- *Contraindications: None in emergency.*
- *Equipment: Self-inflating BVM, appropriately sized mask, O2 supply.*
- *Child and Family Preparation: Explain the need for assisted ventilation.*
- *Positioning and Monitoring:* Sniffing position unless spinal injury. Monitor respiratory rate and chest rise.

Procedure Steps:

1. Position head (Head tilt and chin lift, jaw thrust if trauma).
2. Apply mask: nose to chin seal, by E and C clamp technique.
3. Squeeze bag: 1 breath every 3–5 s.
4. Reassess chest rise and oxygen saturation.

Post-procedure Care:

- Monitor ventilation adequacy (chest rise, SpO_2, ETCO2).
- Assess for rescuer fatigue during prolonged use.
- Maintain oxygen delivery and monitor for air leaks or gastric distension (consider passing orogastric or nasogastric tube to avoid over distention of stomach.

Monitoring:

- Pre-procedure: Baseline SpO_2, ETCO2 and respiratory rate.
- During Procedure: Continuous monitoring of chest rise, SpO_2, ETCO2 and ventilation rate.
- Post-procedure: Regular reassessment of ventilation quality and oxygenation.

Documentation:

- Procedure Details: Indication, technique used, ventilation rate, and oxygen settings.
- Response: Airway patency, chest rise, SpO_2, ETCO2, and respiratory rate.
- Adverse Events: Air leaks, gastric distension, or inadequate ventilation.
- Family Communication: Explanation of assisted ventilation and monitoring.

Needle Thoracostomy

Procedure Description: Always do in assistance with a team

- Needle thoracostomy is an emergency procedure used to relieve a tension pneumothorax — a life-threatening condition where trapped air in the chest compresses the lungs and heart. By inserting a needle into the pleural space, pressure is rapidly released, allowing the lung to re-expand and restoring vital circulation. For primary care providers, recognizing tension pneumothorax early and performing needle decompression without delay can be lifesaving, especially when advanced care or transport is not immediately available.

Importance:

- Rapidly relieves life-threatening pressure in the chest, preventing cardiovascular collapse and restoring ventilation.

Procedure Steps:Always do in assistance with a team

1. Identify the site (2nd intercostal space (ICS) mid-clavicular or 5th ICS mid-axillary).
2. Prepare the area with antiseptic.
3. Insert a 14–18G cannula just above the rib at a 90° angle.
4. Aspirate air until pressure is relieved.
5. Secure the cannula in place.

Role of Primary Care Provider:

- Prepare equipment and maintain a sterile field.
- Position the patient (supine or semi-upright).
- Continuously monitor vital signs (HR, RR, SpO_2, ETCO2).
- Support family by explaining the purpose and outcome.

Monitoring:

- Pre-procedure: Baseline HR, RR, SPO2 and $ETCO_2$.
- During Procedure: Continuous monitoring of HR, RR, SpO_2, ETCO2 and signs of distress.
- Post-procedure: Regular reassessment of respiratory status and oxygen saturation. Monitor for bleeding or air leak from the insertion site.

Post-procedure Care:

- Monitor for clinical improvement and decreased respiratory distress.
- Assess the puncture site for bleeding or air leakage.
- Prepare for definitive chest tube placement.
- Reassess vital signs frequently.

Documentation:

- Procedure Details: Site, size of cannula.
- Clinical Response: Air release, patient stability.
- Complications: Bleeding, obstruction.
- Family Communication: Explain the procedure and outcome.

Finger Thoracostomy

Procedure Description:Always do in assistance with a team

- Finger thoracostomy is an emergency procedure used to quickly relieve a tension pneumothorax when chest tubes or advanced equipment may be delayed. After making a small incision in the chest, the provider uses a finger to open the pleural space, allowing trapped air to escape and the lung to re-expand. It is a rapid, reliable method that restores ventilation and circulation in critically unstable patients. For primary care providers in resource-limited or prehospital settings, timely finger thoracostomy can be lifesaving when needle decompression is insufficient or ineffective.

Importance:

- Provides immediate decompression of tension pneumothorax.

Procedure Steps: Always do in assistance with a team

1. Identify the site (4th/5th Intercostal space -ICS mid-axillary).
2. Make a small incision over the ICS.
3. Bluntly dissect through intercostal muscles.
4. Penetrate the pleura and insert a gloved finger to assess lung re-expansion.
5. Cover with a sterile dressing.

Role of Primary Care Provider:

- Assist with positioning (supine, arm raised).
- Prepare sterile instruments and maintain a sterile field and wear appropriate PPE.
- Support the patient emotionally and explain the procedure to family.

Monitoring:

- Pre-procedure: Baseline HR, RR, SPO2 and $ETCO_2$.
- During Procedure: Monitor respiratory effort, lung sounds, and oxygenation.
- Post-procedure: Continuous monitoring of respiratory rate, oxygen saturation, and signs of bleeding or air leak.

Post-procedure Care:

- Monitor for signs of respiratory improvement.
- Observe for bleeding or air leakage.
- Prepare for formal chest tube placement.
- Reassess respiratory rate and oxygen saturation.

Documentation:

- Procedure Details: Site, technique used.
- Clinical Response: Lung re-expansion, respiratory status.
- Complications: Bleeding, injury to vessels.
- Family Communication: Explain the procedure and expected outcome.

Chest Tube Insertion

Procedure Description: Always do in assistance with a team

- Chest tube insertion is a critical procedure used to drain air, blood, or fluid from the pleural space to allow the lung to re-expand and restore normal breathing. It is essential in cases of pneumothorax, hemothorax, or severe chest trauma. For primary care providers, understanding when a chest tube is needed and initiating the procedure when trained can stabilize a child's breathing, improve oxygenation, and prevent life-threatening respiratory collapse while arranging definitive care.

Importance:

- Restores lung expansion and improves oxygenation by removing trapped air or fluid.

Procedure Steps: Always do in assistance with a team

- Identify the insertion site (usually 5th ICS mid-axillary).
- Prepare the area with sterile technique.
- Make a small incision and bluntly dissect down to the pleura.
- Insert the chest tube and secure it with sutures.
- Connect to the drainage system and confirm placement.

Role of Primary Care Provider:

- Assist with equipment setup and sterile preparation.
- Position the patient (supine or lateral, arm raised).
- Hand sterile instruments to the physician.
- Reassure and support the patient and family.

Monitoring:

- Pre-procedure: Baseline HR, RR, ETCO2, SpO_2.
- During Procedure: Continuous monitoring of oxygen saturation and respiratory effort.
- Post-procedure:
  - Monitor chest tube output and ensure patency.
  - Regularly check for air leaks and dressing integrity.
  - Assess for pain, respiratory effort, and oxygenation.

Post-procedure Care:

- Monitor drainage system for air leaks and patency.
- Reassess pain, provide comfort, and ensure tube security.
- Regularly monitor vital signs, especially oxygen saturation.
- Maintain suction and ensure dressing integrity.

Documentation:

- Procedure Details: Site, tube size, drainage system.
- Output: Type and volume of drainage (air, blood).
- Complications: Air leak, tube displacement.
- Family Communication: Explanation of tube purpose and care instructions.

Circulation Skills

Intraosseous (IO) Access

General description and Anatomical Considerations:Intraosseous (IO) access is a life-saving technique that allows rapid delivery of fluids and medications directly into the bone marrow when intravenous (IV) access is difficult or delayed. For critically ill infants and children, especially those in shock, cardiac arrest, severe dehydration, or trauma, IO access provides a fast, reliable route to resuscitation. It can be established within seconds, works even when veins are collapsed, and ensures that essential medications reach circulation immediately. For primary care providers, being able to recognize when IO access is needed and initiating it early can significantly improve survival during emergencies by preventing delays in critical treatment.

- The tibial plateau is flat and accessible.Other IO insertion sites in children include: • Distal tibia • Proximal humerus (especially in older children) • Distal femur (commonly used in infants and younger children) • Sternum (rare in pediatrics, typically limited to specialized devices and trained providers) These alternative sites ensure rapid vascular access when IV attempts fail, supporting timely resuscitation in critically ill children.
- Growth plates must be avoided.

Preparation:

- *Indications:* Emergency vascular access when peripheral IV access fails.
- *Contraindications:* Fracture, previous IO in the same site, infection.
- *Equipment:* EZ-IO device, appropriate needle size, flush, PPE.
- *Child and Family Preparation:* Explain IO is urgent and temporary.
- *Positioning and Monitoring:* Supine, knee supported. Monitor perfusion.

Role of Primary Care Provider:Always do in assistance with a team

- Preparation: Gather equipment (EZ-IO device, needle, flush, antiseptic). Position patient supine with knee supported. Explain urgency to family.
- During Procedure: Identify site (1–2 cm below tibial tuberosity), clean with antiseptic, insert needle at 90° angle using power driver, and confirm placement by aspiration or flush. Secure the site.

Post-procedure Care:

- Secure and stabilize the IO needle.
- Monitor for infiltration at the site and below the site of insertion, infection, and patency.
- Assess pain and provide analgesia as needed.

Monitoring:

- Pre-procedure: Baseline HR, BP, perfusion.
- During Procedure: Monitor for correct placement and extravasation.
- Post-procedure: Regular checks for patency, complications, and pain.

Documentation:

- Site, size, time, flow confirmation.
- Complications (if any) and response.
- Family communication and education.

Neuro and Orthopedic Skills

Neurological Assessment

Anatomical Considerations.

- Children may have subtle signs of neurological deterioration.
- Opening infant fontanelles allows visual assessment of raised intracranial pressure (ICP).
- The immature nervous system can make standard neurological assessments more challenging, requiring age-adapted techniques.

Preparation.

- *Indications:* All pediatric trauma patients, particularly those with head injury, altered mental status, seizures, or suspected spinal cord injury.
- *Contraindications:* None;this is part of all trauma assessments.
- *Equipment:* Penlight, blood glucose monitor (glucometer), documentation chart.
- *Child and Family Preparation:* Explain that the team will check the child's brain function, pupil response, and blood sugar.
- *Positioning and Monitoring:* If indicated, place the patient in a supine position with cervical spine precautions. Observe signs of neurological compromise (e.g., seizures, decorticate/decerebrate posturing).

Procedure Steps.

1. Assess level of consciousness using the AVPU scale:
   - A = Alert.
   - V = Responds to voice.
   - P = Responds to pain.
   - U = Unresponsive.
2. Alternatively, assess using the Glasgow Coma Scale (GCS) as shown in Table 16.1.

- GCS score range: 3 to 15. A score ≤ 8 indicates a coma and the need for airway protection.

3. Assess pupil size and reactivity using a penlight;check for equal, reactive pupils or signs of fixed/dilated pupil(s).
4. Assess limb movement and tone;note spontaneous movement, purposeful withdrawal from pain, or abnormal posturing.
5. Measure capillary blood glucose to exclude hypoglycemia as a reversible cause of altered mental status.
6. Assess older children's orientation to person, place, and time.

Role of Primary Care Provider:

- *Preparation:* Gather equipment (penlight, glucometer, documentation chart). Explain the assessment purpose to family. Position the child supine with cervical spine precautions if needed.
- *During Procedure:*
  - Assess level of consciousness using AVPU or Glasgow Coma Scale (GCS).
  - Check pupil size and reactivity using a penlight.

Table 16.1 Pediatric Glasgow Coma Scale (pGCS) and its modification in infants

Behavior	Response in children	Response in infants	Score
Eye opening (E)	Spontaneous	Spontaneous	4
	To sound	To sound	3
	To pressure	To pressure	2
	None	No response	1
	Non-testable		NT
Verbal response (V)	Appropriate words or social smile, fixes, and follows	Coos and babbles	5
	Cries but consolable	Irritable cries	4
	Persistently irritable	Cries in response to pain	3
	Restless, agitated	Moans in response to pain	2
	None	No response	1
	Non-testable	Non-testable	NT
Best motor response (M)	Obeys commands	Spontaneous purposeful movements	6
	Localizing	Withdrawal to touch	5
	Normal flexion	Withdrawal to pain	4
	Abnormal flexion	Responds to pain with decorticate posturing (abnormal flexion)	3
	Extension	Responds to pain with decerebrate posturing (abnormal extension)	2
	None	None	1
	Non-testable	Non-testable	NT

[a]Adapted from James H. E. (1986). Neurologic evaluation and support in the child with an acute brain insult. *Pediatric annals*, *15*(1), 16–22

  - Assess limb movement and tone for symmetry and response.
  - Measure capillary blood glucose to rule out hypoglycemia.
  - In older children, assess orientation to person, place, and time.
- *Post-procedure Care:*
  - Frequent reassessment (every 15 minutes if abnormal).
  - Monitor for signs of neurological deterioration.
  - Elevate the head to 30° if raised ICP is suspected (if no contraindications).
  - Maintain normoglycemia, normoxia, and normocarbia.

Monitoring:

- *Pre-procedure:* Baseline neurological status (AVPU/GCS).
- *During Procedure:* Continuously observe for changes in consciousness, pupil reaction, and motor response.
- *Post-procedure:* Monitor for seizure activity, posturing, or any neurological changes. Reassess GCS or AVPU frequently.

Documentation:

- *Assessment Findings:*
  - *AVPU or GCS Score:* Document numerical score and components.
  - *Pupil Response:* Size and reactivity (e.g., 3 mm, reactive bilaterally).
  - *Motor Response:* Limb movement, tone, and posturing.

  - *Blood Glucose:* Record result based on your local guidelines(mg/dl or mmol/L).
  - *Additional Observations:* Seizure activity, abnormal posturing, or LOC changes.
- *Interventions:* Actions taken and escalation if deterioration noted.
- *Family Communication:* Inform family of findings and care plan.

Cervical Spine Immobilization

General and Anatomical Considerations:Cervical spine immobilization is essential to protect the spinal cord in any child with trauma, altered consciousness, or suspected neck injury. By stabilizing the head and neck, providers prevent further movement that could worsen an existing spinal injury. Early and proper immobilization — using manual stabilization, a cervical collar, and appropriate positioning — reduces the risk of neurological damage and is a crucial first step in pediatric trauma care.

- Large head size in children increases risk of neck flexion injuries.
- Ligamentous injuries may occur without fractures.

Preparation:

- Indications: Suspected cervical spine trauma.
- Equipment: Cervical collar, head blocks, tape.
- Child and Family Preparation: Explain collar is to protect the neck.
- Positioning and Monitoring: Manual in-line stabilization until collar in place. Monitor neurological signs.

Procedure Steps:

1. Apply collar sized from chin to trapezius.
2. Use head blocks and tape to secure.
3. Maintain neutral alignment.

Role of Primary Care Provider:

- Preparation: Gather equipment (cervical collar, head blocks, tape). Prepare the patient and family by explaining that the collar is used to protect the neck.
- During Procedure:
  - Maintain manual in-line stabilization at all times.
  - Apply an appropriately sized cervical collar from chin to trapezius.
  - Secure with head blocks and tape while maintaining neutral alignment.
  - Continuously monitor for neurological signs and changes.

Monitoring:

- Pre-procedure: Baseline neurological status (motor function, sensory function).
- During Procedure:
  - Monitor for compromise in airway, breathing, or circulation.
  - Continuously observe for neurological changes or signs of discomfort.
- Post-procedure:
  - Reassess collar fit and skin integrity.
  - Regularly check neurological status to detect any deterioration.
  - Ensure that the collar is not removed without senior instruction.

Post-procedure Care:
- Stability Maintenance: Keep the neck immobilized, and avoid unnecessary movement.
- Skin Integrity: Regularly check under the collar for pressure areas or skin breakdown.
- Patient Comfort: Ensure the collar is not causing discomfort or respiratory compromise.
- Communication: Explain the importance of immobilization to both the child and family.

Documentation:
- Procedure Details:
  - Time applied and collar size.
  - Position and alignment maintained.
- Neurological Assessment:
  - Findings before and after collar application.
  - Any signs of neurological compromise or changes.
- Skin Integrity Check: Document any redness, pressure sores, or discomfort.
- Family Communication: Record information provided and any questions addressed.

Pelvic Binder Application

General and Anatomical Considerations:Pelvic binder application is a rapid way to stabilize a suspected pelvic fracture and reduce life-threatening bleeding. In children with high-energy trauma, a binder helps close the pelvic ring, limit internal blood loss, and improve circulation until definitive care is available. Early application by primary care providers can be lifesaving and should be done as soon as a pelvic injury is suspected.
- Binder must compress over greater trochanters (not iliac crest).
- Children have open growth plates to consider.

Preparation:
- *Indications:* Suspected pelvic fracture with hypotension.
- *Equipment:* Commercial or improvised pelvic binder.
- *Child and Family Preparation:* Explain binder stops bleeding from pelvis.
- *Positioning and Monitoring:* Supine, minimal movement. Monitor vitals and perfusion.

Procedure Steps:
1. Place binder beneath patient using log-roll or lift.
2. Center over greater trochanters.
3. Secure snugly to provide compression.
4. Avoid over-tightening.

Role of Primary Care Provider:
- Prepare equipment (commercial or improvised binder).
- Explain to family the binder's role in stopping bleeding.
- Position the patient supine with minimal movement.

Procedure Steps:

1. Log-roll or lift patient to place binder under hips.
2. Center binder over greater trochanters (not iliac crest).
3. Secure snugly without over-tightening.
4. Continuously monitor vital signs and perfusion.

Monitoring:

- Pre-procedure: Baseline HR, BP, perfusion.
- During Procedure: Monitor for hemodynamic stability and signs of discomfort.
- Post-procedure: Regularly assess vital signs, perfusion, and neurovascular status.

Post-procedure Care:

- Monitor for improvement in shock.
- Maintain binder position and stability.
- Leave binder in place until imaging and surgical review.

Documentation:

- Application Time: Record time and anatomical level.
- Patient Response: Improvement in vitals and perfusion.
- Complications: Signs of ischemia or compartment syndrome.
- Family Communication: Explanation and reassurance given.

Limb Splinting

General and Anatomical Considerations:Limb splinting is essential to stabilize fractures or severe sprains, reduce pain, and prevent further injury. By immobilizing the affected bone or joint, splinting minimizes movement, protects blood vessels and nerves, and helps control swelling. For primary care providers, early and proper splinting improves comfort, maintains alignment, and prevents complications while arranging definitive treatment.

- Growth plates and small joints require careful padding.

Preparation:

- *Indications:* Suspected or confirmed fractures.
- *Contraindications:* None.
- *Equipment:* Box/Kendrick/Thomas splint, bandages, scissors.
- *Child and Family Preparation:* Explain the need for immobilization.
- *Positioning and Monitoring:* Support injured limb. Monitor CMS (circulation, motor, sensation).

Role of Primary Care Provider:

- Gather equipment (splint, bandages, padding, scissors).
- Explain to the child and family that immobilization is necessary to protect the injury.
- Support the injured limb while preparing.

Procedure Steps:

1. Assess limb alignment and neurovascular status (CMS):
   - Circulation (pulse, capillary refill).

   - Motor function (ability to move digits).
   - Sensation (touch and pain response).
2. Apply Splint:
   - Immobilize the joint above and below the injury.
   - Pad all bony prominences to prevent pressure sores.
3. Secure Splint:
   - Bandage without excessive tightness.
   - Reassess CMS after securing.

Monitoring:
- Pre-procedure: Baseline CMS assessment.
- During Procedure: Continuously monitor for pain, swelling, and distal circulation.
- Post-procedure: Reassess CMS every 15 minutes initially, then hourly.

Post-procedure Care:
- Elevate the limb to reduce swelling.
- Regularly check for pressure points and comfort.
- Adjust the splint if there are signs of circulatory compromise.

Documentation:
- Procedure Details: Type of splint used and injury description.
- CMS Findings: Before and after splint application.
- Patient Comfort: Pain level and stability.
- Complications: Any signs of neurovascular compromise.
- Family Communication: Information provided and follow-up instructions.

OPA insertion checklist for primary care providers

Task	Done	Not done	Comments
Assess anatomical considerations (large tongue, floppy epiglottis)	☐	☐	
Gather equipment (OPA, tongue depressor, PPE)	☐	☐	
Explain airway protection to the family	☐	☐	
Position patient supine, neutral neck	☐	☐	
Baseline monitoring (SpO_2, heart rate)	☐	☐	
Select the correct OPA size (mouth to jaw angle)	☐	☐	
Displace the tongue with the depressor and insert OPA (curve-facing tongue)	☐	☐	
Monitor airway patency and ventilation during procedure	☐	☐	
Reassess airway patency and oxygenation post-insertion	☐	☐	
Monitor for gagging, vomiting, or obstruction	☐	☐	
Maintain suction readiness for secretions	☐	☐	
Educate caregivers on airway care and potential complications	☐	☐	
Document indication, OPA size, patient response, and adverse events	☐	☐	

NPA insertion checklist for primary care providers

Task	Done	Not done	Comments
Assess anatomical considerations (narrow nasal passages, adenoids)	☐	☐	
Gather equipment (NPA, lubricant, PPE)	☐	☐	
Explain airway protection to the family	☐	☐	
Position patient supine, neutral neck	☐	☐	
Baseline monitoring (SpO_2, respiratory effort)	☐	☐	
Select appropriate NPA size (nostril to tragus)	☐	☐	
Lubricate the NPA tip with a water-based lubricant	☐	☐	
Gently insert NPA along the nose floor	☐	☐	
Monitor for airway patency and ventilation during the procedure	☐	☐	
Reassess airway patency and oxygenation post-insertion	☐	☐	
Monitor for bleeding, obstruction, or displacement	☐	☐	
Educate caregivers on airway care and potential complications	☐	☐	
Document indication, NPA size, patient response, and adverse events	☐	☐	

BVM ventilation checklist for primary care providers

Task	Done	Not done	Comments
Assess anatomical considerations (small face, short nose)	☐	☐	
Gather equipment (BVM, appropriately sized mask, O_2 supply)	☐	☐	
Explain assisted ventilation to the family	☐	☐	
Position patient in sniffing position (unless spinal injury suspected)	☐	☐	
Baseline monitoring (SpO_2, respiratory rate, chest rise)	☐	☐	
Apply mask with nose-to-chin seal and jaw thrust if trauma is suspected	☐	☐	
Squeeze the bag to deliver breaths (1 every 3–5 s)	☐	☐	
Monitor for effective chest rise and adequate ventilation	☐	☐	
Reassess airway patency and oxygenation post-ventilation	☐	☐	
Monitor for air leaks or gastric distension	☐	☐	
Educate caregivers on potential complications and ventilation care	☐	☐	
Document indication, technique, ventilation rate, and patient response	☐	☐	

Needle Thoracostomy Checklist

Task	Done	Not done	Comments
Preparation: Gather necessary equipment for needle thoracostomy	☐	☐	
Patient and family education about needle thoracostomy procedure	☐	☐	
Position the patient appropriately	☐	☐	
Monitor vital signs before, during, and after the procedure	☐	☐	
Perform needle thoracostomy as per standard protocol	☐	☐	
Monitor for complications and adverse effects	☐	☐	
Provide post-procedure care and reassess the patient	☐	☐	
Document the procedure, patient response, and any complications	☐	☐	

Finger thoracostomy checklist

Task	Done	Not done	Comments
Preparation: Gather necessary equipment for finger thoracostomy	☐	☐	
Patient and family education about finger thoracostomy procedure	☐	☐	
Position the patient appropriately	☐	☐	
Monitor vital signs before, during, and after the procedure	☐	☐	
Perform finger thoracostomy as per standard protocol	☐	☐	
Monitor for complications and adverse effects	☐	☐	
Provide post-procedure care and reassess the patient	☐	☐	
Document the procedure, patient response, and any complications	☐	☐	

Chest tube insertion checklist

Task	Done	Not done	Comments
Preparation: Gather necessary equipment for chest tube insertion	☐	☐	
Patient and family education about the chest tube insertion procedure	☐	☐	
Position the patient appropriately	☐	☐	
Monitor vital signs before, during, and after the procedure	☐	☐	
Perform chest tube insertion as per standard protocol	☐	☐	
Monitor for complications and adverse effects	☐	☐	
Provide post-procedure care and reassess the patient	☐	☐	
Document the procedure, patient response, and any complications	☐	☐	

Intraosseous (IO) access checklist

Task	Done	Not done	Comments
Preparation: Gather necessary equipment for intraosseous (IO) access	☐	☐	
Patient and family education about intraosseous (IO) access procedure	☐	☐	
Position the patient appropriately	☐	☐	
Monitor vital signs before, during, and after the procedure	☐	☐	
Perform intraosseous (IO) access as per standard protocol	☐	☐	
Monitor for complications and adverse effects	☐	☐	
Provide post-procedure care and reassess the patient	☐	☐	
Document the procedure, patient response, and any complications	☐	☐	

Neurological assessment checklist

Task	Done	Not done	Comments
Preparation: Gather necessary equipment for neurological assessment	☐	☐	
Patient and family education about neurological assessment procedure	☐	☐	
Position the patient appropriately	☐	☐	
Monitor vital signs before, during, and after the procedure	☐	☐	
Perform a neurological assessment as per standard protocol	☐	☐	
Monitor for complications and adverse effects	☐	☐	
Provide post-procedure care and reassess the patient	☐	☐	
Document the procedure, patient response, and any complications	☐	☐	

Cervical spine immobilization checklist

Task	Done	Not done	Comments
Preparation: Gather necessary equipment for cervical spine immobilization	☐	☐	
Patient and family education about cervical spine immobilization procedure	☐	☐	
Position the patient appropriately	☐	☐	
Monitor vital signs before, during, and after the procedure	☐	☐	
Perform cervical spine immobilization as per standard protocol	☐	☐	
Monitor for complications and adverse effects	☐	☐	
Provide post-procedure care and reassess the patient	☐	☐	
Document the procedure, patient response, and any complications	☐	☐	

Pelvic binder application checklist

Task	Done	Not done	Comments
Preparation: Gather necessary equipment for pelvic binder application	☐	☐	
Patient and family education about pelvic binder application procedure	☐	☐	
Position the patient appropriately	☐	☐	
Monitor vital signs before, during, and after the procedure	☐	☐	
Perform pelvic binder application as per standard protocol	☐	☐	
Monitor for complications and adverse effects	☐	☐	
Provide post-procedure care and reassess the patient	☐	☐	
Document the procedure, patient response, and any complications	☐	☐	

Limb splinting checklist

Task	Done	Not done	Comments
Preparation: Gather necessary equipment for limb splinting	☐	☐	
Patient and family education about limb splinting procedure	☐	☐	
Position the patient appropriately	☐	☐	
Monitor vital signs before, during, and after the procedure	☐	☐	
Perform limb splinting as per standard protocol	☐	☐	
Monitor for complications and adverse effects	☐	☐	
Provide post-procedure care and reassess the patient	☐	☐	
Document the procedure, patient response, and any complications	☐	☐	

PTRM for PCP Quick Reference Guide 17

Jabeen Fayyaz
and Muhammed Elhady Muhammed Elgasim

Practical Checklist for Pediatric Trauma Triage and Transport

Initial Rapid Assessment: Pediatric Assessment Triangle (PAT)

- *Appearance:*
  - Mental status: Alert? Interactive?
  - Muscle tone: Limp/lethargic?
  - Eye contact or purposeful movement?
- *Work of Breathing:*
  - Nasal flaring/retractions?
  - Abnormal sounds (gasping, stridor)?
  - Posture (tripoding, head bobbing)?
- *Circulation to Skin:*
  - Color: Pale/cyanotic/mottled?
  - Capillary refill: >2–3 seconds?
  - Temperature: Cool extremities?
- *Action:*
  - ≥2 abnormal components → *red* (immediate intervention)
  - 1 abnormal component → *yellow* (urgent monitoring) (Figs. 17.1 and 17.2).

J. Fayyaz (✉)
Department of Pediatrics, SimKIDS Simulation Program, Learning Institute, The Hospital for Sick Children, Toronto, ON, Canada
e-mail: jabeen.fayyaz@sickkids.ca

M. E. M. Elgasim
Medical Educator and Emergency Medicine Specialist—Cork University Hospital, Cork, Ireland

N. T. Rai (ed.), *Pediatric Trauma Resuscitation Manual (PTRM) for Primary Care Providers*, https://doi.org/10.1007/978-981-95-4979-5_17

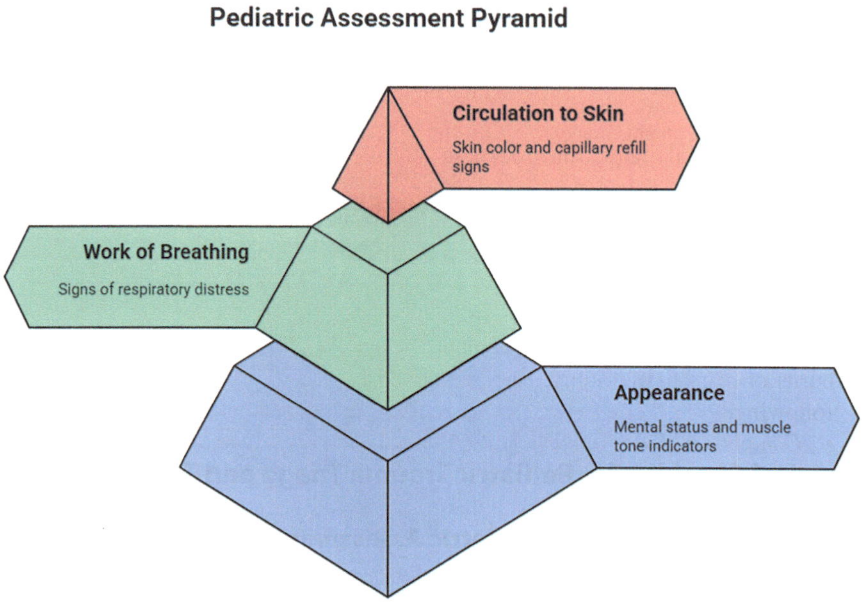

Fig. 17.1 Pediatric assessment pyramid. (Figure illustrated using AI tools with Napkin AI, 2025)

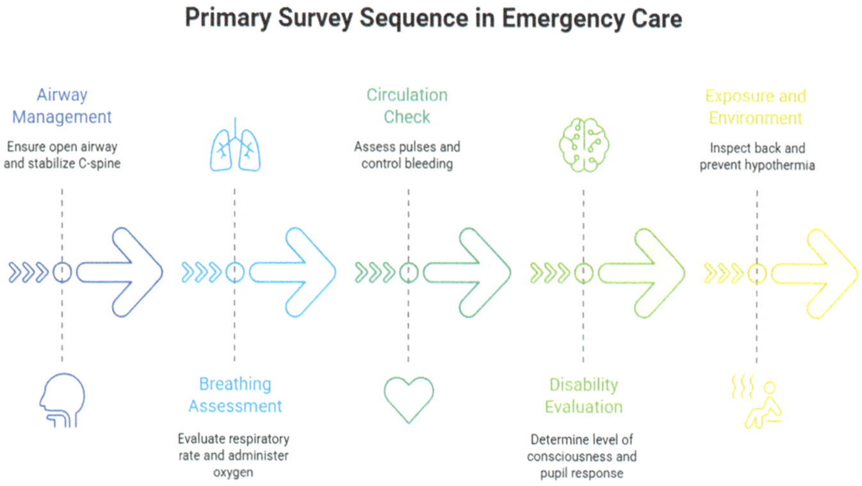

Fig. 17.2 Primary survey sequence in emergency care. (Figure illustrated using AI tools with Napkin AI, 2025)

Primary Survey (ABCDE)

Component	Checklist actions
A: Airway + C-spine	Open airway (jaw thrust if trauma)clear secretions (suction)cervical collar + spine immobilization
B: Breathing	Respiratory rate/depthadminister high-flow O_2 (non-rebreather mask) prepare BVM ventilation if SpO_2 <90%
C: Circulation	Central/peripheral pulsescontrol bleeding (direct pressure/tourniquet)IV/IO access → 10–20 mL/kg crystalloid bolus for shock till blood products arrive
D: Disability	Pediatric AVPU: Alert Voice Pain Unresponsive Pupil check (unequal/dilated?)
E: Exposure/ environment	Log-roll to inspect backwarming blankets (prevent hypothermia) Check blood glucose + core temperature

Triage Categorization

Category	Criteria	Action
Red	GCS ≤8, shock, respiratory failure	*Life-saving interventions + rapid transport*
Yellow	Stable ABCs + fractures/moderate injuries	*Splinting, pain control, close monitoring*
Green	Walking, minor wounds	*First aid + delayed treatment*
Blue/ black	Non-survivable injuries/deceased	*Palliative care/confirm death*

High-Risk Flags (Up-Triage to Red)

- GCS ≤13, SBP <70–80 mmHg (age-based), falls >10 ft., ejection from vehicle, penetrating injuries.

Pre-Transport Stabilization

- *Airway:* Intubate if GCS ≤8 or respiratory failure.
- *Breathing:* Secure O_2/ventilation; confirm ET tube position.
- *Circulation:* Second IV/IO access if ongoing shock.
- *Disability:* Recheck GCS; maintain C-spine immobilization.
- *Exposure:* Document all injuries; cover with warm blankets.

Transport Strategy

- 🚑*Scoop and Run:* Time-critical cases (e.g., TBI, uncontrolled hemorrhage).
- ⏳ *Stand and Play:* Stabilize shock/inotrope support before transport.

Transport Preparation

Team:
- Doctor + PALS-trained nurse + paramedic/driver.

Equipment checklist:
- *Airway Bag:* ET tubes, laryngoscope, suction, BVM.
- *Drugs:* Epinephrine, mannitol, analgesics.
- *Monitors:* Pulse oximeter, ECG, BP cuff.
- *Trauma Kit:* Cervical collar, splints, sterile dressings.

Communication protocol (SBAR): SBAR is a structured communication tool; Situation, Background, Assessment, Recommendation, that helps healthcare providers share critical information quickly and clearly. Using SBAR improves teamwork, reduces errors, and ensures everyone understands the patient's condition and the next steps. For primary care providers, SBAR is especially valuable during handovers, emergency calls, or when escalating care to a specialist or higher-level facility.
- **S**ituation: *"11M, GCS 7, head injury, unstable."*
- **B**ackground: *"Unhelmeted cyclist struck by pole."*
- **A**ssessment: *"Intubated, fluid-resuscitated, unequal pupils."*
- **R**ecommendation: *"Need neurosurgery; ETA 20 mins."*

During Transport

- *Continuous Monitoring:* HR/RR/SpO_2/BP q5–10min; GCS trends.
- *Interventions:*
  - Repeat fluid boluses if shock persists.
  - Manage seizures (benzodiazepines).
- *Documentation:* Log vitals, interventions, and clinical changes.

Handover at Receiving Facility

Structured tool (I-PASS): I-PASS is a structured handover tool; Illness severity, Patient summary, Action list, Situation awareness and contingency plans, and Synthesis by receiver—that ensures safe and consistent transfer of patient information. It reduces communication errors, supports shared mental models, and improves continuity of care. For primary care providers, I-PASS strengthens handovers between clinics, emergency services, and hospitals, especially during high-risk transitions.

1. **I**llness severity: "Critical, GCS 7."
2. **P**atient summary: *"MOI, interventions, CT findings."*
3. **A**ction list: *"Urgent neurosurgery, repeat CT."*
4. **S**ituational awareness: *"BP dropping; needs vasopressors."*
5. **S**ynthesis: Receiver confirms understanding.

Documents to transfer:

- Consent forms, transport records, imaging CDs.

Pediatric-Specific Considerations.

- *Anatomy:* Large head → rigorous C-spine protection.
- *Physiology:* High hypothermia risk → Aggressive warming.
- *Dosages:* Use Broselow tape for drugs/fluids.
- *Family:* Update parents; involve in decisions.

Crisis Resource Management and Disaster Preparedness in Pediatric Trauma

Immediate Response: Crisis Resource Management (CRM) Principles (Fig. 17.3)

CRM principles	Key practices
Situational awareness: Situational awareness is the ability to understand what is happening around the patient, recognize early signs of deterioration, and anticipate what might happen next. It helps providers notice subtle changes, respond quickly to risks, and make safer clinical decisions. Strong situational awareness improves teamwork, prevents errors, and is essential in fast-moving pediatric emergencies.	Scan for safety threats Assess resource availability Identify team positions Identify key equipment (airway kits, IV access, monitors) Monitor patient influx and crowding
Anticipation and planning: Anticipation and planning involve thinking ahead about what a patient may need next and preparing for potential complications before they occur. For primary care providers, this means having equipment ready, organizing tasks, and mentally rehearsing next steps. Good anticipation improves efficiency, reduces delays in care, and keeps children safer during emergencies.	Prepare for high-risk scenarios (e.g., pneumothorax, shock) based on the mechanism of injury Pre-set airway tools (BVM, suction), fluids (20 mL/kg), and analgesics
Leadership and roles: Leadership and clear role assignment ensure that every team member knows exactly what they are responsible for during an emergency. Effective leadership keeps the team organized, reduces confusion, improves communication, and ensures that critical tasks—airway, breathing, circulation—are completed quickly and safely. For primary care providers, strong leadership and defined roles are essential for coordinated, high-quality pediatric resuscitation.	Assign a team leader Define roles clearly: Airway manager, circulation/IV access, vitals monitor, documentation
Effective communication: Effective communication means sharing information clearly, calmly, and concisely so the entire team understands the patient's status and the plan. It reduces misunderstandings, supports teamwork, and improves patient safety. For primary care providers, strong communication is essential during emergencies, handovers, and any situation where quick decisions are needed.	Use closed-loop communication (e.g., "Meena, administer O_2…" → "O_2 applied, saturation rising") Use SBAR format for updates: Situation, background, assessment, recommendation

(continued)

CRM principles	Key practices
Avoid fixation errors: Avoiding fixation errors means not getting stuck on one diagnosis, task, or idea when the patient's condition is changing. It helps providers step back, reassess, and stay open to new information. For primary care teams, avoiding fixation keeps decision-making flexible, reduces mistakes, and ensures timely recognition of deterioration in pediatric emergencies.	Reassess ABCDE every 5 minutes Avoid focusing only on one injury Delegate tasks when needed to maintain situational flexibility

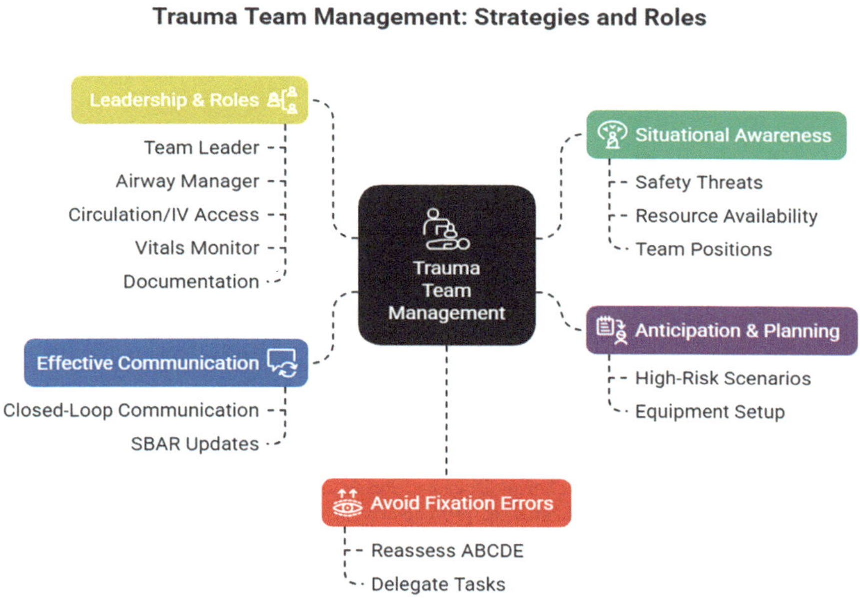

Fig. 17.3 Trauma team management: strategies and roles. (Figure illustrated using AI tools with Napkin AI, 2025)

Disaster-Specific Triage: Jumpstart System (Fig. 17.4)

Category	Criteria	Action
Red (immediate)	Not walking, abnormal breathing, no pulse, or altered mental status	*Life-saving interventions NOW*
Yellow (delayed)	Walking or breathing normally after repositioning airway; responsive	*Stabilize; treat within 2 hrs*
Green (minor)	Walking, minor injuries	*Delayed care; self-care if possible*
Black (expectant)	No breathing after repositioning airway; no pulse	*Palliative care/confirm death*

Post-Disaster Three Actions

a. *Debrief Team: A debrief team allows providers to pause after a clinical event to reflect on what went well, what was challenging, and what can be improved. It strengthens communication, enhances learning, and supports emotional well-being. For primary care providers, regular debriefing builds stronger teams and improves the quality and safety of pediatric care.*
   - Discuss three *strengths* and three *improvements* in response.
   - Address emotional distress.

b. *Patient Follow-up: Patient follow-up ensures continuity of care by checking on a child's recovery, reviewing treatment plans, and identifying any complications early. It strengthens safety, builds trust with families, and helps primary care providers confirm that the child is improving as expected or needs additional support.*
   - Track infections/nutritional needs in displaced children.
   - Facilitate family reunification and mental health support.

c. *System improvement: System improvement means using lessons from patient care and team performance to make changes that strengthen safety, workflow, and overall clinical quality. For primary care providers, this may include updating protocols, improving communication processes, or revising equipment readiness. Small, consistent system improvements lead to better outcomes and a safer environment for children and families.*
   - Advocate for pediatric disaster policies.
   - Restock pediatric emergency kits (include: ET tubes, IO needles, diapers, comfort items).

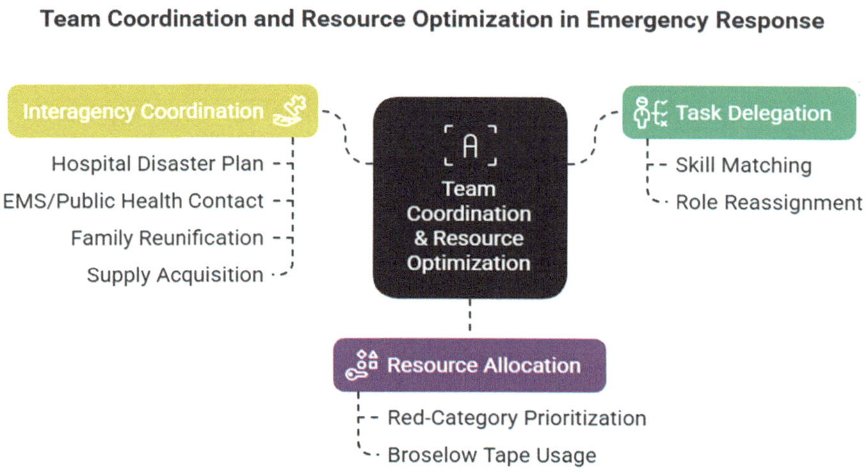

Fig. 17.4 Team coordination and resource optimization in emergency response. (Figure illustrated using AI tools with Napkin AI, 2025)

Pediatric-Specific Disaster Preparedness

- *Equipment Readiness: Ensuring pediatric-sized equipment is available, organized, and immediately accessible is essential during disasters. Children require different airway tools, vascular access devices, medication doses, and monitoring equipment than adults. Regular checks, color-coded systems, and pre-packed pediatric kits help teams respond quickly and safely in high-stress situations. Pediatric equipment readiness prevents delays, supports accurate care, and improves outcomes during mass-casualty or emergency events.*
  - Stock child-sized supplies:
    - Airway: Uncuffed ET tubes (size 3.0–5.5), pediatric BVMs.
    - IV/IO: 22–24G catheters, intraosseous needles.
    - Splints, cervical collars.
- *Training Drills: Regular pediatric-focused disaster drills allow teams to practice their response, identify gaps, and build confidence in managing large-scale emergencies. Drills improve coordination, communication, and decision-making, ensuring providers are prepared to care for children effectively when real disasters occur.*
  - Conduct *simulations* every 6 months:
    - MCI triage (JumpSTART).
    - CRM principles under stress.
- *Family Preparedness: Supporting families in disaster planning helps ensure children stay safe during emergencies. This includes educating caregivers on emergency contacts, medication lists, grab-and-go kits, and plans for children with special healthcare needs. When families are prepared, children experience fewer delays in care, reduced stress, and better outcomes during disasters.*

- Educate parents on:
  - Emergency contacts.
  - Evacuation plans.
  - "Go bags" (meds, medical records, comfort items).

ER Evaluation of Pediatric Trauma

Immediate Preparation and Triage: Rapid pediatric triage helps identify the sickest children first and ensures resources are used where they are most needed. Early preparation; such as organizing teams, assigning roles, and setting up pediatric equipment, supports fast, accurate decision-making. Effective triage allows primary care providers to stabilize critically ill children quickly and direct others to appropriate care pathways during a disaster.

Component	Details
Prehospital phase	Control external bleeding Immobilize the spine Gather MOI, time of injury, age, and vital signs Transport to trauma-capable facility
Hospital phase	Activate trauma team; assign roles Warm the room and prepare the pediatric airway kit Prewarmed fluids and notify support services
Triage (color-coded)	Red: Life-threatening Yellow: Urgent but stable Green: Minor injuries Black: Deceased/unsalvageable

Primary Survey (ABCDE): The ABCDE approach helps providers rapidly identify and treat life-threatening issues in children during emergencies. It focuses on Airway, Breathing, Circulation, Disability, and Exposure, guiding a structured assessment that keeps care organized and timely. For primary care providers, using ABCDE ensures no critical step is missed and supports safer, more effective stabilization of pediatric patients in disaster or emergency situations.

Component	Details
A: Airway + C-spine	Assess for stridor/gurgling Secure airway using jaw thrust + MILS Suction and use adjuncts Assist to intubate if GCS ≤ 8 Apply a C-collar post airway control
B: Breathing	Assess chest rise, jugular venous distension, and emphysema Provide O_2, assist in decompressing tension pneumothorax if suspected Avoid PPV before chest tube

Component	Details
C: Circulation	Identify shock signs, control bleeding Access IV/IO Give a 10–20 mL/kg fluid bolus till blood products arrive Use eFAST and ask for TXA MTP if bleeding persists
D: Disability (neuro)	Use pGCS/AVPU Check pupils Maintain oxygenation Ask for mannitol/hypertonic saline for herniation Ask for help if seizures
E: Exposure/ environment	Fully undress and inspect Prevent hypothermia with warming measures Check glucose and core temperature

Adjuncts to Primary Survey: Adjuncts support and refine the ABCDE assessment by providing additional information that guides immediate care. These include tools such as pulse oximetry, blood glucose checks, bedside ultrasound, ECG monitoring, and point-of-care tests. For primary care providers, using these adjuncts helps confirm diagnoses, identify hidden problems, and ensure timely interventions during pediatric emergencies.

Component	Details
Critical diagnostics	eFAST, CXR, pelvic X-ray, ABG (lactate/base deficit)
Monitoring	Foley (urine output goals), ECG (blunt chest injury), capnography (ETT confirmation)

Transfer Decision: Making an early transfer decision ensures that critically ill or injured children are moved to the right level of care without delay. It involves recognizing when a child needs resources beyond what is available locally, stabilizing them, and arranging safe, timely transport. For primary care providers, clear transfer decisions improve outcomes by getting children to definitive care as quickly and safely as possible.

Component	Details
Indications for transfer	Neurosurgical emergencies, uncontrolled hemorrhage, and inadequate facility
Pre-transfer actions	Stabilize ABCDE. Give SBAR handover: Situation, background, assessment, recommendation

Secondary Survey: The secondary survey is a head-to-toe assessment performed after life-threatening conditions are addressed. It includes a full physical exam, focused history, and targeted investigations to identify any hidden injuries or conditions. For primary care providers, the secondary survey ensures no important problem is missed and guides ongoing management in pediatric emergencies.

Component	Details
History (AMPLE)	Allergies, meds, past illnesses, last meal, events of injury
Head-to-toe exam	Assess head (CSF leak), chest (crepitus), abdomen (tenderness), extremities (deformity), and back (spinal tenderness)
Pain management	Use age-appropriate analgesics

Post-Resuscitation and Definitive Care: After a child is stabilized, post-resuscitation care focuses on maintaining airway, breathing, and circulation while preventing complications. This includes monitoring, reassessing frequently, managing pain, and addressing underlying causes. Definitive care involves transferring the child to the appropriate facility or specialty service for ongoing treatment. For primary care providers, strong post-resuscitation care ensures safer transitions and better recovery for critically ill children.

Component	Details
Continuous monitoring	Reassess ABCDE every 5–15 min. Repeat eFAST, monitor vitals
Definitive care	OR for surgical needs, ICU for ongoing care
Team dynamics	The leader coordinates; uses closed-loop communication

Airway and Breathing Management in Pediatric Trauma

Immediate Assessment: Pediatric Airway Red Flags

Anatomical Considerations in Children.

- *Narrow airway:* Minor edema = major obstruction risk.
- *Large tongue/occiput:* Supine positioning may cause airway blockage.
- *Short trachea:* Increases risk of mainstem (usually right) bronchial intubation.

Signs of Impending Airway Compromise.

- *Stridor/hoarseness* → Laryngeal trauma.
- *Gurgling sounds* → Blood/vomitus in airway.
- *Snoring* → Decreased GCS, loss of pharyngeal tone.
- *Complete silence* → Critical obstruction—act immediately!

Work of Breathing: What to Watch For.

- *Tachypnea > 40/min,* nasal flaring, grunting, intercostal or sternal retractions.
- *Asymmetric chest rise* → Suspect pneumothorax.
- *Paradoxical movement* → Suspect flail chest.

Airway Management: Stepwise Approach (Fig. 17.5)

Steps	Actions	Key notes
1	Cervical spine protection	Manual in-line stabilization (MILS); use a towel under the trunk (infants) or the shoulders (children)
2	Clear and secure airway	Suction (10Fr for infants, Yankauer for older kids); use OPA if unconscious; avoid NPA in suspected skull fracture
3	High-flow oxygen	15 L/min via non-rebreather; target SpO_2 ≥95%
4	Assist in preparing for intubation	Check ETT size (cuffed: Age/4 + 3.5); ketamine 0.25–2 mg/kg IV; rocuronium 1.2–1.6 mg/kg IV; pre-oxygenate
5	Assist in intubation	Blade: Miller (infants), mac (children); ETT depth = age/2 + 12 cm; confirm with bilateral breath sounds, capnography
6	Assist in surgical airway	<12 years, needle cricothyroidotomy; ≥12 years, surgical cricothyroidotomy

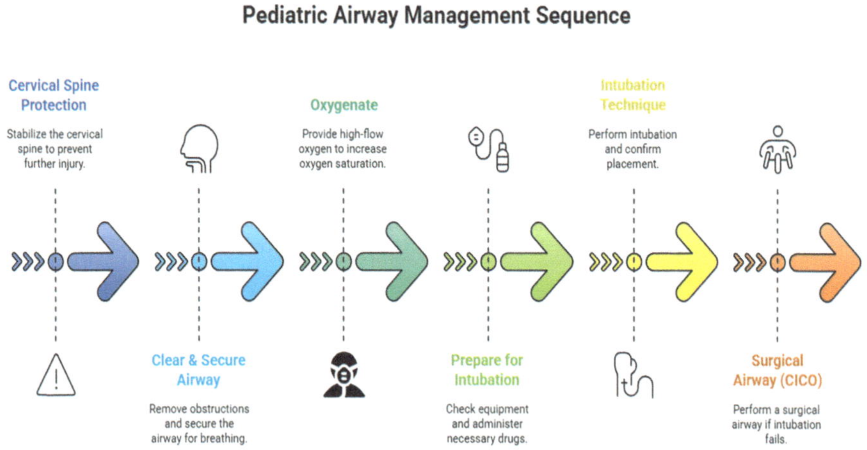

Fig. 17.5 Pediatric airway management sequence. (Figure illustrated using AI tools with Napkin AI, 2025)

Breathing Management (Fig. 17.6)

Steps	Actions	Key notes
1	Assess thorax	Look (symmetry, wounds, cyanosis); listen (air entry, heart sounds); feel (crepitus, hyper-resonance)
2	Identify life threats	TWELVE-C mnemonic for neck signs: **T**racheal deviation **W**ounds **E**mphysema (subcutaneous) **L**aryngeal tenderness **V**enous distension **E**sophageal injury **C**arotid swelling Listen Reduced air entry → pneumothorax Muffled heart sounds → suspect pericardial tamponade Feel Subcutaneous crepitus → rib fracture Hyper-resonance → tension pneumothorax
3	Ask the physician and assist to intervene if necessary	Needle decompression → chest tube (tension pneumothorax); three-sided dressing + chest tube (open pneumothorax); PPV (flail chest)
4	Assist with ventilation support	BVM: 250 mL (infants), 500–1500 mL (children); rate = 20/min; I:E = 1:3; avoid over-ventilation in TBI

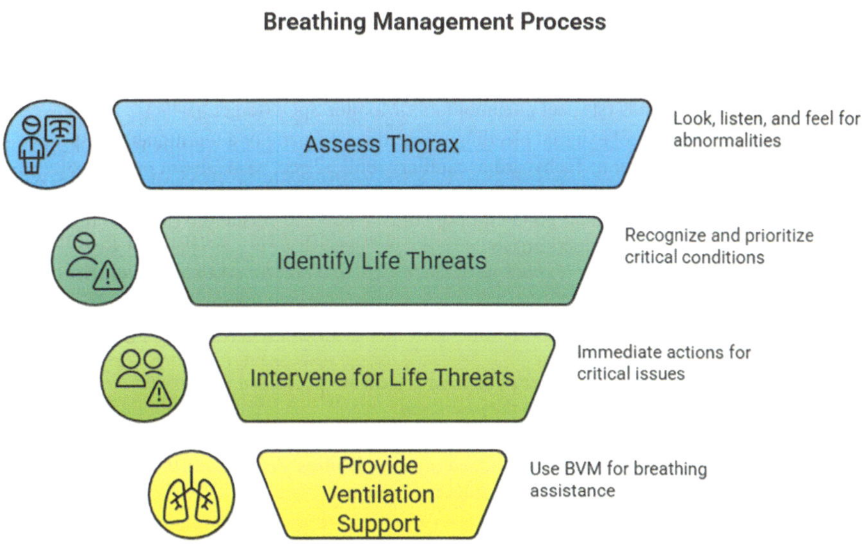

Fig. 17.6 Breathing management process. (Figure illustrated using AI tools with Napkin AI, 2025)

Pediatric-Specific Safety Alerts

- *Act fast:* Hypoxia progresses rapidly in children.
- *Use Broselow tape:* For accurate size and dose estimates.
- *Avoid:*
  - Nasal intubation in suspected skull base fractures or head trauma.
  - Excessive PEEP in suspected pneumothorax.
- *Airway burns?* Intubate early—swelling progresses quickly.

Hemorrhagic Shock Management

Immediate Primary Survey (ABCDE): In hemorrhagic shock, the ABCDE approach ensures life-threatening issues are identified and treated without delay. Providers rapidly assess Airway and support breathing, evaluate Circulation for signs of severe blood loss, check Disability for mental status changes, and fully Expose the patient to locate bleeding sources. Using ABCDE keeps care organized and helps stabilize the child quickly while preparing for urgent hemorrhage control.

Component	Key actions and red flags
A: Airway with C-spine protection	Immobilize the cervical spine with collar/manual stabilizationClear the airway using suction if needed and perform jaw thrust *Red flag: GCS ≤ 8 → prepare for intubation*
B: Breathing and oxygenation	Administer high-flow O_2 via a non-rebreather maskAssess work of breathing: Retractions, grunting, nasal flaringAuscultate for unequal breath sounds (suspect pneumothorax)Monitor SpO_2 (target ≥94%)
C: Circulation and hemorrhage control	Control external bleeding using direct pressure or a tourniquetAssess perfusion: Tachycardia, capillary refill >2 sec, weak/absent pulses, cold/mottled skinSecure IV/IO access x2 (large-bore preferred)Fluid resuscitation: 10–20 mL/kg bolus of isotonic crystalloid (NS/RL),till the blood products arrive *Red flag: If shock persists, prepare a blood transfusion (O-negative if unknown)*
D: Disability (neuro)	Perform AVPU or GCS assessmentCheck pupil size and reactivityTest blood glucose *Red flag: Seizures or falling GCS → urgent neuro intervention might be needed; inform the physician*
E: Exposure/environment	Fully undress the patient for a complete exam; log-roll to inspect the spine and backCheck for hidden injuries: Bruises, deformitiesPrevent hypothermia: Warm room, use blankets

Secondary Survey (after Stabilization): Once the child's airway, breathing, and circulation are supported, a detailed head-to-toe secondary survey helps identify hidden injuries and ongoing sources of blood loss. This includes a focused history, complete physical exam, and targeted investigations such as ultrasound or X-rays. For primary care providers, the secondary survey ensures no critical injury is missed and guides further treatment in hemorrhagic shock.

- *History:* AMPLE (allergies, meds, past illness, last meal, events).
- *Head-to-toe exam:*
  - Abdomen (tenderness, bruising, → suspect internal bleed).
  - Pelvis (instability? → do not compress).
  - Limbs (deformities, pulses).
- *Bedside tests:*
  - ABG (lactate >2 mmol/L → shock; base deficit < −4).
  - FAST scan if available (free fluid?)

Resuscitation Essentials: Early and aggressive resuscitation is key to managing hemorrhagic shock. This includes securing IV or IO access, giving fluid boluses judiciously, initiating blood products when available, and controlling external bleeding. Providers should monitor vital signs closely, reassess frequently, and correct hypothermia to prevent worsening shock. Effective early resuscitation stabilizes circulation and improves survival in children with significant blood loss.

For Shock Persisting After 10–20 mL/kg Crystalloid:
- *Transfuse blood* (10–20 mL/kg PRBCs).
- *Tranexamic Acid (TXA):* 15 mg/kg IV (max 1 g) within 3 h of injury.
- *Activate Massive Transfusion Protocol (MTP) if:*
  - >40 mL/kg blood products needed in 24 h
  - Use a *1:1:1 ratio* (PRBCs/FFP/platelets).

Monitoring During Transport:
- Reassess *q5-15min*: HR, CRT, BP, RR, SpO_2, AVPU.
- Urine output goal: *1–2 mL/kg/hr* (infants/children).
- *Deterioration signs:* Rising lactate, falling GCS, anuria (Fig. 17.7).

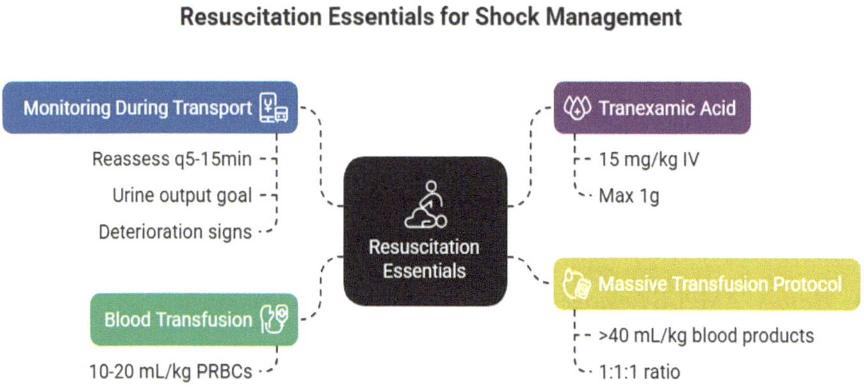

Fig. 17.7 Resuscitation essentials for shock management. (Figure illustrated using AI tools with Napkin AI, 2025)

Special Considerations

- *Pediatric Red Flags:*
  - Altered mental status (drowsiness) *without* hypotension.
  - Tachycardia + cold extremities = early shock!
  - Abdominal bruising + tachycardia → internal bleed until proven otherwise. Pediatric Red Flags Altered mental status without hypotension: Children can lose significant blood volume before their blood pressure drops. A drowsy or irritable child may be in early shock even if their BP appears normal. Tachycardia with cold extremities = early shock: Fast heart rate plus cool, pale hands and feet signal poor perfusion. This is often the earliest and most reliable sign of pediatric shock. Abdominal bruising with tachycardia → suspect internal bleeding: Bruising on the abdomen after trauma especially with a high heart rate should be treated as internal hemorrhage until proven otherwise.
- *Resource-Limited Tips:*
  - Use intraosseous (IO) access if IV fails.
  - Warm fluids to prevent hypothermia.
  - Family presence for child calming (if safe). Resource-Limited Tips Use IO access if IV fails: Do not delay resuscitation. IO access provides rapid, reliable vascular access for fluids and medications. Warm fluids to prevent hypothermia: Cold fluids worsen shock. Even simple warming methods help stabilize the child. Family presence for calming (if safe): A familiar face reduces fear, improves cooperation, and supports more effective resuscitation in children.

Pediatric Head and Maxillofacial Trauma : In pediatric head and facial trauma, the ABCDE approach helps identify life-threatening problems quickly. Secure the airway early, as swelling, bleeding, or facial fractures can rapidly obstruct breathing. Assess breathing and ventilatory effort closely, and evaluate circulation for signs of shock or ongoing bleeding. Check disability by monitoring mental status and pupil response, and fully expose the child to identify hidden injuries. A structured ABCDE survey ensures prompt stabilization and prevents secondary brain injury.

Immediate Primary Survey (ABCDE)

Component	Detailed actions
A: Airway with C-spine protection	Manual in-line stabilization (assume C-spine injury in all head/facial trauma)Clear airway via jaw-thrust maneuver (avoid head-tilt) Suction blood, vomit, or tooth fragments (avoid nasal suction if anterior fossa fracture)Listen for gurgling/stridor—Sign of obstructionPosition infant with shoulder roll (due to large occiput) for neutral alignment
B: Breathing and oxygenation	Administer high-flow O_2 via non-rebreather maskMonitor for aspiration (blood in airway) or signs of chest traumaElevate head 30° if no spinal injury—Helps reduce intracranial pressure (ICP)
C: Circulation and hemorrhage control	Apply direct pressure on bleeding facial or scalp woundsCheck for signs of shock: Tachycardia, prolonged capillary refill time (>2 sec), weak pulsesEstablish IV/IO access, and administer warm isotonic fluid bolus (20 mL/kg) if hypovolemic
D: Disability (neuro assessment)	Use AVPU or pediatric GCS: AVPU: Alert, responds to voice, pain, unresponsive? Pediatric GCS ≤8 → prepare for intubation. Check pupils for size, symmetry, and reactivity (unequal = possible herniation)Assess limb movement: Asymmetry or posturingCheck blood glucoseAsk for help if seizures occur: Position safely; give anticonvulsants if recurrent
E: Exposure/ environment	Log-roll to inspect back and scalp—Palpate for depressions or boggy swellingLook for CSF leaks (clear drainage from nose/ear → suspect basilar skull fracture)Check for raccoon eyes or Battle's sign (late bruising over the mastoid)Prevent hypothermia—Cover with warm blankets (especially the head in infants)

Injury-Specific Actions

Red Flags Requiring Urgent Referral.

- GCS ≤13 or deteriorating AVPU.
- Unequal pupils/posturing.
- Open/depressed skull fracture.
- CSF leak.
- Persistent vomiting/seizures.
- Facial deformity with airway/vision threat (Fig. 17.8).

Maxillofacial Injury Management

Injury type	Immediate actions
Mandibular fracture	NPO (nothing by mouth) Support the jaw → avoid manipulation
Nasal fracture	*No nose-blowing* (risk of orbital emphysema) Ice packs, upright position
Orbital fracture	Check vision/eye movement → *diplopia?* *Avoid pressure on the eye*
Dental avulsion	Rinse tooth in saline → store in *milk/saline* Control bleeding with gauze
Soft tissue injury	Clean with saline → pressure for bleeding Tetanus prophylaxis if dirty wound

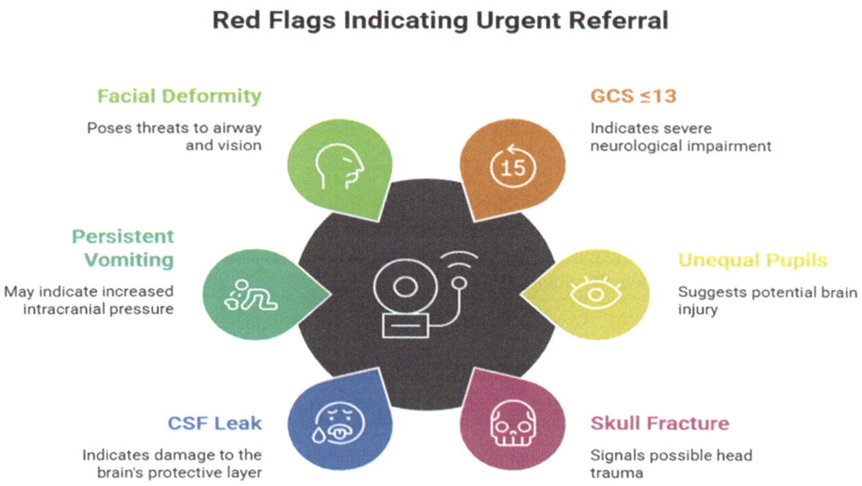

Fig. 17.8 Red flags indicating urgent referral. (Figure illustrated using AI tools with Napkin AI, 2025)

Ongoing Monitoring and Preparation for Transfer

Neurological Monitoring Schedule

- *q15–30 min* for first 2 hours → HR, BP, RR, SpO_2, pGCS, pupils,
- *Hourly* once stable → watch for Cushing's triad (bradycardia, hypertension, irregular breathing).

Documentation Essentials

- *Mechanism of injury* (e.g., fall height, impact object).
- *Timeline:* Injury → arrival → interventions.
- *Vitals/pGCS trends.*
- *SBAR handover* (for referral):
  - **S**ituation: "6yo M, fall from 2nd floor, facial swelling, pGCS 11".
  - **B**ackground: "No LOC initially, vomited ×2 en route".
  - **A**ssessment: "Suspect ZMC fracture + TBI, airway risk".
  - **R**ecommendation: "Urgent CT + maxillofacial consult".

Transfer Preparation

- *Stabilize airway* → intubate if pGCS ≤8 or airway threat.
- *Spinal immobilization:* Collar + spine board.
- *Accompanying kit:* O_2, suction, emergency meds (anticonvulsants).
- *Family briefing:* Explain the reason for the transfer and further plan.

Pediatric Neck Trauma Management

Immediate Primary Survey (ABCDE)

Component	Detailed actions
A: Airway with C-spine protection	Assume C-spine injury—Manual in-line stabilization Listen for stridor, hoarseness, gurgling → signs of airway compromiseSubcutaneous emphysema → possible aero-digestive tract injury *Do not* remove impaled objects—Stabilize with gauze/tape *Assist in preparing for difficult airway*: Have a video laryngoscope and surgical airway kit readyAvoid paralytics if laryngeal injury is suspected
B: Breathing	Administer high-flow O_2 via a non-rebreather maskCheck for tracheal deviation or asymmetric chest riseMonitor SpO_2 continuously
C: Circulation and hemorrhage control	Apply direct pressure to visible bleeding sites—Never use blind clamping Watch for expanding hematoma or pulsatile bleeding—These are hard signs for surgical interventionSecure two large-bore IVs, and give warm crystalloid bolus (10–20 mL/kg) if shock is suspected and till blood products arrive
D: Disability (neuro)	C-spine exam: Check for midline tenderness or deformity Assess using pGCS or AVPUCheck pupils for asymmetryEvaluate limb movement and sensations—Weakness or numbness suggests spinal cord injury
E: Exposure/ environment	Identify zone of injury: Zone I (clavicles → cricoid): Risk to vascular/mediastinal structures Zone II (cricoid → mandible): Most common; accessible for surgery Zone III (mandible → skull base): Risk to vascular/cranial nerve injuries Log-roll the patient to inspect the posterior neck and spine Prevent hypothermia—Cover the patient appropriately

Red Flags and Injury-Specific Actions

Hard Signs Requiring Immediate Surgery
- Airway obstruction
- Expanding/pulsatile hematoma
- Active hemorrhage
- Hemoptysis/hematemesis
- Subcutaneous emphysema

Blunt trauma is suspected if
- Clothesline injury, strangultion, high-impact collision
- Hoarseness, dysphagia, focal neuro deficit

Foreign Body Management
- *Stabilize* in situ (gauze/tape support)
- *Never remove pre-hospital* (risk of exsanguination)
- It is only advised to remove *only in OR* with a vascular surgeon

Pediatric Thoracic Trauma Management

Immediate Primary Survey (ABCDE) (Fig. 17.9)

Component	Assessment and actions
A: Airway protection	Ensure patent airway—Suction if neededListen for stridor or gurgling—Signs of obstructionMaintain C-spine precautions if the mechanism suggests risk
B: Breathing assessment	Observe for asymmetric chest movement or paradoxical breathingAuscultate: Diminished or absent breath sounds—Suspect pneumothorax Palpate for crepitus—Indicates subcutaneous emphysemaAdminister high-flow O_2 via a non-rebreather maskMonitor SpO_2 continuously
C: Circulation and shock signs	Check capillary refill (>2 sec = delayed)Assess for jugular venous distension—May indicate tamponade or tension pneumothoraxPalpate pulses: Weak or absent radial pulse = hypovolemiaSecure two IV/IO linesPrepare and administer warmed crystalloid bolus (10–20 mL/kg till blood products will arrive)
D: Disability (neuro)	Assess neurological status using AVPU or pediatric GCSCheck for pupil asymmetryPerform a blood glucose test
E: Exposure/ environment	Inspect chest for signs of injury: Sucking wounds → open pneumothorax Ecchymosis → underlying contusion Crepitus → rib fracture Log-roll to examine the backPrevent hypothermia with warm blankets

Critical Reminders:
1. *Children hide PTX:* Absent breath sounds may be the only sign—no rib fractures needed.
2. *Pain control = ventilation:* Unrelieved pain → splinting → atelectasis.

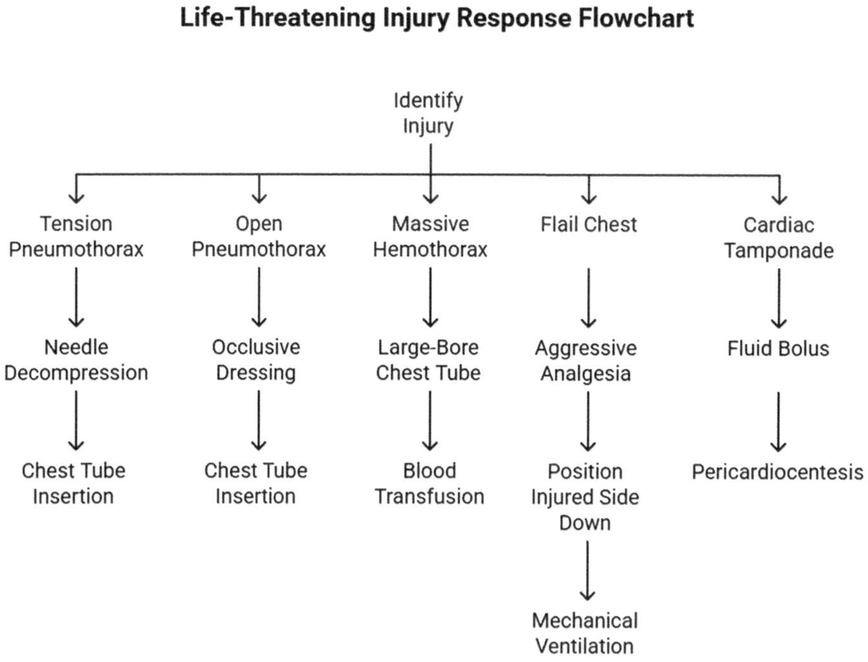

Fig. 17.9 Life-threatening injury response flowchart. (Figure illustrated using AI tools with Napkin AI, 2025)

Pediatric Abdominal and Pelvic Trauma

Immediate Actions (Primary Survey—ABCDE)

Component	Immediate actions
Airway	Maintain cervical spine protection if high-risk mechanism (e.g., MVC, fall >1.5 m)Clear secretions using suction if needed
Breathing	Administer high-flow O_2 if SpO_2 <94% or respiratory distressAssess for pneumothorax: Unequal breath sounds, hypoxia
Circulation	Control external bleeding with direct pressure. Look for shock signs: Tachycardia (HR > age norm), delayed capillary refill (>2 sec), pallorEstablish IV/IO access, and give a 10–20 mL/kg warmed crystalloid bolus. Give blood products if shock persists
Disability	Assess neurological status using AVPU/pGCSCheck pupils for size/reactivity and measure blood glucose
Exposure/ environment	Log-roll to inspect the back and pelvis for injuriesPrevent hypothermia by covering the patient with warm blankets

Red Flags for Abdominal/Pelvic Injury

Clinical Signs:
- Tachycardia + tachypnea *without hypotension* (early compensated shock).
- Abdominal tenderness/guarding (esp. LUQ/RUQ/flank).
- Seatbelt sign, handlebar bruise, or pelvic instability.
- Vomiting, distension, or peritonitis (rigidity, rebound).
- Blood at urethral meatus (suspect pelvic fracture).

High-Risk Mechanisms:
- High-speed MVC, bicycle handlebar impact, fall >3 m.
- Penetrating trauma (stab/gunshot), blast injury.

Diagnostic Steps

1. *Bedside Tests:*
   - *Pelvic compression test:* Gentle pressure to assess instability.
   - *Urinalysis:* Microscopic hematuria → suspect renal injury.
2. *Imaging (If Stable):*
   - *X-rays:* Chest (pneumothorax), pelvis (fractures).
   - *CT abdomen/pelvis:* Gold standard for internal injuries.
3. *Labs:*
   - Trauma panel: Hb, lactate, base deficit, amylase/lipase, LFTs.
4. *Analgesia:*
   - IV paracetamol (15 mg/kg) or cautious opioids (avoid masking peritonitis).
5. *Antibiotics:*
   - IV ceftriaxone + metronidazole for penetrating/open injuries.

Key Pediatric Considerations.
- *Non-accidental Trauma:* Suspect if:
  - Inconsistent history, delayed presentation, or patterned bruises.
  - Fractures in non-ambulatory infants (e.g., rib fractures).
- *Pelvic Binders: Must cover greater trochanters* (not waist) to reduce pelvic volume.

In children, normal BP does not rule out shock! Tachycardia + delayed capillary refill are early warnings.

Pediatric Spinal Trauma Management

Immediate Actions (Scene/Arrival)

1. *Ensure scene safety.*
2. *Manual in-line stabilization (MILS):*
   - Hold head in neutral position (no traction).
   - Maintain until C-spine is cleared by imaging/expert.

3. *Rapid ABCDE assessment:*
   - *Airway:* Open with jaw thrust (protect C-spine), suction secretions.
   - *Breathing:* Check RR, O_2 sat, chest symmetry. *If O_2 sat < 94%*, give high-flow O_2.
   - *Circulation:* Monitor HR, BP, and capillary refill. *If shock*, secure IV/IO access, and control bleeding.
   - *Disability:* Assess AVPU/pGCS, pupils.
   - *Exposure:* Log-roll (four-person team) to examine back; maintain alignment.
4. Immobilize:
   - Apply a *pediatric-sized cervical collar* (measure chin-to-shoulder).
   - Use *modified spine board* (occipital recess/padding for infants).

Primary Survey (Life Threats)

Step	Key actions
Airway	MILS during intubation if needed
Breathing	Treat tension pneumothorax (needle decompression → chest tube)
Circulation	Control hemorrhage (tourniquets if needed). Avoid fluid overload
Disability	Document GCS/AVPU. *If GCS ≤ 8*, prepare for intubation
Exposure	Log-roll to inspect spine. Keep warm (prevent hypothermia)

Red Flags:
- Altered mental status, focal neuro deficits, respiratory distress, hypotension.
- *High-risk mechanisms:* MVC >60 km/h, falls >1.5 m, diving, non-accidental trauma.

Secondary Survey (Detailed Exam)

1. *History (AMPLE):*
   - Allergies, medications, past medical, last meal, events of injury.
2. *Head-to-Toe Exam:*
   - *Head:* CSF leaks, raccoon eyes, Battle's sign.
   - *Neck:* Tenderness, deformity, tracheal deviation.
   - *Chest/abdomen:* Bruising, asymmetry, distension (perform eFAST).
   - *Pelvis/extremities:* Instability, pulses, deformities.
   - *Back:* Log-roll to palpate the spine.

Diagnostics and Imaging

- *X-rays:* AP/lateral C-spine if GCS >14, neck pain, or high-risk mechanism.
- *CT C-spine:* If GCS ≤8, focal deficit, or intubated.
- *PECARN Imaging Criteria:*
  - *CT:* GCS 3–8, abnormal ABC, neuro deficits.
  - *X-ray:* GCS 9–14, neck pain/tenderness.

Special Pediatric Considerations

- *Cervical Collar Sizing:*
  - Measure neck circumference or chin-to-shoulder distance.
  - *Avoid if:* Fixed deformity, swelling, or neuro worsening.
- *Spine Board:* Pad under shoulders/occiput in infants (prevents neck flexion).

Key Reminders

- *Reassess frequently:* Deterioration can occur late.
- *Avoid oversedation:* May mask neuro deficits.
- *Prevent secondary injury:* Hypotension, hypoxia, hyperglycemia.

Pediatric Extremity Injury Management

Immediate Actions (Primary Survey—ABCDE)

Component	Detailed actions
Airway with C-spine protection	Maintain cervical spine immobilization if the mechanism suggests spinal risk (e.g., high-speed MVC, fall >1.5 m) Clear the airway using jaw thrust and suction secretions
Breathing	Administer high-flow O_2 if SpO_2 <94% or signs of respiratory distress Assess for pneumothorax: Unequal breath sounds, hypoxia
Circulation and hemorrhage control	Control bleeding: Apply direct pressure. If uncontrolled, use a tourniquetIdentify shock signs: Tachycardia, delayed capillary refill (>2 sec), pallor *hypotension is a late sign* Establish IV/IO access, and give a 10–20 mL/kg crystalloid bolus till the blood products arrive
Disability (neuro)	Assess AVPU or GCS. If GCS ≤8, plan for intubationCheck pupils for size and reactivity Measure blood glucose
Exposure/ environment	Log-roll the patient to inspect the back and limbs for injuries Prevent hypothermia: Cover with warm blankets

Secondary Survey (Focused Extremity Assessment)

1. *Inspect and Palpate:*
   - *Skin:* Swelling, bruising, deformity, open wounds.
   - *Bones:* Tenderness over growth plates (distal radius, tibia)/joints.
   - *Compare:* Bilaterally for asymmetry.
2. *Neurovascular Check (Critical!)*

1. *Red Flags for Compartment Syndrome (5 P's):*
   - Pain disproportionate to injury.
   - Pallor/paresthesia/paralysis.
   - Pulselessness (late).
   - *Also* anxiety, agitation, ↑ analgesia demand (***3 A's***).

Assessment	Method
Pulses	Radial, dorsalis pedis (*absent* =? *Compartment syndrome*)
Capillary refill	>2 seconds = poor perfusion
Sensation	Light touch, pain in distal dermatomes
Motor function	"Wiggle toes/fingers"; grip strength

Injury-Specific Management

1. *Fractures:*
   - *Splint:* Immobilize the joint above/below the injury.
     - *Upper limb:* Sugar-tong (forearm), thumb spica (thumb).
     - *Lower limb:* Posterior ankle splint.
2. *Open Wounds/Fractures:*
   - Cover with saline-soaked sterile gauze.
   - *Ask for antibiotics:* IV ceftriaxone + metronidazole.
   - *Ask for tetanus:* Update if incomplete/unknown history.
3. *Pain Control:*
   - Mild: Paracetamol (15 mg/kg) or ibuprofen (10 mg/kg).
   - Severe: IV morphine/fentanyl (0.05–0.1 mg/kg).
   - *Avoid NSAIDs* if compartment syndrome is suspected.

Referral and Handover

Emergent Referral (<24 h):
- Open fractures.
- Neurovascular compromise.
- Compartment syndrome.
- Salter-Harris III-V fractures.

Pediatric-Specific Considerations.
- *Non-accidental Trauma:* Suspect if:
  - Fracture in a non-ambulatory infant (e.g., femur in <1 year).
  - Multiple injuries in different healing stages.

In children, absence of deformity does not rule out fracture. Always assess growth plates and neurovascular status!

Pediatric Burn Management

Immediate Actions (First 5 Min)

1. *Stop Burning Process:*
   - Remove clothing/jewellery (*cut around adherent fabric*).
   - *Irrigate* with *cool running water* for 20 min (avoid ice).

2. *Protect the Airway:*
   - Suspect inhalation injury if:
     - Facial burns, singed nasal hairs, soot in the mouth.
     - Hoarseness/stridor, enclosed-space fire.
   - Administer *high-flow O_2* via a non-rebreather mask.
3. *Prevent Hypothermia:*
   - Cover *unburnt* areas with warm blankets.
   - Keep room temperature > 30 °C.

Primary Survey (ABCDE)

Step	Key actions
Airway	Intubate early if signs of obstruction (hoarseness, stridor)
Breathing	Check for chest burns restricting movement; monitor SpO_2 (note: Normal in CO poisoning)
Circulation	IV access (through unburnt skin if possible)
Disability	Check AVPU, blood glucose (hypoglycemia risk)
Exposure	Fully expose child → assess burns; cover with clean dry sheet

Critical Signs Requiring Emergent Transfer:
- Inhalation injury.
- Full-thickness burns.
- Burns >10% TBSA, face/hands/genitals.
- Electrical/chemical burns.
- Suspicion of non-accidental trauma.

Burn Assessment and Resuscitation

1. *Estimate TBSA:*
   - Use the *Lund and Browder chart* (Fig. 13.2).
   - *Exclude superficial burns* (only partial/full thickness count).
2. *Fluid Resuscitation* (if TBSA >15% or signs of shock):
   - *Modified Parkland Formula:*
     - *Half in first 8 h* (from injury time), rest over 16 h.
     - Use *Ringer's lactate.*
   - *Add maintenance fluids* (with dextrose) for children <30 kg.
   - *Target urine output:* 1 mL/kg/hr.
3. *Ask for Pain Control:*
   - IV fentanyl (1–2 μg/kg) or intranasal opioids.
   - Avoid IM injections (Fig. 17.10).

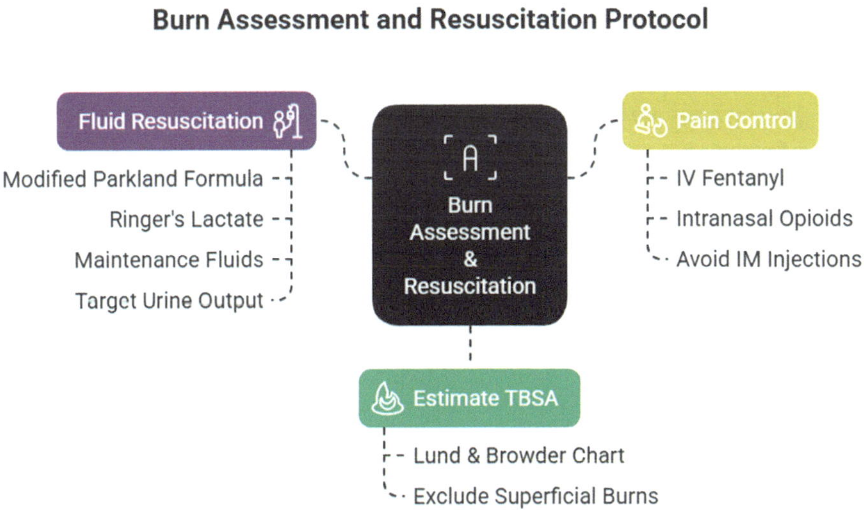

Fig. 17.10 Burn assessment and resuscitation protocol. (Figure illustrated using AI tools with Napkin AI, 2025)

Wound Care and Infection Prevention

1. *Initial Dressing:*
   - Cover with *non-adherent gauze* (e.g., Vaseline-impregnated).
   - *Do not apply ice, toothpaste, oils, or home remedies.*
2. *Blister Management:*
   - Debride large/tense blisters; leave small intact blisters.
3. *Topical Agents:*
   - Apply *silver sulfadiazine* (avoid if sulfa allergy) or *mupirocin*.
4. *Tetanus Prophylaxis:*
   - Update if incomplete/unknown.

Referral and Transfer Preparation

Refer to the Burns Center if:
- TBSA >10%.
- Full-thickness burns.
- Face/hands/genitals/joints involved.
- Inhalation/electrical/chemical burns.
- Suspicion of non-accidental trauma.

Pre-transfer Checklist:
- Ask for a secure airway, IV access, and analgesia.
- Cover wounds with a *clean, dry cloth* (*no elaborate dressings*).
- Document:

  - Mechanism, time of injury.
  - TBSA/depth (Lund and Browder chart).
  - Fluids/meds given.
- Handover using *MIST*:
  - **M**echanism (e.g., "Flame burn in garage").
  - **I**njuries (e.g., "Circumferential leg burns, 23% TBSA").
  - **S**igns (e.g., "HR 135, SpO_2 99%").
  - **T**reatment (e.g., "IV fluids started, fentanyl given").

Key Reminders

- *Children are not small adults:*
  - Higher risk of shock (capillary leak), hypothermia, and hypoglycemia.
  - Use *pediatric-specific formulas* (Modified Parkland) and charts (Lund and Browder).
- *CO poisoning:* Normal SpO_2 is misleading; treat with 100% O_2 if suspected.
- *Circumferential burns:* Monitor for compartment syndrome; may need escharotomy.

Stop the burn, cool the skin, cover the child, calculate fluids, and call for help

GPSR Compliance

The European Union's (EU) General Product Safety Regulation (GPSR) is a set of rules that requires consumer products to be safe and our obligations to ensure this.

If you have any concerns about our products, you can contact us on ProductSafety@springernature.com

In case Publisher is established outside the EU, the EU authorized representative is:

Springer Nature Customer Service Center GmbH
Europaplatz 3
69115 Heidelberg, Germany

Batch number: 10557707

Printed by Printforce, the Netherlands